HEALTH CARE

OPERATIONS AND SUPPLY

CHAIN MANAGEMENT

HEALTH CARE

OPERATIONS AND SUPPLY

CHAIN MANAGEMENT

Operations, Planning, and Control

JOHN F. KROS
EVELYN C. BROWN

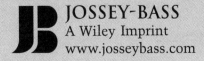

JOSSEY-BASS
A Wiley Imprint
www.josseybass.com

Published by Jossey-Bass
A Wiley Imprint
One Montgomery Street, Suite 1200, San Francisco, CA 94104-4594—www.josseybass.com

Jossey-Bass books and products are available through most bookstores. To contact Jossey-Bass directly call our Customer Care Department within the U.S. at 800-956-7739, outside the U.S. at 317-572-3986, or fax 317-572-4002.

Wiley publishes in a variety of print and electronic formats and by print-on-demand. Some material included with standard print versions of this book may not be included in e-books or in print-on-demand. If this book refers to media such as a CD or DVD that is not included in the version you purchased, you may download this material at http://booksupport.wiley.com. For more information about Wiley products, visit www.wiley.com.

Library of Congress Cataloging-in-Publication Data

Kros, John F.
    Health care operations and supply chain management : operations, planning, and control / John F. Kros, Evelyn C. Brown.—First edition.
        pages   cm
    Includes bibliographical references and index.
     ISBN 978-1-118-10977-9 (pbk.); ISBN 978-1-118-41884-0 (ebk.);
     ISBN 978-1-118-41610-5 (ebk.); ISBN 978-1-118-43367-6 (ebk.)
        1. Health facilities—Business management.   2. Health services administration.   I. Brown, Evelyn C., 1966-   II. Title.
    RA971.3.K767   2013
    362.1068—dc23

                                                                    2012033935

Printed in the United States of America

FIRST EDITION
PB Printing   10 9 8 7 6 5 4 3 2 1

CONTENTS

TABLES AND FIGURES

LIST OF TABLES

LIST OF FIGURES

PREFACE

The health care field is a complex industry with numerous players, from end-user patients to insurance companies to large medical facilities. Health care facilities move large numbers of patients through many processes while attempting to maintain the proper supply of medical products as well as health care experts to complete the required care. Although generally viewed as a service-based industry, the health care field faces some of the most complex operations and supply chain challenges of any industry.

In today's world of government spending cuts and health care reform, health care facilities must closely monitor their operations and determine ways to improve their efficiency in order to survive. Gone are the days of unlimited supplies, carefree spending, and billing Medicare or Medicaid for hospital-acquired conditions. Health care facility managers face two daunting tasks: first, they must change the mind-set and culture of the health care workers, including the doctors; second, they must implement data-driven decision making across all areas of their facilities.

Many of the behaviors and practices that occur in health care facilities are done simply because "that's the way it has always been done." This practice of doing things one way because it is the only way they have ever been done can be costly.

National health expenditure data obtained from the website of the Center for Medicare and Medicaid Services (CMMS) (www.cmms.gov/home/rsds.asp) indicate that total health expenditures in the United States will exceed $4.6 billion by 2020, with these expenditures accounting for almost 20 percent of the U.S. gross domestic product by that time. Figure P.1 and Figure P.2 were generated using CMMS data for 2005 through 2020. Data for the years 2009–2020 are projections only.

Not only are health expenditures in general on the rise, but supply chain costs in the health care industry are also taking a toll on health care facilities'

FIGURE P.1 Graph of Projected Health Expenditures

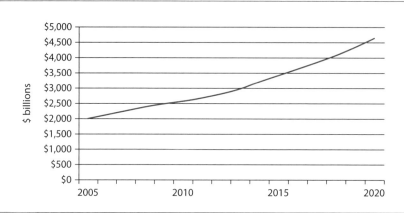

FIGURE P.2 Health Expenditures as a Percentage of Gross Domestic Product

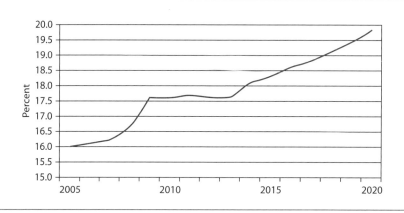

budgets. Research conducted at the University of Arkansas indicates that revamping the supply chain in the health care industry can reduce costs significantly (Nachtmann and Pohl 2009). The results of this research indicate that, among those companies completing the research survey, the average health care provider spends more than $100 million annually on supply chain operations. For most of these organizations, that is about one-third of their annual budgets (Nachtmann and Pohl 2009).

Supply chain costs are not the only area impacting health care settings. Many operational errors are costing hospitals and patients lots of money each year. For example, there are hundreds of cases each year of surgeons mistakenly leaving a sponge, tool, or other object inside a patient (known as a retained foreign body). Research indicates this happens in over 12 percent of surgeries (Gamble 2008), and each instance can cost up to $50,000 (Jaspen 2008).

Another costly operational issue is nosocomial infection, better known as hospital-acquired infection. Obviously, people who are ill have reduced resistance to fungal and bacterial infections, and thus there is a risk that hospital patients will acquire infections if rooms, equipment, and instruments are not kept clean and sanitary. During the decade of the 1990s, hospital-acquired infections increased the U.S. health care system's annual cost between $4.5 and $5.7 billion each year (Graves 2004). During this same time period, the average cost per infection was almost $14,000, with surviving patients experiencing an average cost increase of $40,000 (Stone, Larson, and Kawar 2002). More recent cost figures indicate that the annual cost of these infections had grown to exceed $6.5 billion by 2002 (Graves 2004).

Sponges left in patients and hospital-acquired infections are just two examples of operational challenges facing health care facilities, and both are preventable. Through the application of systematic, thorough procedures, the occurrence of these errors can be greatly reduced. Data clearly indicate that the cost of these mistakes is exorbitant. Health care managers must find a way to focus personnel on making changes that will reduce these errors, thus saving the facility money and improving the well-being of its patients.

Experience has shown that with health care operations, removing the barriers that reinforce the "that's the way it has always been done" mind-set can offer tremendous financial benefit. As an example, consider a small surgery clinic where minor surgical procedures are performed. If the clinic manager permits the doctors to perform surgery in the surgical room of their choice, then fewer than 60 surgeries per day can be performed. If the clinic manager schedules each surgery in the next available surgical room, assuming all rooms contain the same surgical equipment, then over 75 surgeries per day can be performed. By not allowing the doctors to pick and choose the rooms in which they operate, a 25 percent increase in throughput can be realized (Centeno and Dodd 2011). The assigning of surgical rooms in this logical manner also reduces patient wait time, which should lead to improved patient satisfaction.

PURPOSE OF THIS BOOK

This book is intended to be a foundational resource for teaching the utilization of operations and supply chain management (OSCM) in health care management and administration. The text should arm health care facility managers and health care operations analysts with the type of data collection and analysis skills required to realize where and how operational efficiencies can be realized. From understanding supply chains (Chapter 1) and financial aspects of health care operations (Chapter 2), to best practices in scheduling (Chapter 14) and inventory management (Chapter 15), this book takes a comprehensive look at health care operations.

It illustrates concepts and techniques that many health care facilities may have heard of but may have not yet adopted or have not fully implemented. These concepts and techniques are all in areas that are considered leading edge in the operations and supply chain management discipline.

The book introduces the operations and supply chain management concepts in health policy and administration while incorporating the features and functions of Microsoft Excel where appropriate. It provides real data and examples from health care settings to assist in the understanding of the main concepts contained in each chapter.

A strength of this work is that it is organized differently from other textbooks within this category. One main differentiator is the addition and inclusion of supply chain management material to the traditional health care operations topics. Over the past 10 years, the health care industry has driven a trend to modify the traditional operations curriculum by adding supply chain content and including topics such as lean and six sigma. The integration of Excel and spreadsheet models throughout the operations and supply chain material also makes this work unique. The chapters provide material on how to use Excel as a tool within health care operations and supply chain management.

Real-world case examples within the context of health care administration highlight the use of Excel as a valuable decision-making tool for students and health care executives. The work provides novel features such as:

- Leading-edge concepts and techniques that many health care facilities may have heard of but not yet adopted or not fully implemented (e.g., the push lately for training in six sigma and lean).

- Real data and examples from health care settings to assist in the understanding of the main concepts contained in the text.

- Employing Excel as a powerful analytical tool to assist managers in the investigation of their operational setting using data-driven techniques and speaking to the interpretation/communication of the results.

INTENDED AUDIENCE

Students and practitioners using this book come from a variety of backgrounds and have different levels of understanding of many concepts it covers. For this reason, we provide details at the introductory level, assuming little or no quantitative background. Readers who desire more detail on certain topics will find the chapters' references to be valuable sources of additional information and depth.

The text can be employed in undergraduate health administration programs, nursing programs, business programs with health care certificates or concentrations, and maybe even some engineering courses with a bent toward improving health care processes and delivery.

On a graduate level, the text would lend itself to areas such as pharmacy administration, nursing and nursing administration, health information administration, MBA programs with health care certificates or concentrations, and health informatics.

Undergraduate as well as graduate health care administration students will find the text an excellent educational resource. In addition, practicing health policy and health administration managers can also use the book as a reference for day-to-day problem solving. The text helps these students and practitioners realize the importance of sound operations and supply chain management.

ORGANIZATION OF THIS BOOK

The book is organized into four major parts: Strategy, Process Design and Analysis of Health Care Operations, Managing Health Care Operations Quality, and Planning and Controlling Health Care Operations.

Part I begins with an introduction to supply chains and their role in health care operations (Chapter 1). This is followed by chapters that detail financial (Chapter 2) and managerial (Chapter 3) aspects of health care operations.

Part II provides examples of the proper use of data and statistical tools for operations improvement (Chapter 4) and includes numerous tools for problem solving and decision making (Chapter 5). Oftentimes, operations improvements require one to be able to pose what-if scenarios and evaluate alternatives. Simulation (Chapter 6) is introduced as a tool for this type of helpful yet inexpensive analysis.

Just as goods must flow efficiently through a production facility, proper patient flow (Chapter 7) can contribute significantly to a health care facility's efficiency. Additionally, patient flow is affected by facility layout and design (Chapter 8).

Part III is devoted to quality, which has also become imperative for health care facilities to survive in today's competitive market. Managing quality (Chapter 9) and quality control and improvement (Chapter 10) are topics that health care operations managers must understand if they are to create and maintain a reputation for outstanding service at their facility.

Part IV begins with the concepts of a lean enterprise (Chapter 11), which are also important when it comes to maintaining a competitive edge. Application of lean concepts to a service industry such as health care can have dramatic impacts on patient satisfaction and cost of care.

It is not always possible for all types of health care facilities to accurately forecast demand for their services; however, a good understanding of basic forecasting concepts and techniques (Chapter 12) can enable facilities to provide better care by ensuring that appropriate numbers of resources, such as beds and workers, are available.

Health care managers, like all managers, must be able to apply best practices in project management (Chapter 13), scheduling (Chapter 14), and inventory management (Chapter 15). These three topics are covered in the book's final chapters.

USE OF EXCEL IN HEALTH CARE OPERATIONS

Throughout the text, we have included numerous examples of how to utilize MS Excel to solve health care operations problems. It is critical that the reader take advantage of the Excel instructions and examples, as most health care settings will not have or be able to afford specialized software for problem solving and optimization. Excel is a simple yet powerful tool that is available on most PCs encountered in the workplace. Excel's ease of use and widespread availability may make its solutions more acceptable to management. Physicians and other health care workers are likely to have used Excel previously, so explaining the derivation of solutions may be simpler in the context of Excel.

In Chapters 2 and 3, financial analysis is performed using Excel. Examples involving the construction of balance sheets, operating statements, and statements of cash flows are illustrated. Calculations of financial ratios within a spreadsheet are also shown. Finally, the format for activity based costing methods is illustrated using an Excel template.

Chapter 4 includes an example of how Excel can be used to perform required statistical analyses. In addition to presenting the construction of histograms and Pareto diagrams using Excel's Data Analysis add-in package, the Data Analysis add-in is used to test hypotheses using analysis of variance (ANOVA). Excel is also used to construct box-and-whiskers plots and tornado diagrams.

In Chapter 5, problem solving and decision making are accomplished using Excel. The chapter presents construction of payoff tables along with the use of decision criteria via a spreadsheet, and shows expectation calculations using relative references within Excel. In addition, the construction of decision trees as well as sensitivity graphs is presented.

A queuing example in Excel is utilized in Chapter 6. The example walks the student through the creation of arrival times and services times based on a given distribution and the calculation of wait time, system time, and server idle time for each entity that enters the system. It also explains how to calculate summary statistics such as average wait time, average number waiting in line, and server utilization.

Due to the content of Chapters 7, 8, and 9, Excel examples are not employed in those chapters.

Examples of using Excel to aid in quality control are included in Chapter 10. Specifically, the chapter provides Excel templates for the construction of statistical process control charts and the calculation of capability ratios and indices.

Chapter 11 did not lend itself to Excel examples.

Forecasting using Excel is demonstrated through examples in Chapter 12. Excel's Data Analysis add-in is again employed in calculating moving averages, exponential smoothing models, linear regression (simple and multiple) models, and correlation coefficients. Excel templates are presented for error calculations related to the forecasting models.

In Chapter 13, an Excel example is used to demonstrate resource leveling. Additional Excel examples are included to assist with the development of a critical path method (CPM) model and two types of Gantt charts. There is also an Excel example for the Program Evaluation and Review Technique (PERT).

Applications of using Excel for scheduling and capacity management are given in Chapter 14. Johnson's rule for sequencing is presented in spreadsheet format along with the construction of Gantt charts. In addition, an Excel template is constructed to illustrate the center of gravity facility location technique.

In Chapter 15, inventory analysis is performed using Excel. An example involving calculation of the economic order quantity (EOQ) is included to demonstrate how total annual cost can be reduced if the order quantity is set to the EOQ value. The chapter also includes an Excel example on ABC inventory management.

OTHER PEDAGOGICAL FEATURES

In addition to the step-by-step discussions of how health care operations problems are solved using Excel, each chapter includes end-of-chapter exercises that address the material covered in that section. Most of these exercises include the replication of examples from that chapter. The purpose is to provide students an immediate reference with which to compare their work and determine whether they are able to correctly carry out the procedure involved. Data for all the exercises are included on the web at www.josseybass.com/go/.

A supplemental package available to instructors includes all answers to the section exercises. In addition, the supplemental package will contain exam questions with answers and selected Excel spreadsheets that can be used for class presentations, along with suggestions for presenting these materials in a classroom. However, the book can be effectively used for teaching without the additional supplemental material.

Users who would like to provide feedback, suggestions, corrections, examples of applications, or whatever else can e-mail John at krosj@ecu.edu. The website for additional resources and information is www.josseybass.com/go/krosbrown.

Please feel free to contact John and provide any comments you feel are appropriate.

ACKNOWLEDGMENTS

As always, this effort would not have been possible without the support and guidance of numerous colleagues, friends, family, and all those poor souls who had to listen to us bounce ideas off of them, or for that matter anyone who just had to listen to us!

Many people contributed to this book as it now appears. In particular, several outstanding health care professionals from Vidant Rehab Services—Rhonda Joyner, Laura Helms, and Paul Heath—contributed by letting us pick their brains and by providing numerous operations and supply chain examples for us to draw from as we worked together to address the operational challenges their rehabilitation facility faces each day. In addition, Sallie Gough of Med Direct provided critical patient flow information to us when we were just beginning our efforts in the health care arena.

John thanks his wife Novine and his daughters Samantha and Sabrina for always being by his side and encouraging him in the special way they do when the light at the end of the tunnel starts to dim. At present Samantha is 10 years old and always reminds John that she loves him and maybe someday he will be as cool as Justin Bieber. Sabrina is 8 years old and tells John that she expects great things from the East Carolina University Pirates, the Texas Longhorns, and the Nebraska Cornhuskers football teams as well as the Virginia Cavaliers. John would like to say thank you to Novine, Samantha, and Sabrina and that he loves them very much. He also must thank his parents, Bernie and Kaye, who have always supported him, even when they didn't exactly know what he was writing about.

For patiently putting up with John's long-winded descriptions of case study problems and end-of-chapter exercises, a big thanks to the boys over at Manland. Numerous outstanding real-life examples from their own personal health care–related trials and tribulations were imparted to me, whether I wanted them or not, during Thursday card nights.

Evelyn thanks her parents, Betty and Dan Brown, for all of their support throughout her education and her career in academia.

John and Evelyn thank all of those who received email attachments, Dr Pepper–stained hard copies, or random sheets of paper scribbled with half-blown ideas. We appreciate all your input or, for that matter, the simple fact that you took time to look at our work and listen to our ramblings. We specifically would like to thank Scott Bankard, David Z. Cowan, and Soroush Saghafian for feedback on the initial plan and approach of the book. We would also like to thank Asoke K. Dey, Christopher A. Harle, and Echu Liu, who contributed thoughtful and constructive comments on the draft manuscript.

And finally, to anyone we have forgotten to mention, thank you very much.

John F. Kros, PhD
Evelyn C. Brown, PhD

REFERENCES

Centeno, M., and H. Dodd. 2011. "Scheduling Short, Medium, and Long Surgical Procedures: Effects of the Schedule Mix." *Proceedings of the 2011 Institute of Industrial Engineers Annual Conference*, Reno, NV. Available at www.cmms.gov /home/rsds.asp.

Gamble, K. 2008. "No Sponge Left Behind." Health Care Informatics. Available at www.healthcare-informatics.com/article/no-sponge-left-behind.

Graves, N. 2004. "Economics of Preventing Hospital Infection." *Emerging Infectious Diseases* 10(4). Available at wwwnc.cdc.gov/eid/article/10/4/02–0754.htm.

Jaspen, B. 2008. "Technology Cuts Risk of Surgical Sponges: Objects Left in Patients Expensive to Remove." *McClatchy-Tribune Regional News*, January. Available at www.bcbs.com/news/national/technology-cuts-risk-of-surgical-sponges-objects-left -in-patients-expensive-to-remove.html.

Nachtmann, H., and E. Pohl. 2009. "The State of Healthcare Logistics: Cost and Quality Improvement Opportunities." Center for Innovation in Healthcare Logistics, University of Arkansas.

Stone, P., E. Larson, and L. Kawar. 2002. "A Systematic Audit of Economic Evidence Linking Nosocomial Infections and Infection Control Interventions, 1990–2000." *American Journal of Infection Control* 30:145–152.

THE AUTHORS

JOHN F. KROS

John F. Kros is a professor of marketing and supply chain management in the College of Business at East Carolina University in Greenville, North Carolina. He is a coauthor of *Statistics for Health Care Professionals: Working with Excel.* Dr. Kros is active in research within the medical community through partnerships at Vidant Medical (formerly University Health Systems and Pitt County Memorial Hospital), the Brody School of Medicine, and the East Carolina University Student Health Center. He teaches operations and supply chain management and spreadsheet modeling.

Dr. Kros's research areas include simulation/process analysis, quality control, and applied statistical analysis. He has published in numerous journals including *Interfaces*, the *Journal of Business Logistics*, *Quality Engineering*, *Quality Reliability Engineering International*, *Computers and Operations Research*, and the *Journal of the Operational Research Society*.

He holds a bachelor of business administration degree from the University of Texas at Austin, a master of business administration from Santa Clara University, and a PhD in systems engineering from the University of Virginia.

Before joining academia, Dr. Kros was employed in the electronic manufacturing industry by Hughes Network Systems (HNS), Germantown, Maryland. HNS is a major manufacturer of electronic circuit boards, DSS satellite dishes, cellular phone and switching equipment, high-speed cable modems, and network computer satellite systems.

EVELYN C. BROWN

Dr. Brown is a professor in the Department of Engineering at East Carolina University. She teaches courses in principles and methods of systems engineering and system optimization.

Dr. Brown's work has been published in journals such as the *International Journal of Production Research*, *Computers and Industrial Engineering*, *Omega— The International Journal of Management Science*, *IEEE Transactions on Evolutionary Computation*, and *Engineering Applications of Artificial Intelligence*.

Dr. Brown earned a BS in mathematics from Furman University, an MS in operations research from North Carolina State University, and a PhD in systems engineering from the University of Virginia.

Prior to employment at East Carolina, she taught for seven years at Virginia Tech, where her research focused on applications of genetic algorithms, particularly to grouping problems. Before becoming a full-time academician, she worked for Nortel Networks in Research Triangle Park, North Carolina, as an operations researcher and project manager.

HEALTH CARE

OPERATIONS AND SUPPLY

CHAIN MANAGEMENT

PART I

STRATEGY

CHAPTER 1

HEALTH CARE OPERATIONS AND SUPPLY CHAIN STRATEGY

LEARNING OBJECTIVES

➠ Understand why the management of operations and supply chains is important to the health care profession.

➠ Understand the role that purchasing, logistics, and vendor-managed inventory play in health care.

➠ Understand the meaning of efficient and effective operations and supply chain management.

(Continued)

⟹ See how the management of operations and supply chains relates to health care.

⟹ Understand the competitive dimensions of operations and supply chain strategy within health care.

⟹ Know what measures are used to evaluate the operations and supply chain management function.

⟹ Understand what the bullwhip effect is and how it applies to health care.

HEALTH CARE OPERATIONS AND SUPPLY CHAIN MANAGEMENT

The operations and supply function in hospitals has historically been viewed as having a limited scope, many times falling under the term *materials management*. However, over the past decade progressive hospitals have adopted and adapted the concepts of the broader topic of supply chain management (SCM). The combination of operations with supply chain management presents a more expansive and robust view than the subarea of materials.

Definitions of Supply Chain Management

Experts in the field often define *supply chain management* as the sum total of parties involved, directly or indirectly, in fulfilling a customer request.

Two of the most prominent professional supply chain management organizations in the world define supply chain management as follows:

The Institute for Supply Management defines supply management as "the identification, acquisition, access, positioning, management of resources and related capabilities the organization needs or potentially needs in the attainment of its strategic objectives."

The Council for Supply Chain Management Professionals defines supply chain management as the function that "encompasses the planning and management of all activities involved in sourcing and procurement, conversion, and all logistics management activities. Importantly, it also includes coordination and collaboration with channel partners, which can be suppliers, intermediaries, third party service providers and customers."

These definitions are very broad and contain customer-centric concepts, as they also consider new product identification and development, marketing, operations, distribution (channels), finance, and customer service as part of supply chain management.

These definitions can be applied to health care operations and/or systems to include the flow of products and associated services to meet the needs of the health care provider and system and the patients served.

Operations and Supply Chain Management Applied to Health Care

In turn, the nature of this book is quite different from the traditional operations text that may focus more on products and manufacturing from a perspective such as the automaker Ford, or a high-technology firm such as Hewlett-Packard, or a continuous processing company such as Alcoa.

This text addresses the broader picture of operations and supply chain management tasks: not only the sourcing of materials, but also forecasting demand, developing and employing simulation models, discussing quality management tools and techniques, and the management of projects within health care. All of these topics will be applied to the health sector. Knowledge of these tasks will assist the health care professional and act as a building block for operations and supply management excellence.

Given the unique nature of the health care profession, the hospital operations and supply chain manager most often has relationships with a wide variety of organizations that connect suppliers to the health care organization. These relationships extend to group *purchasing* organizations, distributors, third-party service providers, information managers, and transportation support staff.

Health Care Operations and Supply Chain Management in Action

It is said that when times are good, expansion plans, future investments, and revenue growth are the focus points in most industries. However, during down times, all organizations scrutinize spending. Economic crises hit all industries, including the health care sector. Adjustments are made, such as private practices being closed, hospital operating margins being squeezed, and many nonclinical jobs getting cut.

So what do hard times mean for health care industry supply chain managers? It appears that in an attempt to usher in supply chain efficiencies and shape a healthier bottom line, clinicians, executives, and others are now more ready than ever before to listen to their supply chain managers.

It has been shown that supply chain managers' importance has been heightened as a result of recent estimates showing that average hospital profit margins are down. It is very possible that health care supply chain executives at large health care organizations are responsible for hundreds of millions of dollars in spending per year. The best supply chain managers seek input for all levels in the health care organization, from physicians to nurses to pharmacists. Many times those employees demand products and services without any notion of potential costs or impacts to the operating atmosphere.

Of late, it appears that health care supply chain managers are beginning to look at other industries for assistance. Many health care organizations are looking to inject talent from those who have not been in the health care industry and can be tapped for new ideas.

The bottom line is sometimes summarized as follows:

- Executive leadership [is] beginning to include the supply chain as a key contributor to a healthy bottom line.

- Executives are looking for supply chain managers outside of the industry to run their health care supply chains.

- A shift from tactical to strategic models is occurring.

- As the supply chain becomes more efficient, supply chain managers are being asked to bring efficiencies to other spending areas of a health care network.

—From "Troubled Times Magnify Health Care Supply
Chain Manager's Role," Knowledge@W.P. Carey

PURCHASING, LOGISTICS, AND
VENDOR-MANAGED INVENTORIES

Supply costs are on average around 30 to 40 percent of total operating costs in most hospitals (Kehoe, December 2011 issue of *Healthcare Facilities Management*). In the recent past, many health care organizations were not focused on managing the supply chain, but relied on external entities called group purchasing organizations (GPOs) to negotiate all of their contracts (e.g., Novation and Premier).

Internal as well as external operations of a health care organization are encompassed by the *logistics* function. Externally, the distribution of health care products is a great challenge for the global logistics system. Firms such as Baxter, Cardinal, or even UPS act as third-party logistics providers (3PLs) since many health care organizations do not support their own logistics network. However, internally, health care logistics has organization-specific needs of purchasing, warehousing, transport logistics, and collaboration. Many health care organizations choose health care logistics software to help in these areas.

It can be said that the health care industry has been reluctant to follow the lead of manufacturing by adopting just-in-time (JIT) inventory and logistical systems. However, the health care industry has begun to understand the benefits of JIT. By using bar code technology of medical products for faster delivery, reduced medical errors, and prevention of fraud and abuse, health care professionals see tangible benefits. Using a health care logistics software system can cut operation costs and result in lower patient care costs. Streamlining operations with suppliers through effective use of e-commerce can result from applying health care logistics tools. Efficient health care logistics systems can also reduce internal labor costs.

The health care field is positioning itself for increased use of JIT inventory and logistical systems. In addition, review of the contractual agreements with GPOs and third-party logistics providers is paramount for the improvement in spend management. This can be witnessed anecdotally as those contracts become increasingly complex and tight budgets demand better control of costs. More health care organizations are being asked to isolate, track, and manage third-party spending (e.g., electronic invoicing and auditing thereafter). Also, more collaboration is occurring as those vendors bring solutions such as JIT inventory management to the table. One manner in which JIT inventory management is being manifested in health care organizations is through the use of vendor-managed inventory systems.

The Vendor-Managed Supply Chain

Vendor-managed inventory (VMI) is one technique that has become popular for addressing the areas isolating and tracking inventory. VMI and VMI systems have been in use in the retail industry for a decade. VMI has the capability to forecast a hospital's demand for supplies and can help eliminate the problem of over-stocking costs. In turn, demand ultimately drives the product ordering and replenishment cycles. Hospitals should focus on supply demand management in particular.

VMI allows the supplier (typically a distributor) to respond to the hospital's immediate supply needs as determined by the hospital's own consumption data. Orders are generated on the basis of an economic order quantity (EOQ; covered in Chapter 15). EOQ takes into account factors such as safety stock, lead time, seasonality, and demand created by exceptional circumstances. As a result, the hospital is able to reduce its in-house inventory and lower its order management costs.

The VMI software usually resides with the health care distributor (e.g., Cardinal) because of the benefits that a distributor can gain from the economies of scale (i.e., running the VMI application across multiple health care facilities). The arrangement is also attractive to a distributor as a means to better understand its own demand for supplies and in turn more efficiently manage its own inventory and order processes.

EFFICIENCY, EFFECTIVENESS, AND VALUE

Technology investment, acquisitions, and major expansion are all ways health care professionals could enhance their current operation. However, innovations in operations and the supply chain tend to be reliable and are generally low-cost. Currently, those studying within the health care profession are well positioned to develop innovative operations and supply chain–related ideas.

This book provides the reader with the concepts and tools now being employed at the best health care organizations in the world. These concepts and tools allow those organizations to develop efficient and effective operations and supply chain areas. Efficiency is defined as performing a task at the lowest possible cost or with the least amount of resources. One goal of an efficient health care facility is to provide a quality service by using the smallest input of resources possible.

Effectiveness, in turn, means doing the correct things to assist the customer/patient and bring the most value to the organization. Value could be profit if the health care organization is a for-profit entity, or value could be helping the most people possible if the organization is a nonprofit or not-for-profit entity.

As a health care provider tries to maximize efficiency and effectiveness at the same time, a conflict may be created between the two goals. This is a typical trade-off in the health care world, as providers wish to do the best for the most but are still constrained by limited resources. At a health care facility, being effective means helping as many patients as possible to get the proper health care. However, being efficient in that same arena means minimizing the amount spent with each patient and using the least amount of resources to help the patient.

Value comes from both of these goals being optimized. It may sound odd in a health care setting that we are talking about value, but think on this: What would happen if a patient went to a health care facility for an earache and got the best care ever but it took three days to actually be seen? The experience was highly effective but not efficient, to say the least. However, if a patient received attention very quickly but no one even looked in the patient's ear regarding the pain, the experience would have been highly efficient but not very effective. The value for the patient would be low in each of these cases.

Health care professionals must provide value, and that value comes from the combination of effectiveness and efficiency within the health care organization. Smart management of resources, operations, and the health care supply chain can lead to high levels of value.

A Brief History of Health Care Supply Chain Management and the Association for Healthcare Resource and Materials Management

The Association for Healthcare Resources and Materials Management (AHRMM) began in the early 1950s as part of the American Hospital Association. Over the past 60 years, the Association has continually grown and reinvented itself to become the leading professional organization for the health care resource and materials management field. A brief history is presented here to illustrate how the organization developed into a vital part of the health care supply chain industry.

- Early 1900s—The first health care group purchasing organization (GPO) is formed.

- 1929—Baylor University Hospital in Dallas, Texas, introduces the first monthly hospital insurance plan.

- 1940s—Employer-based health insurance grows as World War II begins.

- 1950—The Naval School of Healthcare Administration is established to provide training in health care administration and financial and materials management.

- 1951—The Association for Healthcare Resource & Materials Management begins on September 19 in Chicago.

- 1962—AHRMM's first annual conference is held.

- 1975—AHRMM's name is changed to the American Society for Hospital Purchasing and Materials Management (ASHPMM) to more accurately reflect the emergence of materials management systems in the hospital industry.

- Early 1980s—The prospective payment system is instituted by Medicare.

- 1983—ASHPMM becomes the American Society for Hospital Materials Management (ASHMM) to reflect changes in the health care field.

- 1983—The term *diagnosis-related group* (DRG) is implemented.

- Late 1980s—Reduced reimbursements to health care providers lead to hospital consolidation, increased use of GPOs, and the development of vendor-managed inventory control programs.

- The mid-1990s bring the Efficient Healthcare Consumer Response (EHCR), the Health Insurance Portability and Accountability Act (1996), and the Ambulatory Payment Classification Act (1999).

- 1998—ASHMM officially changes its name to the Association for Healthcare Resource & Materials Management (ARHMM).

- 2000—The Certified Materials & Resource Professional (CMRP) program is introduced.

- Early 2000s—More health care organizations begin developing relationships with third-party logistics providers (3PLs) and implementing collaborative planning, forecasting, and replenishment (CPFR) agreements with suppliers.

- 2009—AHRMM continues its mission to partner with other health care professionals, and in conjunction with GS1 Healthcare US creates and releases the "Standardization Stat!" video promoting awareness of the issues of standardization in the health care supply chain.

—From the Association for Healthcare Resource &
Materials Management website (www.ahrmm.org)

Why Study Health Care Operations and Supply Chain Management?

Besides the notion of creating value by optimizing both effectiveness and efficiency, there are five other reasons to study health care operations and supply chain management.

1. Approximately 45 percent of a health care organization's total operation expenses are made up of supplies, pharmaceuticals, consumables, and physical plant (e.g., equipment, transportation networks, etc.). With that said, it is critical to understand the operational and supply chain aspects of the organization to ensure effective and efficient management of those expenses.

2. A health care education is incomplete without an understanding of modern approaches to managing health care operations and the supply chain. There is much talk of health care reform, and at the operations and supply chain management level these initiatives draw heavily on total quality control principles, process design and reengineering, statistical data analysis, and inventory control, to name four.

3. The underlying concepts of operations and supply chain management provide a systematic method of observing, documenting, and analyzing health care organizational processes.

4. Operations and supply chain management tools interface with many other functions within the health care industry. All health care professionals, whether doctors, nurses, or administrators, must plan work, control quality,

and ensure productivity of the individuals under their supervision. All health care employees, from surgeons to janitorial staff, must know how to effectively and efficiently perform their jobs.

5. Career opportunities in the health care profession are ever expanding, and now more than ever before, health care employees are being asked to perform their jobs more efficiently and effectively. The management of operations and the supply chain becomes even more important with this new emphasis.

COMPETITIVE DIMENSIONS OF HEALTH CARE

Although not quite as broad as, say, retail, health care customers do have choices regarding the services and products they purchase. Obviously health care customers include patients, but customers can also include vendors and third-party providers. In the case of patients, some primarily listen to their family doctor or health care provider whereas others may purchase services from third-party providers (e.g., walk-in or doc-in-the-box services). Some patients are interested in cost only, and certain health care organizations may cater to these customers. In contrast, vendors or third-party providers may not have as broad a choice in where their services are needed. They may have to compete directly on price or speed of delivery, both of which may be dictated by another party (e.g., a hospital, an in-home patient, the state, or U.S. government). In fact, there are a number of competitive dimensions that health care providers must address.

Health care providers do establish *competitive dimensions*, which may include these four areas:

1. Cost or price—lower-priced or free services such as a free clinic.

2. Quality of service—delivery of outstanding services such as the Mayo Clinic.

3. Speed of delivery—delivery of the service quickly such as a minor medical facility.

4. Support after the service—excellent support after the service has been rendered, such as technical sales help regarding medical equipment (e.g., insulin pumps).

Competitive Dimensions of Health Care and Trade-Offs

It becomes apparent after perusing the competitive dimensions that it may be impossible for one health care organization to excel simultaneously on all the dimensions at once. This notion is central to the concept of operations and supply chain strategy. Trade-offs exist between any and all of these competitive dimensions. In turn, the organization must decide on which performance parameters are critical to success and concentrate resources on those areas.

A good example of this type of trade-off is when a health care organization wishes to focus on speed of delivery (i.e., see patients as quickly as possible) but also wants to be flexible (i.e., be able to see any and all types of patient problems). A trade-off usually must be made. Minor medical facilities may do a better job at providing speedy service but they cannot handle major medical issues such as brain surgery.

Likewise, high quality is generally traded off with lower cost. A strategic position is not sustainable unless an organization makes compromises with other positions. The notion of a trade-off is just this: when more of one item necessitates less of another.

Some health care organizations have attempted to provide choices to their patients by straddling different dimensions. For example, a large trauma one health care facility (i.e., full service, high quality) may build an off-site emergency department to handle less severe or acute patient problems and in turn deliver on speed or lower cost. However, organizations must be aware that straddling is a risky strategy and many ill-fated attempts have been abandoned (e.g., discount LASIK eye centers delivered on speed and price, but were flawed regarding post-op support).

Measures to Evaluate the Operations and Supply Chain Management Function

Although health care has not been put under the microscope as minutely as have publicly held business entities, that time has almost come to an end. Monitoring, assessing, and improving a health care organization's performance, specifically in regard to operations and supply chain management, are becoming commonplace in today's competitive world.

Key performance indicators (KPIs) are data-driven measures that can range from improving patient safety practices to reducing variability of supply utilization to reducing overall health care costs. KPIs are an important part of taking a proactive approach to running a health care organization. KPIs are generally used to benchmark a health care provider's performance compared to other similar providers in the marketplace.

It can be said that when the organization understands exactly what care is being provided by whom, what resources are consumed, the total cost of that care, and the resulting outcomes, then an organization can establish benchmarks, capture feedback, and implement changes to achieve continuous improvement in patient outcomes as well as cost control. The following list gives a number of KPIs for a typical health care organization. KPIs are discussed in more detail in Chapter 11 on lean concepts in health care.

Standard KPIs may include:

- In-house infection rates

- Prime-time utilization

- Estimated case time duration and accuracy

- Emergency room throughput

- Mean emergency room wait time

- Average inventory and inventory turns

THE BULLWHIP EFFECT IN HEALTH CARE

The *bullwhip effect* can be defined as the instance where orders to a supplier tend to have larger variance than sales to the buyer (i.e., demand distortion), and the distortion becomes amplified (i.e., variance amplification) as it propagates upstream in the supply chain.

The inability of the health care industry to predict demand leads to a wide range of these types of upstream inefficiencies. In general, inventory piles up, inventory turns go down, inventory becomes obsolete, and in turn costs increase. The health care industry has not fully investigated the cost of these inefficiencies.

For example, in a manufacturing setting the bullwhip effect results in higher levels of inventory and shortages. However, in the health care industry it leads to lower levels of throughput, higher operating costs, and longer patient waits. In turn, the causes of these problems must be addressed by employing initiatives and strategies for minimizing the bullwhip effect.

Strategies for Minimizing the Bullwhip Effect

Strategies for minimizing the bullwhip effect can be categorized in five areas: reduction of uncertainty, reduction of variability, development of strategic partnerships, realignment of incentives, and improved coordination within the supply chain. Each of these areas is detailed next.

1. *Reduction of uncertainty.* Reducing uncertainty throughout the supply chain is a main driver of minimizing or even eliminating the bullwhip effect. Timely and consistent data delivery assists in eliminating the duplication of effort.

2. *Reduction of variability.* The use of good forecasting methods alleviates variability. Minimizing variability helps reduce the overall bullwhip effect.

3. *Development of strategic partnerships.* Strategic partnerships have the ability to change the manner in which information is shared. In turn, better information can help minimize the bullwhip effect. In the case of hospitals, the hospital administration could forge strategic alliances with medical specialists. Although this might not eliminate the bullwhip effect, it will in part reduce the effect.

4. *Realignment of incentives.* Incentives are pervasive throughout the supply chain. In addition, each supply chain entity appears to be evaluated and rewarded based on different criteria. This disparity leads to a lack of coordination and meaningful information sharing and in turn exacerbates the bullwhip effect. These evaluation and reward systems should be modified to stress cooperation across stages.

5. *Improved coordination within the supply chain.* In points 1 to 4 the themes of reducing uncertainty and variability and improving information exchange play into the final area of improved coordination within the supply chain. Improved coordination across the supply chain has the ability to bring about improvements in the other four areas and in turn improvements in the bullwhip effect.

TABLE 1.1   Major Causes of the Bullwhip Effect

Bullwhip Effect Causes	Contributing Factors to the Effect	Remedies to Minimize the Effect
I. Inadequate or nonexistent forecasting methods and/or poor update of forecasts	• Lack of forecasts and/or the reluctance to share forecast information • Lack of planning and implementation based on forecasts (i.e., winging it)	• Adopt a forecasting method and use it. • Inform your suppliers what your forecast is and update the data.
II. Lack of information sharing and coordination across the supply chain	• Incompatible information technology systems across the supply chain • Lack of motivation or poor incentives for sharing information • A culture of not sharing information	• Develop strategic partnerships that encourage information sharing. • Align incentives to encourage data/forecast sharing.
III. Management practices (e.g., batching, parking preferences)	• Batching due to high transportation costs • Limited resource allocation due to high cost of one entity in the supply chain (e.g., high cost of surgeon's visits)	• Use lean practices to reduce the setup cost, transaction cost, and/or transportation cost. • Implement systemwide objectives to modify the measurement and evaluation system to align it with the overall strategic plan.

Adapted from Kannan Sethuraman and Devanath Tirupati, "Evidence of Bullwhip Effect in Healthcare Sector: Causes, Consequences and Cures," *International Journal of Services and Operations Management* 1, no. 4 (2005): 372–394.

Table 1.1 summarizes the major causes of the bullwhip effect, notes some contributing factors to the bullwhip effect, and recommends some remedies for minimizing the effect.

SUMMARY

This chapter has discussed the overall importance of operations and supply chain management to the health care profession. It proposed definitions of supply chain management, including several by the most prominent professional supply chain groups in the world. It described operations and supply chain management applications to the health care industry. Nachtmann and Pohl 2009 provide additional information on the state of logistics in health care; Schneller et al. 2006 provide a strategic overview of managing health care supply chains.

Furthermore, the roles of purchasing, logistics, and vendor-managed inventory (VMI) were detailed. The chapter discussed vendor-managed supply chains along with the software that accompanies VMI.

The notions of efficiency, effectiveness, and value were reviewed, as well as reasons to study health care operations and supply chain management, such as the large impact on operating expenses, understanding how operations and supply chain management interface into the bigger picture, documenting and analyzing health care organizational processes, and finally career opportunities.

Competitive dimensions of health care were given. Cost, quality, speed, and support may all be advantages that health care organizations compete on. The chapter discussed trade-offs between and within each dimension.

Key performance indicators (KPIs) such as average inventory or mean emergency room wait time are examples of measures to evaluate operations and supply chain management within an organization.

Finally, the bullwhip effect was defined and related to the health care industry. The chapter concluded with strategies for minimizing the bullwhip effect, as well as causes and contributing factors.

KEY TERMS

bullwhip effect

competitive dimensions

key performance indicators

logistics

purchasing

supply chain management

vendor-managed inventory

DISCUSSION QUESTIONS

1. Discuss what health care supply chain management is and how it compares to operations.

2. Discuss why operations and supply chain management must be studied at the same time.

3. What role does purchasing play in a health care organization?

.4. What role does vendor-managed inventory play in a health care organization?

5. Discuss efficiency, effectiveness, and value regarding health care organizations.

6. What are the competitive dimensions of operations and supply chain management in a health care organization?

7. What measures should be used to evaluate the operations and supply chain management functions within a health care organization?

8. What is the bullwhip effect, and how does it apply to health care?

MINICASE: THE BULLWHIP EFFECT IN HEALTH CARE ORGANIZATIONS

Blue County Memorial Hospital (BCMH) is one of the largest health care organizations in eastern North Carolina. It serves the eastern one-third of North Carolina and maintains a 500-bed facility offering 24/7 acute medical and surgical care. The health care facility has over 30,000 patient admissions a year, and its average length of stay (LOS) is about four days.

The health care facility is organized by specialty and staffed with qualified MDs, physician assistants (PAs), nurses, and technicians. BCMH contains 12 operating rooms, all with state-of-the-art equipment, numerous wards for postoperative care, and related ancillary services (rehabilitation, testing labs, etc.). The operating room department has a large challenge in that it must manage and allocate equipment and staff so that surgeries can be performed effectively but also in the most efficient manner possible. In all, the assignment of equipment and staff is a difficult job.

State regulations require threshold levels for nurse-patient ratios, and not meeting these thresholds may lead to underutilization of available capacity. In turn, the size and mix of staff are critical decisions for the workforce planners. Overstaffing, understaffing, or unbalanced staffing leads to issues with quality of care and increased patient cost. BCMH meets its staffing requirements with a mix of permanent staff and an on-call group of part-time staff available on short notice. There is also temporary staffing that occurs for nurses with six-month to one-year contracts. Overall, the hospital's staffing needs have been met by

60 percent permanent staff, 35 percent temporary staff, and 5 percent on-call staff.

BCMH provides services to patients, and in turn those patients, either through insurance or by direct payments, reimburse BCMH for services provided. Although many services are provided, surgery is one area where BCMH adds value and garners profits. However, surgery demands numerous resources, including equipment and staff (surgeons, nurses, technicians, etc.). BCMH is also responsible for preoperative care and postoperative care. Insufficient capacity in any area (surgery, postoperative wards, etc.) can lead to surgical procedures being turned away or to higher costs if accepted when over capacity.

Slotting is used for planning and scheduling purposes. Each area within BCMH is broken up in half-day slots, meaning there are 14 slots per week. Slot planning and scheduling is conducted about once a quarter (once every three months). A plan is developed in consultation with surgeons; demand for surgical procedures varies little from year to year, but the demand does have a seasonal component, making some quarters busier than others. In addition, some specialties have peak demands whereas other specialties have very stable demand.

The slotting and planning process also encompasses the staffing of nurses. The labor cost of nurses for surgery is one of the largest and most controllable operating costs. Nursing staffing plans are prepared each month for a month's time frame and two weeks in advance. The nursing schedule is frozen one day in advance and then resource requirements are matched based on the upcoming surgeries. This type of planning is efficient for day-to-day operations but gives limited flexibility in terms of the permanent staff, temporary staff, and on-call staff. The nurse scheduler must many times rely on temporary staff or on-call staff when demand changes occur in the short term. Subsequently, BCMH must meet its nursing needs from outside, and in monetary terms the outside staff costs more, as higher rates are paid to the outside staff. In addition, the staffing in preoperative and postoperative wards is done in a similar fashion.

Is it possible that BCMH could experience the bullwhip effect? What items can be identified that would exacerbate the bullwhip effect at BCMH? How does variability from all areas impact BCMH? Can the use of temporary workers benefit BCMH but also be detrimental at the same time?

REFERENCES

Association for Healthcare Resource & Materials Management website (www.ahrmm.org).

Kehoe, Bob. 2011. "Quality Measurement Tools and Collaboration Drive Success." *Healthcare Facilities Management*, 45–48.

Nachtmann, Heather, and Edward A. Pohl. 2009. "The State of Healthcare Logistics: Cost and Quality Improvement Opportunities." Center for Innovation in Healthcare Logistics, University of Arkansas, July.

Schneller, Eugene S., Larry R. Smeltzer, and Lawton Robert Burns. 2006. *Strategic Management of the Health Care Supply Chain.* Hoboken, NJ: John Wiley & Sons.

Sethuraman, Kannan, and Devanath Tirupati. 2005. "Evidence of Bullwhip Effect in Healthcare Sector: Causes, Consequences and Cures." *International Journal of Services and Operations Management* 1 (4): 372–394.

"Troubled Times Magnify Health Care Supply Chain Manager's Role." January 28, 2009, in Knowledge@W.P. Carey (http://knowwpcarey.com).

CHAPTER 2

FINANCIAL ASPECTS OF HEALTH CARE OPERATIONS AND SUPPLY CHAIN MANAGEMENT

LEARNING OBJECTIVES

⟹ Describe three financial statements and what they measure.

⟹ Understand the basic financial ratios and metrics for health care operations and supply chain management.

⟹ Know what time value of money is and how it is used.

⟹ Understand break-even and crossover analysis.

HEALTH CARE FINANCE AND OPERATIONS/SUPPLY CHAIN MANAGEMENT

Health care organizations interact in a unique financial environment. To get an understanding of how operations and supply chain management (SCM) can benefit the organization, it is important to discuss financial statements, specifically how revenues and costs impact these documents. To many health care professionals, accounting or finance courses were not requirements for their field of study. However, to improve a health care organization's operations and supply chain, a health care professional must understand the basics of:

- The three main financial statements.

- What financial ratios for health care operations are, why they are used, and how to interpret them.

- Know what time value of money is and how to use it.

- What break-even analysis and crossover analysis are.

How Do Health Care Providers Get Paid?

Fee-for-service (FFS) was in a sense the original reimbursement method, in which health care providers were paid directly for every service performed. FFS is relatively unused today, representing only a small percentage of an average hospital's total revenue. From the payer or reimbursement prospective, there are problems with FFS. For example, hospitals see them as incentives to perform more services. From strictly an accounting perspective, it may be said that the greater the utilization or number of procedures or resources utilized, the greater the potential reimbursement. Most health care providers and payers are not in favor of this approach, as there is not an alignment of reimbursement around incentives.

In the era of FSS, health care organizations were on a cost-plus reimbursement system. Cost-plus systems literally are characterized by actual costs being covered plus a small profit margin. The system reimburses actual costs plus this profit margin regardless of the total cost to deliver services. It can be said that before the 1980s, when revenue was almost unlimited, there was no need for cost efficiencies or fiscal discipline in spending or utilization patterns.

1980s Health Care Legislation

The early 1980s brought about legislation that introduced a different payment system, the prospective payment system. The legislation, the Tax Equity and Fiscal Responsibility Act, made major changes in Medicare reimbursement practices. Prospective payment is a methodology by which fee schedules are calculated based on treatment type or illness classification. The fees are paid in advance of the treatment without regard to actual costs incurred. Prospective payment systems resulted in the end of most cost-plus pricing by health care organizations.

As health care organizations moved past the 1980s, there have been continued financial pressures. During this time, health care organizations have endured a variety of reimbursement systems. The vast majority of these systems were aimed at reducing costs and improving financial stewardship. Capitation is one system that emerged. Capitation is a system in which financial risk of care is transferred to physicians and away from health plans or insurers, by limiting payments to a fixed-dollar amount. Standard primary care capitation reimbursed the health care provider on a per-member per-month basis, akin to a flat payment being made per capita to a defined population over a certain period of time. Capitation tended to be used in the early 1990s more than today.

Introduction of the Diagnosis-Related Group

Today, the most popular payment system employed is a classification system referred to as diagnosis-related group (DRG). DRGs categorize all patients through principal and secondary diagnosis, procedures provided, age, sex, and a number of other factors. Commercial insurers and payers use the system because it is very comprehensive regarding classification. Medicare also requires the use of DRGs. Payment rates are set based on the patient's illness and length of time required to treat the illness in the DRG system. Insurers tend to negotiate the rates and establish discounted rates based on market coverage, type of service, and volume of activity. Overall, most health care organizations use a standard fixed reimbursement rate for each type of service performed.

For the health care professional, the financial implications of changes to these reimbursement systems are enormous. Since payments are now set at basically a standard rate, there is pressure on health care organizations to hold costs down below that rate. Therefore, a health care professional must see that the need for managing costs, maximizing productivity, and optimizing resources is of utmost importance. Understanding the three basic financial statements is a good place to start this discussion. The income statement or operating statement, balance sheet, and statement of cash flows are presented next.

INCOME STATEMENT/OPERATING STATEMENT

The *income statement* or *operating statement* (statement of operations) is one of the most important components of a health care organization's financial system. In the case of a for-profit health care organization an income statement is developed, whereas when speaking of a not-for-profit health care organization, a statement of operations is developed. Table 2.1 juxtaposes the major sections of the two financial statements.

As some health care organizations operate as not-for-profit entities whereas some operate as for-profit entities, the term *operating statement* will be used for both types in this chapter.

The operating statement tracks revenues (monies coming into the organization), expenses (monies going out of the organization), and margins (e.g., gross or operating). The basic principle behind the operating statement is:

$$\text{Profit} = \text{Revenue} - \text{Expenses}$$

Figure 2.1 displays a basic health care organization's operating statement.

TABLE 2.1 For-Profit and Not-for-Profit Health Care Financial Statements

For-Profit Health Care Organization	Not-for-Profit Health Care Organization
Income Statement	**Operating Statement**
Revenues	Unrestricted Revenues, Gains, and Other Support
− Expenses	− Expenses
Operating Income	*Operating Income*
+ Other Income	+ Other Income
Operating Earnings before Income Taxes	Excess of Revenues, Gains, and Other Support over Expenses
− Income Taxes	+ Other
Net Income	*Increase in Unrestricted Net Assets*

FIGURE 2.1   Operating Statement for a Health Care Organization

	A	B	C
1	**Sample Not-For-Profit Healthcare Organization,**		
2	**Operating Statement, December 31, 201X and 201Y**		
3	*Revenues, Gains, and Other Support*	**201X**	**201Y**
4	Net Patient Service Revenue	$68,125	$63,154
5	Premium Revenue	$8,920	$8,760
6	Other Revenues	$2,081	$4,170
7	Net Assets Released from Restriction Used for Operations	$240	$0
8	*Total Revenues, Gains, and Other Support*	$ 79,366	$ 76,083
9			
10	*Expenses*		
11	Salaries and Benefits	$43,120	$39,950
12	Medical Supplies and Drugs	$21,226	$17,697
13	Insurance	$6,471	$6,821
14	Depreciation and Amortization	$3,826	$3,424
15	Interest	$1,402	$1,460
16	Provision for Bad Debts	$800	$1,040
17	Other Expenses	$1,600	$1,040
18	*Total Expenses*	$ 78,444	$ 71,432
19			
20			
21	*Operating Income*	$922	$4,651
22	Other Income		
23	Investment Income	$3,120	$2,420
24	*Excess of Revenues over Expenses*	$ 4,042	$ 7,071
25			

Four distinct areas exist on the operating statement presented in Figure 2.1. Those areas are:

1. Revenues, Gains, and Other Support

2. Expenses

3. Operating Income

4. Excess of Revenues over Expenses

Each of these areas is discussed next.

Revenues, Gains, and Other Support

The revenue of a health care organization is garnered by providing patient services, the sale of assets for more than their book value (i.e., selling an asset for a gain), and other revenues such as contributions. In the case of a for-profit entity this line item would just be referred to as revenues.

Figure 2.1 displays these revenues in cells A3 through C5. Column A contains the monikers for the operating statement, while columns B and C contain the actual numbers. Column A is referred to in this example only to assist with reading the entire statement, but is excluded from discussion hereafter. The revenue categories are as follows:

- Net Patient Service Revenue (refer to cells A3 through C3) encompasses revenues earned from patient care less the amount of items such as contractual discounts or exclusions.

- Premium Revenue (refer to cells A4 through C4) is revenues earned from sources such as capitated contracts.

- Other Revenues (refer to cells A5 through C5) are derived from sources such as support services or contributions.

Expenses

Expenses are associated with the levels of resources employed to generate revenue. These expenses can include salaries, supplies, and insurance, to name just a few. Only Depreciation and Amortization, Provision for Bad Debts, and the Other Expenses categories are explained next, as the other categories are self-explanatory. This section is almost identical for both a for-profit and a not-for-profit health care entity.

- The Depreciation and Amortization category (refer to cells A13 through C13) is the accounting measure for the use of longer-lived assets (e.g., physical plant, durable equipment, etc.) during a defined period.

- Provision for Bad Debts (refer to cells A15 through C15) is an estimate of the amount of money owed to the organization that it has decided it will not be able to collect (i.e., think bill collector calling).

- Other Expenses (refer to cells A16 through C16) are in a catch-all category for any expenses that are not easily encapsulated within the other expense categories.

Operating Income

Operating income is the difference between Total Revenues, Gains, and Other Support (cells A7 through C7) and Total Expenses (cells A17 through C17). To calculate operating income, you subtract expenses from the total revenues.

This is the measure of income earned resulting from health care operations. In the case of a for-profit entity this is simply revenues less expenses.

Excess of Revenues over Expenses

Excess of Revenues over Expenses (cells A23 through C23) is sometimes referred to as net income or even the bottom line. However, in a not-for-profit health care entity, this is actually not the bottom line in the statement of operations. Formally, there is an emphasis to treat not-for-profit health care entities like their for-profit business cousins. This in turn adds another section to the operating statement called the Change in Unrestricted Net Assets section. For the sake of brevity, this chapter does not detail that section, and the reader can consult the Zelman et al. 2009 text in the references section of the chapter for more information on this topic.

Excess of revenues over expenses is operating income plus any other income. Other income could include items such as investment income, grants, parking fees, or extraordinary items. A health care organization wants to have a positive value for this line item. If the line item is negative, then the organization is losing money (i.e., spending more than it is taking in).

A difference that must be noted here between for-profit and not-for-profit entities is taxes. In the case of a for-profit health care entity, a provision for taxes must be included. In a successful organization, taxes are usually a net outflow from the organization. However, in a not-for-profit entity, tax payments are not required and therefore are not included in the statement of operations.

The operating statement illustrates the inflows of revenues and outflows of expenses within an organization; however, assets, liabilities, and equity must also be discussed. The next section details that statement that brings together assets, liabilities, and equity in what is called the balance sheet.

BALANCE SHEET

Balance sheets traditionally show a summary of an organization's assets, liabilities, and shareholders' equity. However, in the case of not-for-profit health care organizations, net assets replace shareholders' equity since there are no true shareholders. A balance sheet is a snapshot in time that captures what an organization looks like financially at a particular moment (e.g., the end of the quarter or end of the fiscal year).

A balance sheet is made up of three major sections: the heading, the body, and the notes. The heading contains the name of the organization, the name of the statement, and two dates (indicating the time frame). The body contains three sections: assets, liabilities, and net assets (for a not-for-profit entity). Figure 2.2 displays a balance sheet for a not-for-profit health care organization.

FIGURE 2.2   Balance Sheet for a Not-for-Profit Health Care Organization

	A	B	C	D
1	Sample Not-For-Profit Healthcare Organization			
2	Balance Sheet			
3	December 31, 201X and 201Y			
4	**Assets**	201X	201Y	
5	**Current Assets:**			
6	Cash and Cash Equivalents	$ 3,806	$ 4,702	
7	Short-Term Investments	12,669	8,592	
8	Assets Limited to Use	776	1,040	
9	Supplies	1,600	1,600	
10	Prepaid Expenses	536	685	
11	Patient Accounts Receivables-			
12	Net Estimated Uncollectables of $2,000 in 201X and $2,500 in 201Y	12,080	11,355	
13	*Total Current Assets*	31,467	27,974	
14				
15	**Non-Current Assets**			
16	Assets Limited as to Use	15,159	15,873	
17	Less Amount Required to Meet Current Obligations	(776)	(1,040)	
18		14,383	14,833	
19	Long Term Investments	3,744	3,744	
20	Long Term Investments & Cap. Acquisit.	256	416	
21	Properties and Equipment, Net	40,830	40,394	
22	Other Assets	1,356	1,096	
23	*Total Non-Current Assets*	60,570	60,482	
24				
25	**Total Assets**	$ 92,037	$ 88,456	
26				
27	**Liabilities and Net Assets**			
28	**Current Liabilities**			
29	Accounts Payable and Accrued Expenses	4,654	4,306	
30	Estimated Third-Party Payor Settlements	1,714	1,554	
31	Current Portion of Long-Term Debt	1,176	1,400	
32	Deferred Revenues	1,575	1,691	
33	*Total Current Liabilities*	9,120	8,950	
34				
35	**Non-Current Liabilites**			
36	Long-Term Debt, Net of Current Portion	18,515	19,211	
37	Other	3,162	2,533	
38	*Total Non-Current Liabilities*	21,678	21,744	
39				
40	**Total Liablities**	30,798	30,694	
41				
42	**Net Assets**			
43	Unrestricted	56,677	52,959	
44	Temporarily Restricted	1,692	1,976	
45	Permanently Restricted	2,870	2,826	
46	*Total Net Assets*	61,239	57,762	
47				
48	**Total Liabilities and Net Assets**	$ 92,037	$ 88,456	
49				

The name *balance sheet* is derived from the notion that assets must equal liabilities plus net assets (for a not-for-profit health care organization); or in the case of a for-profit health care entity, assets must equal liabilities plus shareholders' equity. The equations then are as follows:

$$\text{Assets} = \text{Liabilities} + \text{Net assets}$$
$$\text{Assets} = \text{Liabilities} + \text{Shareholders' equity}$$

From Figure 2.2 it can be seen that total assets in the year 201X are $92,037 and total liabilities plus total net assets also equal $92,037, hence the name *balance sheet*. Not-for-profit health care organizations used the term *fund balance* instead of *net assets* up until around 1996. Governmental and other not-for-profit entities still use the term.

Assets

The resources an organization owns are considered assets. Assets are recorded at their original cost and are divided into two categories, current assets and non-current assets. In a health care organization, assets are used to provide services to patients and to generate revenues.

Current Assets

This category of asset is defined as assets that will be consumed or used within one year. For a health care organization these are the assets that turn an organization's capacity (e.g., equipment, labs, physical plant) into patient services. Current assets can include the following (see Figure 2.2):

- Cash and Cash Equivalents (refer to cells B6 and C6).

- Short-Term Investments (refer to cells B7 and C7).

- Assets Limited to Use (refer to cells B8 and C8).

- Supplies (refer to cells B9 and C9).

- Prepaid Expenses (refer to cells B10 and C10).

- Patient Accounts Receivable, Net of Estimated Uncollectables (refer to cells B11, B12, C11, and C12).

If an asset can be turned into cash quickly, it is said to be liquid. On the balance sheet, current assets are listed by order of liquidity with the most liquid being listed first. Current assets require special attention due to their liquidity and the potential for them to be mishandled. Hence, special oversight is given.

Noncurrent Assets

Noncurrent assets are assets that will be consumed over periods longer than one year. This category of assets represents costly items and provides the organization with the means to deliver services over time. Noncurrent assets are categorized as follows (see Figure 2.2):

- Assets Limited as to Use (refer to cells B16 and C16).

- Long-Term Investments (refer to cells B19 and C19).

- Properties and Equipment, Net (refer to cells B21 and C21).

- Other Assets (refer to cells B22 and C22).

In the same way that current assets are given special attention, noncurrent assets also are given special attention in that they are costly and take longer periods of time to acquire as well as to manage.

Liabilities

Liabilities are the obligations of a health care organization to pay its creditors. Liabilities are also divided into two categories: current liabilities and noncurrent liabilities.

Current Liabilities

Current liabilities are short-term obligations that due to contractual terms will be paid within one year. Common current liabilities include (see Figure 2.2):

- Accounts Payable and Accrued Expenses (refer to cells B29 and C29).
- Estimated Third-Party Payer Settlements (refer to cells B30 and C30).

- Current Portion of Long-Term Debt (refer to cells B31 and C31).

- Deferred Revenues (refer to cells B32 and C32).

Noncurrent Liabilities

Noncurrent liabilities are longer-term obligations such as mortgages payable or bonds payable that will be paid back over a period of more than one year (refer to cells B36, B37, C36, and C37 in Figure 2.2).

Net Assets

The last category on the balance sheet is net assets. In the case of a for-profit organization, this section is referred to as shareholders' equity. The term *net assets* in the case of a not-for-profit health care organization is assigned to illustrate the interests in the assets of the organization by entities such as the community. The community may include a county or municipality or even a religious organization.

Not-for-profit health care organizations must further categorize net assets into three subcategories defined by restriction level (see Figure 2.2):

1. Unrestricted (refer to cells B43 and C43).

2. Temporarily Restricted (refer to cells B44 and C44).

3. Permanently Restricted (refer to cells B45 and C45).

Net assets that are not restricted by donors are considered unrestricted net assets. If the assets are restricted, then the level of restriction must be noted. An example of a temporary restriction on net assets may be the donation of land by a religious organization with the provision that the health care organization cannot sell the land for three years. In contrast, a permanent restriction would be a person setting up an endowment that stipulates that only the interest from the endowment can be spent while the principal must remain intact.

Many times the net asset section is accompanied by a statement of changes in net assets that details the changes from year to year of unrestricted, temporarily restricted, and permanently restricted net assets. For brevity, this statement is not presented here, and those interested are referred to the references section of this chapter, specifically Data Trends 2008 and Zelman et al. 2009, for more information.

Balance Sheet Notes

In most cases the information presented in the body of the balance sheet is in summary form. Financial notes for the balance sheet are grouped together and presented at the end of the entire financial statement. Additional key information is presented in the notes, and the notes should not be considered unnecessary. Notes contain information such as what specific accounting policies (e.g., last in, first out [LIFO] or first in, first out [FIFO] for inventories) the health care organization employs, how charity care is accounted for, which net assets are restricted and why, and the depreciation method used (e.g., straight-line or double-declining), to name a few items of information covered.

STATEMENT OF CASH FLOWS

The *statement of cash flows* answers the question "Where did our cash go, and where does our cash come from?" Many may think that the operating statement would answer this question, but it does not, at least not fully. The operating statement really tells us how much the organization has earned or lost and what resources were used in that endeavor. The statement of cash flows must be developed to report on how cash flowed out of the organization and how cash flowed into the organization.

The statement of cash flows contains a heading, a body, and ending notes. The same time period that is covered by the operating statement is covered by the statement of cash flows. The body consists for the following sections:

- Cash Flows from Operating Activities

- Cash Flows from Investing Activities

- Cash Flows from Financing Activities

- Net Increase (Decrease) in Cash and Cash Equivalents

Key noncash transactions are also disclosed (e.g., acquisitions of other companies). The form presented here is the indirect method, although a direct method does exist.

Cash Flows from Operating Activities

The inflows and outflows from normal business activities are identified in this section. Since the information needed to determine cash inflows and outflows is

FIGURE 2.3   Statement of Cash Flows for a Health Care Organization

	A	B	C	D
1	Sample Not-For-Profit Healthcare Organization			
2	Statement of Cash Flows			
3	December 31, 201X and 201Y			
4	**Cash Flows From Operating Activities**	201X	201Y	
5	*Change in Net Assets*	$ 3,478	$ 6,493	
6	Adjustements to Reconcile Change in Net Assets to Net Cash Provided by Operating Activities			
7	Extraordinary Loss from Debt Extinguishment	400	-	
8	Depreciation	3,826	3,424	
9	Net Realized Gain and Unrealized Gain on Investments	(360)	(460)	
10	Transfers to Parent	512	2,400	
11	Provision for Bad Debt	800	1,040	
12	Restricted Contributions and Investment Income Received	(44)	(330)	
13	Increase (Decrease) in:			
14	Patient Accounts Receivable	(1,525)	(1,629)	
15	Trading Securities	172	-	
16	Other Current Assets	149	(1,985)	
17	Other Assets	(260)	(193)	
18	Increase (Decrease) in:			
19	Accounts Payable and Accured Expenses	349	543	
20	Estimated Third Party Payor Settlements	161	244	
21	Other Current Liabilites	(116)	(206)	
22	Other Liabilities	630	(102)	
23	*Net Cash Provided by Operating Activities*	8,170	9,239	
24				
25	**Cash Flows from Investing Activities**			
26	Purchase of Investments	(3,015)	(1,720)	
27	Capital Expenditures	(3,782)	(4,688)	
28	*Net Cash Used in Investing Activities*	(6,798)	(6,408)	
29				
30	**Cash Flows from Financing Activities**			
31	Transfers to Parent	(512)	(2,400)	
32	Proceeds from Restricted Contributions/Investments	44	330.4	
33	Payments on Long-Term Debt	(19,760)	(643)	
34	Payments on Capital Lease Obligations	(120)	(80)	
35	Increase in Long-Term Debt	18,080	400	
36	*Net Cash Used in Financing Activities*	(2,268)	(2,393)	
37				
38	Net Increase (Decrease) in Cash and Cash Equivalents	$ (895)	$ 438	
39				
40	Cash and Cash Equivalents at Beginning of Year	$ 4,702	$ 4,263	
41				
42	Cash and Cash Equivalents at End of Year	$ 3,806	$ 4,702	
43				

not usually accounted for formally, the cash flows from operating activities is derived from the change in net assets. Adjustments are then made to convert the change in net asset information into cash flows. Figure 2.3 displays an example of a statement of cash flows.

Adjustments to reconcile the change in net assets to net cash flows can include items such as (see Figure 2.3):

- Depreciation (refer to cells B8 and C8).

- Net Realized and Unrealized Gains from Investments (refer to cells B9 and C9).

- Transfers to Parent (refer to cells B10 and C10).

- Provision for Bad Debt (refer to cells B11 and C11).

- Changes in Patient Accounts Receivable (refer to cells B14 and C14).

- Changes in Accounts Payable and Accrued Expenses (refer to cells B19 and C19).

- Changes in Other Liabilities (refer to cells B22 and C22).

These are just a few of the items that might be included in the operating activities cash flows section.

Cash Flows from Investing Activities

This section of the cash flows statement is derived mostly from changes in the balance sheet, specifically the noncurrent assets section. Cash flows from accounts such as the following are included (see Figure 2.3):

- Sales of Long-Term Investments.

- Purchases of Long-Term Investments (refer to cells B26 and C26).

- Sales of Plant, Property, and Equipment.

- Purchases of Plant, Property, and Equipment (refer to cells B27 and C27).

Sales and purchases are both recorded here whether they be investments or equipment that will be used to generate patient revenue.

Cash Flows from Financing Activities

Financing activities can include items such as proceeds from interest income or long-term debt issuances. Cells B31 through C35 in Figure 2.3 include financing activity. These activities encompass money flows that assist the organization in its everyday operations (e.g., debt to finance operations, interest payments from holding accounts, transfers to or from a parent to aid in making payments or meeting obligations).

Cash and Cash Equivalents at End of Year

Cash and cash equivalents at the end of the year are calculated by adding the Net Increase (Decrease) in Cash and Cash Equivalents to the Cash and Cash

Equivalents at Beginning of Year. The number on the statement of cash flows is the same as the Cash and Cash Equivalents amount on the balance sheet.

In sum, the purpose of the statement of cash flows is to detail where the organization's cash came from and how it was spent during the recording period. Actual cash flows are identified, whereas the operating statement records amounts based on the accrual method or when earnings and resources are used.

BASIC FINANCIAL RATIOS AND METRICS

The previous sections detailed how a health care's financial statements are constructed. This section discusses how the information contained in the operating statement and the balance sheet can be used to gauge the financial health of the organization's operations and supply chain activities.

Some of the most valuable tools to employ when analyzing an organization's financial health are financial ratios. Financial ratios allow a health care professional to get a better look inside the organization's financial performance than one can get just perusing the basic statements. Ratios not only are useful for gauging internal health but also can be compared externally to benchmark against other health care organizations. This section introduces three major financial ratio categories: profitability, liquidity, and asset management ratios.

There are numerous financial ratios that exist. For the sake of brevity, the ratios listed in Table 2.2 from each category will be detailed. Please refer to the references section of this chapter, specifically Zelman et al. 2009, for more information on financial ratios and ratio analysis.

TABLE 2.2 Key Health Care Financial Ratios

Asset Management Ratios	Liquidity Ratios	Profitability Ratios
Inventory turnover	Current ratio	Operating margin
Days in patient accounts receivable	Quick ratio	Return on assets
Case mix index	Average pay period	
Supply expense to net patient revenue	Working capital	
Supply expense to total operating revenue	Days of working capital	
Supply expense to adjusted patient days		
Supply expense to adjusted discharges		

Note: For all ratio calculations, unless otherwise noted, the dollar figures are in thousands ($000).

Asset Management Ratios

Asset management ratios measure how effectively a health care organization is managing its assets. Assets such as inventories, accounts receivable, and supplies are analyzed. In the field of operations and supply chain management, the ratios in this category are among the most important.

Asset management ratios give an operations and supply chain manager an inside look at how the organization's assets are being employed, how quickly they are being turned (used up), and how quickly assets that have been used for patient services are being turned into cash. The pulse of an organization is in a sense measured using asset management ratios. Turns that are too low or receivables that take too long to be converted to cash lead to a sluggish organization and inefficient use of resources (e.g., think about providing service to a patient and immediately receiving payment versus waiting 180 days for the payment).

Inventory Turnover Ratio

The first ratio is the traditional inventory turnover ratio (Equation 2.1). The ratio is:

$$\text{Inventory Turnover Ratio} = \frac{\text{Cost of Goods Sold}}{\text{Average Inventory}} \qquad (2.1)$$

Cost of goods sold (COGS) is found on the operating statement and refers to the cost of the materials and/or supplies that are used to provide services (refer to Figure 2.1, cells B10 and C10). Average inventory is the average of the year-over-year inventory numbers (supplies) and is found on the balance sheet (refer to Figure 2.2, cells B9 and C9). For our earlier example, the inventory turnover ratio (Equation 2.2) is calculated as:

$$\text{Inventory Turnover Ratio} = \frac{\$21,226}{\$1,600} = 13.3 \qquad (2.2)$$

The result, 13.3, is a rough approximation of how often the health care organization's inventory is sold out and restocked or turned over. A turnover ratio of 13.3 would need to be compared with an industry average to gauge if this turnover is considered good or not so good.

Days in Patient Accounts Receivable

Future revenue to be recognized is what accounts receivable (AR) measure. In other words, if a health care organization got paid immediately for all transactions, then AR would be zero. However, health care organizations rarely get paid immediately for services rendered. The more quickly an organization can convert AR to cash, the better. Therefore, days in patient accounts receivable is very important to analyze. Days in patient accounts receivable (Equation 2.3) is calculated as:

$$\text{Days in Patient Accounts Receivable} = \frac{\text{Accounts Receivable}}{(\text{Total Revenue}/360)} \quad (2.3)$$

The number 360 is used as a normalizing factor. It is assumed that a year is 360 days. Accounts receivable can be found on the balance sheet (refer to Figure 2.2, cells B11, B12, C11, and C12) while total revenues can be found on the operating statement (refer to Figure 2.1, cell B6). Therefore, in our previous example, days in patient accounts receivable (Equation 2.4) is then:

$$\text{Days in Patient Accounts Receivable} = \frac{\$12,080}{(\$79,366/360)} = 54.79 \quad (2.4)$$

In other words, it takes the health care organization about 55 days to convert accounts receivable to cash. To benchmark with other health care providers, this number falls right in the middle of the industry range.

Case Mix Index

The case mix index, while not formally a financial ratio, is a very relevant measure to adjust for each individual health care organization's patient complexity and intensity. Overall, the greater a patient's intensity and complexity, the greater the amount of resources such as supplies that will be consumed. The case mix index is a common way to adjust for patient mix differences among health care organizations.

The case mix index is formally calculated by averaging the diagnosis-related group (DRG) weightings for all patients served over the course of the accounting period in question. DRG codes are assigned to all patients. Although DRGs are typically used only for Medicare reimbursement, they can be applied across all costs. The index can be 1, less than 1, or more than 1. If the index is 1, then the hospital being analyzed is equitable regarding patient mix and no adjustment is in order. However, if the index is below or above 1, then there is a mismatch in the hospital's patient mix and an adjustment must be made. The case mix index can be employed for any of the following supply expense ratios when comparing across multiple hospitals.

Supply Expense to Net Patient Revenue

Supply expense to net patient revenue is a widely used ratio for supply expense analysis. This ratio does a good job of measuring internal performance on a period-over-period time frame. If the ratio rises over time, it may be indicating changes in supply management behavior such as changes in consumption, pricing, or suppliers without any changes in patient revenue.

It must be noted that the ratio docs not take into account variations in reimbursement rates or fluctuations in revenue. The health care industry on average has a supply expense to net patient revenue ratio of around 18 percent.

The ratio (Equation 2.5) is calculated as follows:

$$\text{Supply Expense to Net Patient Revenue} = \frac{\text{Supply Expense}}{\text{Net Patient Revenue}} \quad (2.5)$$

As in our previous example, supply expense can be found on the operating statement (refer to Figure 2.1, cell B10); net patient revenue can also be found on the operating statement (refer to Figure 2.1, cells B2 and B3). Therefore, for the example, supply expense to net patient revenue (Equation 2.6) is:

$$\text{Supply Expense to Net Patient Revenue} = \frac{\$21,226}{(\$68,125 + \$8,920)} = 0.28 \quad (2.6)$$

At 0.28 (28 percent), the example health care organization is above the industry level for supply expense to net patient revenue.

Supply Expense to Total Operating Revenue

The relative intensity of supply utilization in support of patient care and daily operations is measured with the supply expense to total operating revenue ratio. This ratio is different from the supply expense to net patient revenue ratio as it includes all revenues, not just those derived from patients. For the health care industry as a whole, better-performing entities have ratios around 13 to 14 percent.

The ratio (Equation 2.7) is calculated as follows:

$$\text{Supply Expense to Total Operating Revenue} = \frac{\text{Supply Expense}}{\text{Total Operating Revenue}} \tag{2.7}$$

As in our previous example, supply expense can be found on the operating statement (refer to Figure 2.1, cell B10); total operating revenue can also be found on the operating statement (refer to Figure 2.1, cell B6). Therefore, for the example, supply expense to total operating revenue (Equation 2.8) is

$$\text{Supply Expense to Total Operating Revenue} = \frac{\$21,226}{\$79,366} = 0.27 \tag{2.8}$$

At 0.27 (27 percent), the example health care organization is above the industry level for supply expense to total operating revenue.

Supply Expense to Adjusted Patient Days

The term *adjusted patient days* refers to the mix of inpatient versus outpatient visits. If a health care facility has an equal mix of inpatient versus outpatient days, then the metric that accommodates this mix of patients is the adjusted patient days. The metric adjusted patient days (Equation 2.9) is calculated as follows:

$$\text{Adjusted Patient Days} = \frac{\text{Total Gross Revenue}}{\text{Total Inpatient Revenue}} \times \text{Number of Patient Days} \tag{2.9}$$

For our example, let's assume the ratio of total gross revenue to total inpatient revenue is 2 and the number of patient days is approximately 60,000. Therefore the adjusted patient days metric is 120,000. Supply expense can be found on the operating statement (refer to Figure 2.1, cell B10).

In turn, the supply expense to adjusted patient days ratio (Equation 2.10) is

$$\text{Supply Expense to Adjusted Patient Days} = \frac{\text{Supply Expense}}{\text{Adjusted Patient Days}}$$

$$= \frac{\$21,226,000}{120,000} = \$177 \qquad (2.10)$$

Note: Here we use the actual supply expense and not the abbreviated ($000) version from the operating statement so units match.

Industry averages of supply expense to adjusted patient days range from $95 to $297. Therefore, the health care organization in our example falls right in the middle of the industry range.

Supply Expense to Adjusted Discharges

Output of a health care organization can be measured by the number of discharges it completes. However, it is well known that some patients require more services than others. For example, severely ill patients may place greater demands on medical records than they would, say, on waiting room staff or on the collections department.

Health care organizations not only provide inpatient services such as those for the severely ill but also produce outpatient services. It can be said that health care facilities with fewer discharges tend to have higher relative rates of outpatient services. If discharges are not adjusted for outpatient services, whatever measure of output is being used could be biased. Therefore, discharges must be adjusted.

Adjusted discharges are in turn utilized as an aggregate indicator of hospital activity. As was previously discussed, adjusted discharges must be calculated to reflect the impact of both inpatient and outpatient volume. In addition, total patient service revenue is the only financial indicator that can be split into inpatient and outpatient components.

The three steps used to calculate adjusted discharges are:

1. Inpatient gross revenue per discharge (Equation 2.11) is calculated as follows:

Inpatient Gross Revenue per Discharge =

$$\frac{\text{Total Gross Inpatient Service Revenue} + \text{Total Gross Inpatient Ancillary Revenue}}{\text{Total Inpatient Discharges}}$$

$$(2.11)$$

2. Outpatient equivalent discharges (Equation 2.12) is then calculated as follows:

$$\text{Outpatient Equivalent Discharges} = \frac{\text{Gross Outpatient Revenue}}{\text{Inpatient Gross Revenue Per Discharge}}$$

$$(2.12)$$

3. Finally, total adjusted discharges (Equation 2.13) is calculated as follows:

$$\text{Adjusted Discharges} = \text{Total Inpatient Discharges} + \text{Outpatient Equivalent Discharges} \quad (2.13)$$

With adjusted discharges calculated and equal to 12,000 (this is an assumption, as no calculations were completed) for our health care example, supply expense to adjusted discharges (Equation 2.14) is calculated as follows:

$$\text{Supply Expense to Adjusted Discharges} = \frac{\text{Supply Expense}}{\text{Adjusted Discharges}}$$

$$= \frac{\$21,226,000}{12,000} = \$1,768$$

$$(2.14)$$

Note: Supply expense can be found on the operating statement (refer to Figure 2.1, cell B10).

The supply expense to adjusted discharges ratio of $1,768 is a bit high compared to the U.S. average of approximately $1,150 for like health care organizations. It must be noted that size of health care facility, patient mix, and case mix all can impact this calculation.

Liquidity Ratios

Health care organizations must be able to meet their cash obligations such as accounts payable (i.e., paying your suppliers). But maintaining liquidity (e.g., acquiring and keeping large amounts of cash on the books) also has its costs. Therefore, health care organizations must balance the need for liquidity with the costs associated with that liquidity.

Liquidity ratios such as the current ratio and the quick ratio measure an organization's ability to meet its cash obligations. Ratios such as average pay period, working capital, and days of working capital also measure an organization's liquidity. These ratios are all investigated in this section.

Current Ratio

The current ratio (Equation 2.15) compares the dollars of current assets to the dollars of current liabilities for an organization.

$$\text{Current Ratio} = \frac{\text{Current Assets}}{\text{Current Liabilities}} \qquad (2.15)$$

In general, current liabilities must be paid off in the next accounting period, and current assets will then be converted into cash during the same time period (if not already cash). Therefore, the higher an organization's current ratio, the greater an organization's liquidity. It must be noted that this interpretation requires that receivables and inventories are properly valued on the balance sheet. For our example, current assets as well as liabilities can be found in Figure 2.2, cells B13 and B33, respectively.

For our health care example, the current ratio (Equation 2.16) is:

$$\text{Current Ratio} = \frac{\$31,467}{\$9,120} = 3.45 \qquad (2.16)$$

The ratio can be interpreted for our example as $3.45 of current assets to pay for each dollar of current liabilities.

Quick Ratio

The quick ratio is very similar to the current ratio but is a stricter measure of liquidity in that it removes inventories from the current assets. Inventories are removed because they are viewed as the least liquid current asset. For health care organizations and in our example, inventories may be considered supplies. For consistency, the term *inventories* will be used in the definition. The quick ratio (Equation 2.17) is calculated as follows:

$$\text{Quick Ratio} = \frac{\text{Current Assets} - \text{Inventories}}{\text{Current Liabilities}} \qquad (2.17)$$

For our example, current assets, inventory, and liabilities can be found in Figure 2.2, cells B13, B9, and B33, respectively.

For our health care example, the quick ratio (Equation 2.18) is:

$$\text{Quick Ratio} = \frac{\$31,467 - \$1,600}{\$9,120} = 3.27 \qquad (2.18)$$

The ratio can be interpreted for our example as $3.27 of current assets other than inventories to pay for each dollar of current liabilities.

Average Pay Period

The average pay period measures the average amount of time that it takes before an organization meets its current liabilities. Put another way, it is the number of days in which cash expenses are outstanding or not currently paid. Higher values of average pay period indicate a lack of liquidity.

Average pay period (Equation 2.19) is calculated as follows:

$$\text{Average Pay Period} = \frac{\text{Current Liabilities}}{(\text{Total Expenses} - \text{Depreciation})/360} \qquad (2.19)$$

For our example, current liabilities can be found on the balance sheet (refer to Figure 2.2, cell B33), whereas total expenses and depreciation can be found on the operating statement (refer to Figure 2.1, cells B16 and B12, respectively).

For our health care example, the average pay period (Equation 2.20) is:

$$\text{Average Pay Period} = \frac{\$9,120}{(\$78,444 - \$3,826)/360} = 44 \tag{2.20}$$

In sum, it takes approximately 44 days to pay off the organization's current liabilities.

Working Capital

Working capital is the difference between current assets and current liabilities. This difference (hopefully positive) is what is turned into cash and used to pay liabilities. This conversion process for a health care organization is driven by working capital from receiving funds to pay invoices to paying providers' salaries.

Working capital (Equation 2.21) is calculated as follows:

$$\text{Working Capital} = \text{Current Assets} - \text{Current Liabilities} \tag{2.21}$$

For our example, current assets and current liabilities can be found on the balance sheet (refer to Figure 2.2, cells B13 and B33), and therefore working capital (Equation 2.22) is:

$$\text{Working Capital} = \$31,467 - \$9,120 = \$22,347 \tag{2.22}$$

Working capital needs to be sufficient to cover the costs of providing services, along with ordering and storing any supplies, but not too large as to become an inefficient use of resources.

Days of Working Capital

Days of working capital is another indicator or how efficiently an organization is able to meet its obligations. Days of working capital (Equation 2.23) is calculated as follows:

$$\text{Days of Working Capital} = \frac{\text{Current Assets} - \text{Current Liabilities}}{\text{Total Revenues}/360} \qquad (2.23)$$

For our example, current assets and liabilities can be found on the balance sheet (refer to Figure 2.2, cells B13 and B33), while total revenues can be found on the operating statement (refer to Figure 2.1, cell B6). In turn, days of working capital (Equation 2.24) is:

$$\text{Days of Working Capital} = \frac{\$31,467 - \$9120}{\$79,366/360} = 101.40 \qquad (2.24)$$

The health care organization has approximately 101 days of working capital.

Profitability Ratios

The impact of operations and supply chain decisions on a health care organization's financial condition are measured by *profitability ratios*. For profit, health care organizations require positive net income to remain viable in the long run. It can be said that profitability ratios are perhaps the most important measures of financial condition. Profitability ratios require some definition of profit, such as profit per dollar of assets or profit per dollar of revenue. Not-for-profit health care organizations also need to measure profitability, but since they are not for profit by mission, their definition of profit will differ from that of for-profit organizations.

For example, profit can be defined on a total basis, including all sources of income, such as contributions. Or profit could be defined as stemming solely from the organization's health care operations. In some cases, profit could be defined either before or after taxes (for investor-owned providers) and either before or after financial costs (interest expense). Finally, profit could also be defined on the basis of simple accounting rules (such as net income), or it can be defined as cash flow (net income plus noncash expenses).

In turn, the many definitions of profit bring many profitability ratios. For brevity, two profitability ratios, operating margin and return on assets, are given here. The reader is referred to the references section at the end of the chapter, specifically Zelman et al. 2009, for a comprehensive list of sources for financial ratio analysis.

Operating Margin

Operating margin is one of the most common ratios for any organization. The formula for operating margin (Equation 2.25) is:

$$\text{Operating Margin} = \frac{\text{Operating Revenue} - \text{Operating Cost}}{\text{Operating Revenue}} \qquad (2.25)$$

For our health care example, operating margin is then calculated as in Equation 2.26, with operating revenue (total revenues) and operating cost (total expenses) found in the operating statement (refer to Figure 2.1, cells B6 and B16):

$$\text{Operating Margin} = \frac{\$79,366 - \$78,444}{\$79,366} = 1.2\% \qquad (2.26)$$

The operating margin for our health care organization is approximately 1.2 percent. While this margin is positive, it is below the 2010 industry average of 3.4 percent ("A Solid Year" 2011).

Return on Assets

Return on assets (ROA) measures total profitability as a percentage of total assets. In other words, it measures an organization's ability to use its assets to generate income. If an organization's ROA is higher, that means it is more productive (financially) using its assets. ROA is calculated as in Equation 2.27, with operating income coming from the operating statement (refer to Figure 2.1, cell B19) and total assets coming from the balance sheet (refer to Figure 2.2, cell B25):

$$\text{Return on Assets} = \frac{\text{Operating Income}}{\text{Total Assets}} \qquad (2.27)$$

For our health care example, ROA (Equation 2.28) is:

$$\text{Return on Assets} = \frac{\$922}{\$92,037} = 1.0\% \qquad (2.28)$$

For our health care example, the ROA is 1 percent, which means that every dollar invested in assets leads to $0.01 in profit.

TIME VALUE OF MONEY

The concept of *time value of money* is important in that money tomorrow is not worth the same as money today. When speaking of money, the time period must be the same for each monetary entity. For example, consider a health care provider that renders services today for $1. One customer pays a dollar as he leaves but another customer asks to be billed later and makes a dollar payment a year later. Those two dollars are in different time periods and hence must be converted to the same time period to compare their values.

A detailed discussion of the time value of money is outside the scope of this book. However, two time value concepts, future value and present value, are briefly illustrated next.

Future Value

It can be said that a dollar today is worth more than a dollar received in the future. If you had the dollar now, you could invest and gain interest and in turn end up with more than a dollar in the future.

Future value (FV) is calculated (Equation 2.29) as follows:

$$FV_n = PV(1 + k)^n \tag{2.29}$$

where,

FV_n = Future value at the end of n periods

PV = Present value or the beginning amount

k = Interest rate that is paid on the account per year

n = Number of periods interest is earned

If we allow $PV = \$100$, $k = 5$ percent or 0.05, and $n = 1$, then the future value is calculated as follows (Equation 2.30):

$$FV_n = PV(1+k)^n = \$100(1+0.05)^1 = \$105 \qquad (2.30)$$

Therefore, if we have \$100 and we invest it at a 5 percent rate per period for 1 period we garner \$105. Present value (PV) works much in the same way but instead of working forward in time we work backward.

Present Value

The process of finding *present value* (PV) is formally called discounting. As previously mentioned, finding a PV is really the reverse of finding an FV. It can be said that if you know the PV you can compound using an interest rate to find the FV; likewise, if you know the FV you can discount using an interest rate to find the PV.

Present value (Equation 2.31) is calculated as follows:

$$PV_n = \frac{FV}{(1+k)^n} \qquad (2.31)$$

The symbol definitions remain the same as in the previous FV example. For example, if we are offered an investment that pays \$127.63 in five years, we can calculate what that investment would be worth today. If we assume a 5 percent interest or discount rate per year, present value (Equation 2.32) is calculated as follows:

$$PV_n = \frac{FV}{(1+k)^n} = \frac{\$127.63}{(1+0.05)^5} = \frac{\$127.63}{1.2763} = \$100.00 \qquad (2.32)$$

Therefore, a payment of \$127.63 in five years is equivalent to \$100.00 today invested at 5 percent for five years. In other words, an investor would be indifferent to being paid \$127.63 in five years or taking \$100.00 and investing it at 5 percent for five years.

Due to space constraints, this is a very abbreviated treatment of the time value of money. The authors encourage the reader to look over the references section at the end of the chapter, specifically Zelman et al. 2009, for more information on the time value of money.

BREAK-EVEN ANALYSIS

To begin discussing *break-even analysis*, the profit equation must first be investigated. The general equation contains three parts: profit, revenues, and costs. The general equation (Equation 2.33) looks like this:

$$\text{Profit} = \text{revenues} - \text{costs} \qquad (2.33)$$

Profit, revenues, and costs are related to the volume of items produced and sold. Each is a function of the volume of items produced, volume of items sold, and the prices of those items. The general equation can be broken down into a mathematical equation detailing the specific relationships that profit, revenues, and costs have to volume.

Cost and Volume Models

The cost of providing a service or a product has two major cost components, fixed and variable costs. Fixed costs are the portions of the total cost that do not depend on the level of volume; fixed costs do not change. Variable costs are the portions of total cost that are dependent on volume. Total cost is the sum of fixed cost and variable cost.

Let's take a private clinic as an example. The clinic knows it will take $100,000 to set up a proposed new outpatient operation. This cost won't change as the number of patients goes up or down. It is considered fixed and is incurred even if no patients are seen. The clinic also knows that it takes $100 in labor and materials to service a patient. Therefore, $100 is the variable cost associated with how many patients are seen. The resulting cost and volume model (Equation 2.34) for seeing x number of patients is written as:

$$\text{Total cost} = \$100,000 + \$100x$$

$$\text{where } x = \text{number of patient consultations} \qquad (2.34)$$

The total cost for the clinic outpatient operations can now be calculated by using Equation 2.34. For example, if the clinic believes it will consult with 100 patients, or $x = 100$, the total cost is calculated (Equation 2.35) as:

$$\text{Total cost} = \$100,000 + \$100(100) = \$110,000 \qquad (2.35)$$

Business analysts and economists use this model to describe how the total costs of a firm change as the volume changes. This is called marginal analysis. In the case of costs, the marginal cost is defined as the rate of change of the total cost with respect to the volume produced, or x in our equation. From the total cost equation, we can see that for each extra patient consultation, the total cost would rise by $100. The marginal cost is equal to the variable cost in this case.

Revenue and Volume Models

Health care professionals must also be concerned with the revenue stream associated with producing products. A model relating revenue and volume produced can be created. Let's use the outpatient clinic example again. The firm realizes $300 for each patient consultation. Therefore, the total revenue (Equation 2.36) for the firm can be written as:

$$\text{Total Revenue} = \$300x \tag{2.36}$$

where x = number of patient consultations.

As in the case of costs, business analysts and economists use this model to describe how the total revenues of a firm change as the volume changes. Once again, this is called marginal analysis. In the case of revenues, the marginal revenue is defined as the rate of change of the total revenue with respect to the volume, or x in our equation. From the total revenue equation, we can see that for each extra patient consultation, the total revenue would rise by $300. In other words, if the firm consults with one more patient it would receive another $300 in revenue.

Profit and Volume Models: Putting It All Together

As we have discussed, profit is made up of revenues minus costs. The last two sections detailed the relationships between cost and volume and between revenue and volume. Since profit is made up of revenues minus costs, then profit must also be related to volume. On the assumption that patients will seek services from the clinic, we can develop an equation for profit based on volume.

As was stated earlier, profit equals revenues minus costs, and if we combine the revenue and cost volume equations, the total profit equation can be written as (Equation 2.37):

$$\text{Total profit} = \text{revenue} - \text{costs} = \$300x - (\$100,000 + \$100x)$$
$$= \$200x - \$100,000 \qquad (2.37)$$

Therefore, we can see that total profit is related to the volume of patient consultations, x.

Break-Even Example

The managers of the clinic's outpatient operation have been asked to figure out how many patient consultations must be made to break even. The term *break-even* refers to the relationship between revenues and costs. Specifically, break-even is the level of sales at which revenue and cost equal each other. After developing the relationship between profit and volume of patient consultations, the managers can answer this question, using the profit equation and some simple algebra.

Using the profit equation just derived (Equation 2.37), let's attempt to find, by trial and error, the break-even point. First let's allow volume of patient consultations to equal 400 (i.e., $x = 400$), and calculate profits as follows (Equation 2.38):

$$\text{Total profit} = \$200(400) - \$100,000 = -\$20,000 \qquad (2.38)$$

The clinic's manager would conclude that at a volume of 400 patient consultations, the clinic would incur a loss of $20,000. This indicates that if the level of patient consultations is at 400 the clinic will lose money.

However, let's assume that the volume of patient consultations is equal to 600 (i.e., $x = 600$); profit is then calculated as follows (Equation 2.39):

$$\text{Total profit} = \$200(600) - \$100,000 = \$20,000 \qquad (2.39)$$

Now you can see that at a level of 600 patient consultations, the clinic would realize a profit of $20,000. Using simple logic, the manager can conclude that the break-even point must lie somewhere between a production and sales level of 400 and a level of 600 patient consultations. We can develop a simple equation to help us find the break-even point of any profit equation. The first step is to set revenue equal to cost. This is done by using the profit equation and setting it equal to 0. The resulting equation is Equation 2.40:

$$\text{Total profit} = \$200x - \$100,000 = 0$$
$$\$200x = \$100,000 \qquad (2.40)$$
$$x = 500$$

The clinic's manager can conclude that the clinic must consult with at least 500 patients to cover all costs and break even.

Graphical Break-Even Solution

This relationship among revenue, cost, and profit can be graphed to show all possible combinations of volume and resulting profits. Figure 2.4 displays this graph along with the firm's break-even point, fixed cost, total cost, total revenue, profits, and losses.

In addition, a general relationship for computing the break-even point can be established. If we allow x to equal the number of units/patients serviced (i.e., the volume) and we allow P to equal the selling price per unit, then total revenue can be written as shown in Equation 2.41:

$$\text{Total revenue} = Px \qquad (2.41)$$

Cost can also be represented in the same manner, where fixed cost is represented by FC and variable cost is represented by a combination of two symbols, V and x. The x is the same x as stated before and represents the number of units produced and sold. The V is equal to the variable cost associated with producing an extra unit. Total cost is written as shown in Equation 2.42:

$$\text{Total cost} = FC + Vx \qquad (2.42)$$

Combining these relationships, we can write total profit as in Equation 2.43:

$$\text{Total profit} = Px - (FC + Vx) \qquad (2.43)$$

The break-even point is calculated by setting total profit equal to zero and solving the resulting equation for x, as in Equation 2.44:

FIGURE 2.4 Graphical Break-Even Analysis

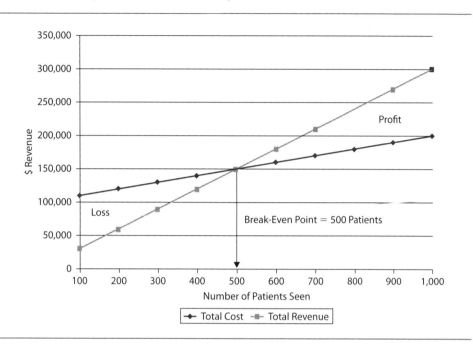

$$\text{Total profit} = 0 = \text{Px} - (\text{FC} + \text{V}x)$$
$$\text{FC} = \text{Px} - \text{Vx} \qquad (2.44)$$
$$\text{FC} = \text{x}(\text{P} - \text{V})$$

Given this relationship, a health care manager who knows the organization's fixed cost, sale price, and variable cost per unit can easily obtain the organization's break-even point.

CROSSOVER ANALYSIS

The clinic manager for the outpatient clinic has been approached by two companies selling two different automated blood-testing machines. The first machine would cost the clinic $5,000 up front (i.e., fixed cost machine 1) while the second machine would cost $2,500 up front (i.e., fixed cost machine 2). Although the first machine costs more up front, it does have a lower cost to run. The variable cost to run the first machine is $5 per blood sample tested whereas the variable cost of the second machine is $12 per blood sample tested.

For the clinic, an analysis of where the two machines cross over, or the unit volume at which the costs of the two machines are equal, needs to be completed. This *crossover analysis* enables the clinic to identify the point (in number of units) where it would be indifferent to the costs generated by the two different machines.

The volume of blood tests performed dictates the long-run cost of each machine. To find the crossover point, the clinic's manager can use the following formula:

$$\text{FC machine } 1 + (\text{VC machine } 1)x = \text{FC machine } 2 + (\text{VC Machine } 2)x$$

where FC = fixed cost, VC = variable cost, and x = number of blood tests.

The clinic is interested in finding the value of x, which equates these two sides of the formula. Solving for x, the formula becomes as follows (Equation 2.45):

$$x = \frac{\text{FC Machine } 2 - \text{FC Machine } 1}{\text{VC Machine } 1 - \text{VC Machine } 2} \qquad (2.45)$$

Using the numbers provided by the clinic manager, the number of blood tests representing the crossover point is then as shown in Equation 2.46:

$$x = \frac{\$2,500 - \$5,000}{\$5 - \$12} \approx 357 \qquad (2.46)$$

At approximately 357 blood tests, the total cost of each of the two machines is equal to the cost of the other. Above and below that volume of blood tests, one machine is preferable to the other. A crossover graph should be developed to assist with this analysis. In addition, the graph will better illustrate the risks involved with choosing one machine over the other.

Crossover Graph

Figure 2.5 depicts the crossover graph for the clinic's blood-testing machine options. It can be seen from the crossover graph that when the clinic performs more than 357 blood tests, the lower-cost machine is machine 1 (e.g., the cost line for machine 1 is lower than that of machine 2 at volumes greater than 357 units). However, if the clinic performs fewer than 357 blood tests, then machine 2 is the better choice (i.e., lower cost).

When the number of blood tests is low (e.g., 50) or when the number of blood tests is high (e.g., 700), the choice of which machine to buy is not difficult. However, when the number of blood tests to perform lies close to the crossover point, then the decision becomes more difficult. In this case, some trade-off and risk analysis must be done.

One way to analyze the problem when the number of units is close to the crossover point is to ask the question: "What happens to the cost of my choice when the opposite of what I thought would happen does in fact happen?" For example, the clinic may believe it will perform around 350 blood tests but then as patients are serviced it ends up performing 450 blood tests. If the clinic was counting on volumes lower than the crossover point and chose machine 2, it ended up performing more blood tests than the crossover point and would have had lower costs if it had chosen machine 1. Some may chalk this up to chance,

FIGURE 2.5 Crossover Graph

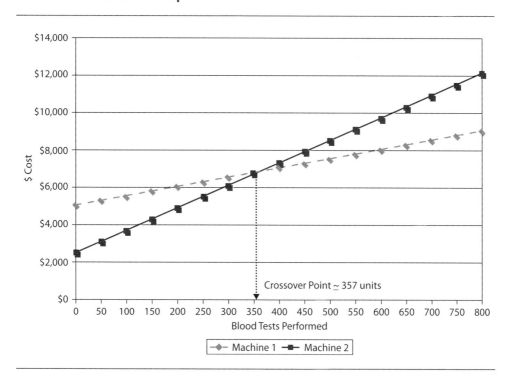

shrug it off, and move on, but if the clinic estimates incorrectly, it could cost it a lot of money in the long run.

So a good question to ask here is: What are the risks of underestimating and/ or overestimating the number of blood tests to be performed? Simply put, if the clinic believes that the number of patients served will grow in the future, it may be willing to take a risk in purchasing machine 1, paying higher costs for volumes lower than the crossover point for a while, but then benefiting from the lower costs of machine 1 when volumes rise above the crossover point. Conversely, if the clinic believes it will not do that many in-house blood tests and in the vast majority of times it performs lower levels of tests and stays below or close to the crossover point, it might be better served by machine 2, as it will offer lower costs below the crossover point. Remember that this analysis assumes that the clinic can forecast the volume of blood tests to be performed with some accuracy. In addition, this basic analysis does not take into account differences in testing quality, speed, or reliability between the two machines.

SUMMARY

Health care organizations interact in a unique financial environment. To get an understanding of how operations and supply chain management can benefit the organization, it is important to discuss financial statements, financial ratios, break-even and crossover analysis, and specifically how revenues and costs impact these documents. For many health care professionals, accounting or finance courses were not requirements for their field of study. This chapter has provided information on finance and accounting from the perspective of a health care organization's operations and supply chain areas.

KEY TERMS

asset management ratios	*fee-for-service*
balance sheet	*future value*
break-even analysis	*income statement*
crossover analysis	*liquidity ratios*

operating statement   *statement of cash flows*

present value   *time value of money*

profitability ratios

DISCUSSION QUESTIONS

Financial Statements

1. Create an operating statement for a not-for-profit hospital given the following list of its revenues and expenses. What would this statement be called for a for-profit hospital?

   - $1,500,000 received as support services and contributions.

   - $10,000,000 earned for patient services.

   - $4,000,000 received from capitated contracts with health maintenance organizations (HMOs).

   - $2,500,000 given in contractual discounts to Medicare and Medicaid patients.

   - $1,000,000 in uncollected debts.

   - $1,000,000 in depreciation and amortization of assets.

   - $4,500,000 in salaries, insurance paid, and utilities.

   - $500,000 in supplies.

   - $2,000,000 in other expenses.

2. Where would each of the following be listed on a balance sheet?

   a. Cash

   b. Parking garage

   c. Accounts payable

   d. Accounts receivable

   e. Bonds payable in four years

   f. Prepaid expenses

3. Create a statement of cash flows for Hospital XYZ, an investor-owned for-profit hospital with 5,000 outstanding shares of stock, for the year 2010 given the following list of activities.

- Began 2010 with $150,000 in cash and cash equivalents.

- Paid dividends of $10 per share.

- Increase in accounts receivable of $10,000.

- Increase in accounts payable of $5,000.

- Sale of neighboring lot for $2,000,000.

- Expansion project costing $1,500,000.

- Issuance of 10-year bonds totaling $5,000,000.

- Purchase of new equipment totaling $4,000,000.

Ratios

4. Hospital XYZ has annual revenues of $100,000,000 and its current accounts receivable is $7,500,000. What is its days in patient accounts receivable, and what does this figure mean?

5. Compute the ratios and metrics given the following information on Hospital XYZ:
   - Current assets: $40,000,000

   - Total assets: $100,000,000

   - Current liabilities: $12,000,000

   - Total liabilities: $45,000,000

   - Annual revenue: $435,000,000

   - Total expenses: $425,000,000

   - Operating income: $10,000,000

   - Inventories: $5,000,000

   - Depreciation: $2,000,000

a. Current ratio

b. Working capital

c. Days of working capital

d. Quick ratio

e. Average pay period

f. Return on assets

g. Return on equity

6. Given the following figures, compute the adjusted discharges for Hospital XYZ.

- Total inpatient discharges: 11,250

- Gross outpatient revenue: $1,000,000

- Inpatient gross revenue per discharge: $14,000

Time Value of Money

7. Hospital XYZ currently has a contract with an HMO that agrees to pay it $5,000,000 at the end of each of the next five years. The hospital has the ability to opt out now to renegotiate, and the new deal has a predicted present value of $21,500,000. Assuming the hospital has a discount rate of 7 percent and the deals differ only in payment structure, what is the present value of the current contract, and which contract should Hospital XYZ choose?

8. Dr. Sanders has just performed a back surgery on his uninsured patient, John, and has billed John for $10,000. They have agreed to set up a financing plan with John paying $2,000 up front and the rest in two years. John will be paying 10 percent annual interest on the unpaid portion of his bill. What amount will be due at the end of the second year?

9. In employment contract negotiations between Dr. Sanders and Hospital XYZ, Dr. Sanders has requested a college fund for his son worth $150,000 12 years from now. The hospital prefers to pay him a discounted value now as a signing bonus for this. Ignoring taxes and assuming Dr. Sanders is confident he can invest at an interest rate of 6.5 percent annually, what would the signing bonus need to be to satisfy Dr. Sanders?

Break-Even/Crossover Analysis

10. What is the marginal cost for a surgeon seeing 250 patients annually with fixed costs of $30,000 per year and total costs of $115,000 per year?

11. Assuming Hospital XYZ has an annual fixed cost of $750,000 and each patient day costs $150 while bringing in $275 in revenue, how may patient days does the hospital need to break even each year?

12. Hospital XYZ is in the market for a new MRI machine and is considering two different products. Machine A costs $20,000 up front and $200 per use. Machine B costs $14,500 up front and $265 per use. At what point do these two machines cross over? Which machine should they choose if their estimated number of uses is 15 over this point? Which machine should they choose if their estimate is 4 under?

REFERENCES

"Data Trends: Supply Chain Benchmarking." 2008. *Healthcare Financial Management* (August).

"A Solid Year: Healthcare Business News and Research." 2011. *Modern Healthcare* at www.modernhealthcare.com/article/20110606/MAGAZINE/110609993#.

Zelman, W. N., M. J. McCue, and N. D. Glick. 2009. *Financial Management of Health Care Organizations: An Introduction to Fundamental Tools, Concepts and Applications.* San Francisco: Jossey-Bass.

CHAPTER 3

MANAGERIAL ACCOUNTING ASPECTS OF HEALTH CARE OPERATIONS AND SUPPLY CHAIN MANAGEMENT

LEARNING OBJECTIVES

⟶ Understand what managerial accounting is and how it is applied to health care organizations.

(Continued)

⏺ Understand what activity-based costing is and how it is applied to health care organizations.

⏺ Understand the implications for health care providers and operational managers regarding financial operations.

MANAGERIAL ASPECTS OF HEALTH CARE OPERATIONS AND SUPPLY CHAIN MANAGEMENT

It has been established that health care organizations interact in a unique financial environment. An understanding of financial statements, specifically how revenues and costs impact these documents, is valuable to a health care professional. However, to improve a health care organization's operations and supply chain, a health care professional must also understand the basics of:

• What managerial accounting is and why it is important to operations and supply chain management (SCM).

• What activity-based costing (ABC) is and its implications for health care organizations.

MANAGERIAL ACCOUNTING

The question "What did it cost?" is a common question in any organization. However, it is especially important in the health care profession, where prices are set by insurers or other third-party payers, or when attempting to assess the financial viability of different programs and services.

When discussing the purchase of supplies or labor, the answer to the question is straightforward. For example, a manager can just look at the invoice or at a salary/wage rate. Also, in the case when an organization provides goods or services that are alike, it is relatively easy to calculate what the good or service costs. Things get complex when an organization provides multiple nonalike goods or services that use differing amounts of resources (i.e., almost every health care provider).

Cost Information and Resource Usage

Cost information for a good or service is used primarily for three purposes: profitability assessments, comparative analyses, and pricing decisions. Health care managers use cost information for one or all of these purposes at different times and under varying decision-making scenarios.

Cost information leads us to the fundamental issue that *managerial accounting* addresses. The use of resources, for what and how much, is what managerial accounting investigates. The recourses investigated include land, labor, and capital.

Measuring as accurately as possible the consumption of these resources associated with producing a good or service is a goal of managerial accounting. As previously mentioned, if an organization provides a single good or service or provides like goods or services, the measurement process is quite easy. All costs could be added together and divided by the number of units or hours of service produced to arrive at a cost per unit. For example, a laboratory that processes only one type of test will have a relatively easy time calculating the full cost of each test.

However, few health care organizations produce a single product or service. Resources consumption is at times unique to a good or service but many times the resource consumption is spread over multiple goods or services. Managerial accounting attempts to identify the factors that influence the use of resources and, in turn, the costs. Managerial accountants seek out what are referred to as *cost drivers*.

Health Care Operations and Supply Chain Management in Action: The ABCs of ABC Costing

As the health care industry has changed, it has become more and more challenging for individual practices to remain profitable. Evaluating the performance of a health care practice with regard to cost is key to ensuring business sustainability. Although appearing to be right in front of the decision maker, accurate cost information is at times hard to obtain or at least decipher.

Manufacturing companies were faced with this same challenge decades ago. They needed to continue to produce high-quality products at low costs but also to eliminate unnecessary costs and plan for change. A methodology referred to as activity-based costing (ABC) was developed to assist in getting a handle on current costs and help plan for changes in future costs.

In general, ABC identifies relationships between activities and the associated resources needed to complete said activity. Costs are then assigned to the resources consumed by the activity. There have been a number of instances in which ABC has been applied to a medical practice.

Cost Data and ABC

It may be assumed that all health care practices have a computerized billing system, but that does not mean costs are easily extracted and analyzed. The value of cost data is that when they are analyzed they can be used for planning purposes to make better decisions in the future.

The accrual basis is the cornerstone of the cost system and must be used to effectively employ ABC. However, many individual health care providers use a cash basis for accounting. One of the first steps these individual health care providers must take is to convert their accounting systems from a cash basis to an accrual basis. Once this step is taken, then the ABC process can be embarked upon.

Cost centers can be identified and are the units through which a health care provider operates. Administration, laboratory, pathology, and surgery are all examples. Providers define their own cost centers. The determination of cost centers will be dependent on how a particular practice operates. ABC analysis provides for areas such as contract negotiation, managed-care cost allocation, and equipment purchases or leases. However, ABC analysis is not static. Continual monitoring and updates must be made as medical processes change.

Cost Drivers

Cost drivers link product and service activities directly to costs. Many costs in a clinic are directly linked to the number of patients seen. Other costs result from the number or complexity of the service provided. In general, there are six cost drivers in most health care organizations. Table 3.1 describes these six cost drivers and gives examples for a health care organization. Note that the classification scheme lists and classifies the activities that cause costs to exist. Costs are not listed by organizational structure.

TABLE 3.1 Six Cost Drivers and Health Care Examples

Cost Driver	Examples
Program—the fixed cost incurred so the health care organization is prepared to provide service	Fixed costs of equipment such as x-ray machines or other fixed costs required to run health care programs (e.g., chairs for waiting room)
Factor prices—the cost per unit of each resource	Price per lab test; hourly wages for lab technician, nurse, or specialist
Efficiency—the number of resource inputs needed for each unit of output	Time and supplies per lab test; time and supplies per rapid strep test; nursing hours per patient
Case type—sometimes called case mix	Appendicitis; gallbladder removal; pneumonia
Volume—the number of patients of each type	10 appendectomies; 5 gallbladder removals; 50 cases of pneumonia
Patient needs—the resources used by a patient of a particular case type	For an appendectomy: three hours in surgery, one day in recovery room, one day of level II nursing care, two tests

Summary of Managerial Accounting Choices

"What did it cost?" is a common question in any organization but the main question for managerial accounting. Cost information for a good or service is used primarily for three purposes: profitability assessments, comparative analyses, and pricing decisions. Cost information leads us to the fundamental issue that managerial accounting addresses.

The use of resources, for what and how much, is what managerial accounting investigates. The recourses investigated include land, labor, and capital. Managerial judgment is involved in the development of a managerial accounting system. Cost drivers must be identified and applied to the various procedures a health care organization provides. Allocation of costs will be determined in part by the choice of the support centers and drivers themselves.

ACTIVITY-BASED COSTING

The roots of *activity-based costing* (ABC) go back to the 1980s and manufacturers' efforts to analyze and eliminate unnecessary costs from their operations. The costing methodology was adopted in other industries throughout the 1990s and into the 2000s, including health care. ABC has continued to evolve, now encompassing time-driven ABC and activity-based management (ABM). It is a common question for many health care professionals to ask how ABC can be applied to their organizations and how it relates to existing costing methods.

ABC proponents are correct in their criticism of traditional hospital costing methods that embody too closely these characteristics:

- No split of direct versus indirect costs.

- Ratios of departmental costs to charges (RCCs).

- Single cost component.

- Cost apportionment based on prices of charge code items.

When costs are developed using these methods, they are most likely inaccurate and difficult to trace. Traceability is crucial in costing. However, when using traditional methods of costing, fixed/variable and *direct cost/indirect cost* distinctions are not evident in the process. In addition, traditional costing makes it almost impossible to analyze the effects of activity changes such as labor rates or hours of lab analysis (refer to earlier discussion on cost drivers). In using traditional costing, overhead is hidden in product costs using general allocations.

ABC makes a concerted effort to tie areas usually thought of as general overhead (e.g., consumable supplies, testing time, etc.) to their own activity measures (i.e., *traceable costs*). ABC's main tenet is to reveal all activities contributing to cost, allowing managers to eliminate activities that do not add value. This notion goes hand in hand with continuous improvement, and thus ABC is often heard in connection with six sigma, lean, reengineering efforts, and improving/optimizing the supply chain.

What Are ABC's Primary Weaknesses?

ABC can be very time-consuming to the organization. The method demands a large volume of data on processes and end services. It has been noted that ABC can transform every manager into an amateur accountant. In turn, those managers become fixed on tracking activity costs, rather than tracking and perfecting the activity itself.

TABLE 3.2 Activities and Cost Drivers for the Nurse's Station

Activity	Cost Driver
Supervision	Number of patients admitted
Delivering nursing care	Weighted patient days
Changing linen and garments	Number of patient days

What Are the Basic Steps of ABC?

Developing the initial ABC model consists of three steps:

1. Determine key activities, resources, related cost drivers, and *cost objectives*/objects of the product or service to be investigated (e.g., activities for a nurse's station).

   For example, Table 3.2 displays the following activities and related cost drivers identified for a typical nurse's station. The cost objects are the three levels of patients the nursing station services: high frequency of care, above-average frequency of care, and average frequency of care.

2. Determine all the resources (with their respective costs) that support the activities and are required to create the end product or deliver the end service. Flowcharting/process mapping works well for this step, and non-value-added activities should be examined here.

3. Collect relevant data concerning costs and physical flow for cost objectives, drivers, and total cost per activity.

Figure 3.1 displays the flowchart/process map and relevant cost data and calculations for the nurse's station example.

Table 3.3 contains the formulas for the cost per unit driver calculations. The actual cost per unit driver is calculated as follows (refer to Figure 3.1):

Given:

Indirect costs = $183,000 (cell B2)
Supervision traceable costs = $63,000 (cell B4)
Nursing care traceable costs = $92,000 (cell C4)
Changing linens and garments traceable costs = $28,000 (cell D4)
Supervision cost driver = Number of patients admitted
Nursing care cost driver = Weighted patient days
Changing linens and garments cost driver = Number of patient days

FIGURE 3.1 Flowchart/Process Map for the Nurse's Station Example

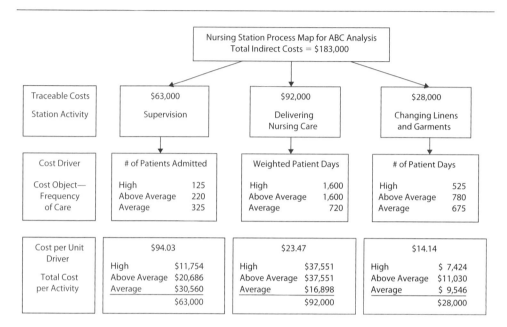

TABLE 3.3 Formulas for the Cost per Unit Driver Calculations

Activity	Cost per Unit Driver	Excel Formulas
Supervision	$= \dfrac{\$63,000}{(125 + 220 + 325)} = \$94.03$	$= \frac{B4}{B11}$ (cell B13)
Nursing care	$= \dfrac{\$92,000}{(1,600 + 1,600 + 720)} = \$23.47$	$= \frac{C4}{C11}$ (cell C13)
Changing linens and garments	$= \dfrac{\$28,000}{(525 + 780 + 675)} = \$14.14$	$= \frac{D4}{D11}$ (cell D13)
	Supervision $= 670$	$=$ SUM(B8 : B10) cell B11
Total	Nursing care $= 3,920$	$=$ SUM(C8 : C10) cell C11
	Changing linens & garments $= 1,980$	$=$ SUM(D8 : D10) cell D11

The cost per unit driver is then multiplied by the associated cost object (high, above average, or average) to find the total cost per activity (see Table 3.4).

The traditional method of assigned indirect costs would yield the results shown in Table 3.5.

Comparing the ABC method to the traditional method, we see that supervision should be charged much more in indirect costs than either nursing care or changing linens and garments. The traditional method would assign each activity

TABLE 3.4 Formulas for the Total Cost per Activity Calculations

Activity	Cost per Unit Driver		Excel Formulas
Supervision	High	= $94.03(125)	= B13(B8) cell B15
	Above Average	= $94.03(220)	= B13(B9) cell B16
	Average	= $94.03(325)	= B13(B10) cell B17
Nursing care	High	= $23.47(1,600)	= C13(C8) cell C15
	Above Average	= $23.47(1,600)	= C13(C9) cell C16
	Average	= $23.47(720)	= C13(C10) cell C17
Changing	High	= $14.14(525)	= D13(D8) cell D15
linens and	Above Average	= $14.14(780)	= D13(D9) cell D16
garments	Average	= $14.14(675)	= D13(D10) cell D17
Total	Supervision	= $63,000	= SUM(B15 : B17) cell B18
	Nursing care	= $92,000	= SUM(C15 : C17) cell C18
	Changing linens & garments	= $28,000	= SUM(D15 : D17) cell D18

TABLE 3.5 Formulas for the Traditional Method of Indirect Cost Assignment

Traditional Costing	Cost Driver Calculations (Excel Formulas)
Annual cost of nurse's station	$183,000 (cell B21)
Total patient days (annually)	2,045 (=SUM(B22:B24)) cell B25
Total cost activity	$$= \frac{\$183,000}{2,045} = \$89.49 \left(= \frac{B21}{B25} \right) \text{ cell B26}$$

the same charge of $89.49 (see Table 3.5). It is apparent from the ABC method that there are dramatic differences in the three activities and how they use resources, and in turn how they should be charged the associated indirect costs.

For more information on activity-based costing applied to the health care industry, see Canby 1995, Helmi and Tanju 1991, Kaplan et al. 2007, and Shields 2001.

SUPPLY CHAIN MANAGEMENT BEHIND THE SCENES: COST DRIVERS AT HOSPITALS

As previously mentioned, concepts of activity-based costing were developed during the 1970s and 1980s, mostly in the manufacturing sector. However, activity-based costing is also widely used in the health care industry.

Cost-Driven Factors to Consider

One study identified approximately 250 activity cost drivers that hospitals should consider, including account management, corporate support, delivery, information technology, interest, line cost, occupancy, order cost, procurement, and staging cost.

Typically, when introducing an activity-based system into a hospital, the accounting team meets with materials management/procurement to develop a pricing schedule based on the hospital's activities. It can be said that many times materials management uses the old cost-plus theory. In turn, there is only so much saving that can ever be realized in that system. Therefore, the discussion focuses on ways to become more efficient and places where savings can be identified. Supplying an area such as the operating room makes up a large share of a health care provider's supply budget. Items such as unnecessary worker movements and behavior are identified and slow-moving inventory items are reduced.

For example, an operating room unit may issue special requests for 100 items a day from the supply manager. In many cases, the supply manager is not prepared for these requests and in turn must perform special supply pulls, staging, and routing procedures. The issue at hand is that there is no penalty for these special requests but the requests pile on unnecessary costs. Surgeons and their teams drive this process most of the time, and if their teams could look for the emergency item before contacting the supply manager or come to an agreement to increase inventory levels at nursing stations, costs could be decreased. ABC analysis aids in identifying these types of behavior and creating incentives to eliminate unnecessary actions and in turn drive down costs.

SUMMARY

A common question in any health care organization is, "What did the service cost?" Cost information is primarily used for three purposes: profitability assessments, comparative analysis, and pricing decisions. Managerial accounting coupled with cost information addresses these three areas. Activity-based costing uses managerial accounting information to identify relationships between activities and the associated resources needed to complete them. Costs are then assigned to the resources consumed by the activity. In all, managerial accounting and, in particular, activity-based costing, are areas that impact a health care organization's success and are necessary for health care professionals to understand.

KEY TERMS

activity-based costing

cost driver

cost objective

direct cost

indirect cost

managerial accounting

traceable cost

DISCUSSION QUESTIONS

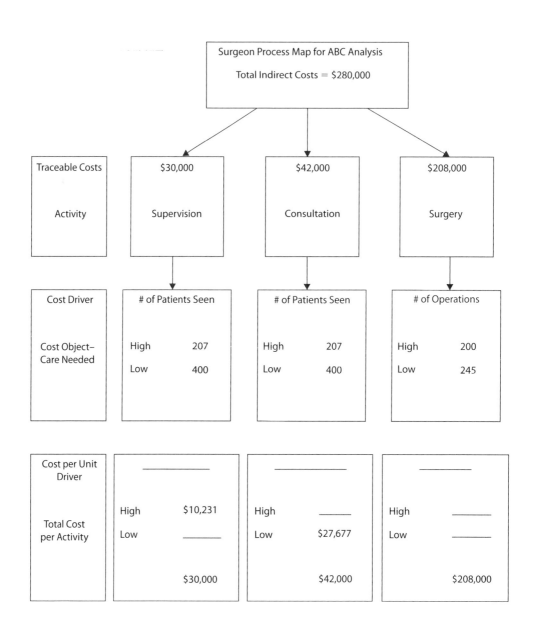

1. Fill in the blanks for the ABC analysis process map.

2. Based on the process map, calculate the assigned indirect costs using the traditional method. Explain the pros and cons of this in comparison to activity-based costing.

3. Using the process map, which activity should be charged the highest amount of associated indirect costs? The lowest?

REFERENCES

Canby, J. B., IV. 1995. "Applying Activity Based Costing to Healthcare Settings." *Healthcare Financial Management* (February): 50–56.

Helmi, M. A., and M. N. Tanju. 1991. "Activity Based Costing May Reduce Costs, Aid Planning." *Healthcare Financial Management* (November): 55–56.

Kaplan, Robert S., and Steven R. Anderson. 2007. *Time-Driven Activity-Based Costing.* Boston: Harvard Business School Press.

Shields, T. 2001. "Hospitals Turning to Activity-Based Costing to Save and Measure Distribution Costs." Downloaded from www.hpnonline.com/inside/2001–11/sb .html.

PART II

PROCESS DESIGN AND ANALYSIS OF HEALTH CARE OPERATIONS

CHAPTER 4

DATA AND STATISTICAL TOOLS FOR HEALTH CARE OPERATIONS IMPROVEMENT

LEARNING OBJECTIVES

➠ Understand graphical methods of data description, specifically histograms.

➠ Understand and calculate measures of central tendency and dispersion.

➠ Use Excel to construct histograms and calculate measures of central tendency and dispersion.

(Continued)

⏺ Calculate and interpret expected values.

⏺ Understand the concept of Pareto analysis.

⏺ Be able to create and interpret box-and-whisker plots.

⏺ Understand and create tornado diagrams.

DESCRIPTIVE STATISTICS FOR DESCRIBING DATA SETS

The acquisition, analysis, and description of data are fundamental tasks managers are challenged with every day. Many health care professionals find themselves inundated with data—at times overwhelmed and unable to glean even the most basic information from important data sets. This chapter provides some simple methods for data organization and description.

The authors wish to stress that, by learning a few basic descriptive and numeric methods of data analysis and presentation, health care professionals can become more efficient and effective problem solvers. This chapter presents graphical and numerical description methods and links the methods together to paint a full picture of the problem at hand.

GRAPHICAL METHODS OF DATA DESCRIPTION

Two graphical methods of data are presented: histograms and relative frequency diagrams. These methods are most commonly used to visually describe real-world data sets. It is vitally important that the student begin to look for links between the two methods and to use both methods to fully paint a picture of the data.

Histograms

Histograms relate the number of occurrences of each event in an event space to each other. Each event is represented on the *x*-axis of the histogram, while the number of times each event occurs is represented on the *y*-axis. Histograms are very common in everyday life. Many people don't use the term *histogram* and instead refer to diagrams depicting the occurrence of events as graphs.

As a student of health care operations and supply chain management (SCM), you have more than likely seen many histograms throughout your studies. An example could be the distribution of diagnosis-related group (DRG) codes for any given day. A histogram for a daily set of DRG codes might look something like Figure 4.1.

Histograms are a straightforward, easy-to-construct method of graphical data description that almost everyone understands. All commercial spreadsheet packages have the capability to construct histograms. A later section in this chapter demonstrates how to create a histogram in Excel.

Relative Frequency Diagrams

Relative frequency diagrams resemble histograms but relate the occurrence of events in terms of probability. Instead of displaying the number of times an event

FIGURE 4.1 Histogram for Daily Recorded DRG Codes

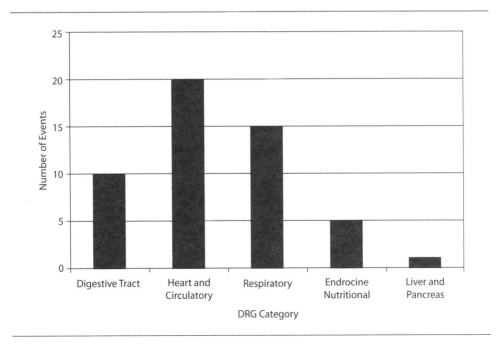

has occurred, a relative frequency diagram displays the percentage of times each event occurred out of the total number of events.

Relative frequency diagrams are used when two groups of similar data need to be compared but may differ in size. For example, as a health care professional you want to know the various percentages of DRG codes that are recorded for a given day. In turn you may wish to compare those percentages to the percentages of those same DRG codes for another day or time period. It would not be helpful to compare the two histograms, because of the difference in magnitude of the sample sets. The medical facility may have thousands of time periods of data, and you may have only one day of data.

Figure 4.2 displays the relative frequency diagram for the DRG coding example. Even though histograms and relative frequency diagrams resemble each other, each type gives a decision maker unique information.

A relative frequency diagram allows the two sets of data to be compared on the basis of a common denominator, percentage histograms, throughout your studies.

Let's go back to the example of the DRG category. Table 4.1 contains the data on the DRG category.

FIGURE 4.2 Relative Frequency Diagram

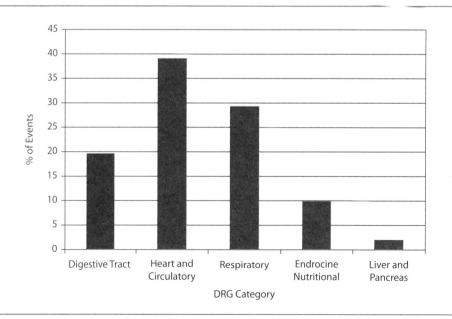

TABLE 4.1   DRG Category Data

DRG Category	DRG Code Amount	Relative Frequency	Percentage
Digestive tract	10	10/51	0.1961
Heart and circulatory	20	20/51	0.3922
Respiratory	15	15/51	0.2941
Endocrine nutritional	5	5/51	0.0980
Liver and pancreas	1	1/51	0.0196
Total	51	51/51	1.0000

To create a relative frequency table, the relative frequency of each event in the event space must be calculated. Column 3 in Table 4.1 performs this operation. In turn, column 4 contains the relative frequency in terms of percentage.

We have noted that the histogram and the relative frequency diagram look very much alike. This is true only because the magnitudes of the numbers are in the same ratios. However, each graph gives a decision maker unique information about the data set being investigated. Most important in the case of the relative frequency diagram is comparability to other data sets.

Is there any other reason why a relative frequency diagram might be used instead of a histogram? It could be because clients tend to understand and respond to percentages better. Would it be possible to use a relative frequency diagram to misrepresent data?

NUMERICAL METHODS OF DATA DESCRIPTION

For a health care professional to become a more effective and efficient problem solver, numerical methods of data description must be mastered. Two types of numerical methods are detailed in this section. They include:

1. Measures of central tendency

2. Measures of dispersion

Health care professionals must employ both measures of central tendency and measures of dispersion to fully describe a problem.

Someone who does not employ both of these measures tells only half the story. Health care professionals can improve their problem solving skills greatly by learning to describe data sets in terms of central tendency and dispersion.

Measures of Central Tendency

Measures of central tendency describe the data set in terms of a single number. Two of the most common measures of central tendency will be detailed:

1. Simple mean

2. Median

Simple Mean

The *simple mean* of a data set is defined as its average. It should be noted that statisticians use the terms *mean* and *average* interchangeably. The formula used to calculate the simple mean is shown in Equation 4.1:

$$\mu = \frac{\sum_{i=1}^{n} x_i}{n} \tag{4.1}$$

where μ = Greek lower case mu, for mean

x_i = individual data point i

n = total number of data points

S = Greek capital sigma, meaning summation

Given the data set 5, 7, 12, 39, 7, the simple mean would be calculated as shown in Equation 4.2:

$$\mu = \frac{\sum_{i=1}^{n} x_i}{n} = (5 + 7 + 12 + 39 + 7)/5 = 14 \tag{4.2}$$

If you are using Excel, the formula to calculate average is: average(number1, number2, . . .).

TABLE 4.2 Common Measures of Central Tendency in Health Care

Use	Description
How long does a patient reside in the hospital?	Average length of stay
How long does someone wait in the ER?	Average ER wait time
What is a patient's average blood pressure?	Average blood pressure readings over time

We encounter and use the measure of simple mean every day. Examples of common occurrences of the simple mean as a measure of central tendency are listed in Table 4.2.

As human beings, we overuse and at times misuse the simple mean as a measure of central tendency. This occurs when the simple mean is calculated from a sample that is biased, either by including extreme values, which we define as outliers, or by not obtaining a large enough sample size.

Look back at our example data set, 5, 7, 12, 39, 7. Is there something that looks out of place? Yes, 39 is large compared to the other values. In fact, it is large enough that it could significantly bias the simple mean upward. Is there something we can do to remedy this? Yes, there is. We can use another measure of central tendency that adjusts for outliers—the median.

Median

The definition of the *median* is the middle value of the data set. The median divides the data set into two equal halves. The median is employed in areas that tend to have outliers of large magnitude or where the data set has known bias. Three real-life examples of where the median is used instead of the simple mean are:

1. Housing prices

2. Health care salaries

3. National income figures

The next time you get a chance, take a look through the real estate section of your local newspaper. It should become obvious that there are some prices that are very, very high in comparison with your average price for a home. These high-priced homes tend to skew or bias the simple mean upward. Therefore, housing price trends are almost always discussed in terms of median and not in terms of simple mean.

Median is calculated according to two rules:

1. If your data set contains an odd number of data points:

   - Order the data points from lowest to highest.

   - Starting from the left and right, count in from each side until you reach the middle data point.

   - This number is the median.

2. If your data set contains an even number of data points:

   - Order the data points from lowest to highest.

   - Starting from the left and right, count in from each side until you reach the two middle data points.

   - Take the average of these two points, and this number is the median.

If we take a look back at our example data set, 5, 7, 12, 39, 7, we can calculate the median. Since the data set contains an odd number of data points, we will use the steps listed under the first set of instructions for calculating median.

Order the data points from lowest to highest: 5, 7, 7, 12, 39.

Starting from the left and the right, count in from each side until you reach the middle data point, 7.

The middle number, 7, is the median for our example. The formula in Excel for median is: median(number1, number2, . . .). Now, let's compare the numbers we obtained for the simple mean and the median.

Comparison of Mean and Median

When we compare the mean of 14 to the median of 7, the difference is significant. The simple mean is skewed upward because of the effect of the data point 39. This does not infer that the median is the correct measure and simple mean is the incorrect measure.

A decision maker must decide which is the more appropriate measure of central tendency to use. If the numbers in our example were actually estimated numbers in tens of thousands of dollars representing housing prices or salaries in an area, an individual using the simple mean might be overstating the actual central tendency by relying on the simple mean. This is the reason real estate agents and the federal government use the median as the measure of central tendency when relaying information on trends in housing prices and salaries.

When was the last time you used a mean to explain a situation or a set of data? Have you ever used the median to describe a set of data or a situation? Look around for examples in everyday life of the use of mean and median. When would a health care professional want to use a mean? A median?

Most Common Measure of Central Tendency

Critical thinking and judgment must be developed when it comes to measures of central tendency. Basically, a decision maker must know where and when to use simple mean and median. However, overwhelmingly we see and use the simple mean in our everyday lives.

As was stated before, we calculate average emergency room (ER) wait times, average prescriptions written, or average health care salaries on a daily basis. Simple mean is the most common measure of central tendency because it is the easiest to compute and the easiest to understand. There are some rules of thumb one should remember before using the simple mean to describe a data set's central tendency. Using these rules of thumb will help avoid the pitfalls of overestimating or underestimating the data set's true central tendency. There are two steps:

1. Do a preliminary scan of the data to identify any outliers (i.e., very large or very small data points with respect to the overall data set).

2. If outliers are found, a few courses of action can be taken:

   • Throw the outlier data points out and use the modified data set to calculate the simple mean, making sure to note somewhere in the final results that the outlier data points were removed.

   • Discount the outliers by some factor and calculate the simple mean using the modified data set, making sure to note the data points that were discounted and the method used to discount them.

   • Calculate both the mean and the median and provide a comparison of the two measures for the client.

Decision makers must decide the most appropriate measure of central tendency to describe data sets. Remember that, as a health care professional, it is your responsibility to determine which measure of central tendency is proper for the data set. The bottom line is: begin to develop your critical thinking and judgment on the issue of central tendency.

Measures of Dispersion

As mentioned earlier, we all see and use measures of central tendency every day in the real world. It is obvious at times, however, that just using central tendency to describe a data set is shortsighted. If we use only the simple mean or median to describe a data set, we have painted only half the picture.

In addition to measures of central tendency, measures of dispersion can be used as measures of risk. The concept of risk will be discussed in later chapters, but decision makers frequently use measures of dispersion to describe the relative risk of a data set and, in turn, the risk of possible alternatives. Overall, measures of dispersion can be used to define and quantify risk.

This section discusses three measures of dispersion:

1. Range

2. Variance

3. Standard deviation (SD)

In addition, examples will be given to help solidify the link between measures of central tendency and measures of dispersion.

Range

We use *range* to describe data sets in our everyday lives. It is common to speak of "high" versus "low" or "the most" versus "the least." The simple range is the difference between two points. The simple range is calculated as follows.

Simple range = High point of data set − Low point of data set

If you are using Excel, the formula would be max(number1, number2, . . .) − min(number1, number2, . . .).

However, statisticians use the term *range* differently—or at least they use a different definition. Instead of the simple range, statisticians generally use what is called the *interquartile range (IQR)* to describe the dispersion of a data set. The statistical definition of IQR is given first and then we discuss its relationship to the simple range measurement.

Definition of Interquartile Range Before the advent of handheld calculators and desktop computers, statisticians needed a quick and easy way to describe data sets with regard to dispersion. Thus the IQR was born. The following are the general rules about calculating IQR. The similarities to the calculation of median will be noted later in the section.

In essence, when calculating the IQR we wish to divide the data into four equal groups and study the extreme points. To calculate the IQR we proceed as follows.

Calculation of Interquartile Range

1. Arrange the data in numerical order.

2. Divide the data into two equal groups at the median.

3. Divide these two groups again at their medians.

4. Label the median of the lower group the first quartile (Q1) and the median of the higher group the third quartile (Q3).

5. The IQR = Q3 − Q1.

These calculations are fairly simple, which makes this measure of dispersion a good back-of-the-envelope calculation that can be used to get a quick view of the makeup of a data set. One can see the direct relation the IQR has to the median. However, decision makers will find that the IQR is not used all that often in real life.

Most health care professionals find it much easier today to use spreadsheet programs to analyze data sets and calculate measures of dispersion. As a result, the use of the IQR has diminished. Other measures of dispersion have become more popular. Variance and standard deviation are two of the most common of these measures and are detailed next.

Definition of Variance

The *variance* of a data set measures the spread from the mean. Many of us use the term *variance* in our everyday lives to describe data sets. Variance is calculated as shown in Equation 4.3:

$$s^2 = \frac{\sum_{i-1}^{n} x_i - \mu}{n - 1} \tag{4.3}$$

Variance measures the spread of the data from the mean. From the earlier example, let's calculate the variance for the following data set: 5, 7, 12, 39, 7.

Let $n = 5$ and $\mu = 14$. Therefore variance is then calculated as shown in Equation 4.4:

$$\begin{aligned}
\sigma^2 &= \frac{(5 - 14)^2 + (7 - 14)^2 + (12 - 14)^2 + (39 - 14)^2 + (7 - 14)^2}{5 - 1} \\
&= (81 + 49 + 4 + 625 + 49)/4 \\
&= 202
\end{aligned} \tag{4.4}$$

The Excel formula for variance is VAR(number1, number2, ...). Standard statistical nomenclature labels variance as σ^2. However, statisticians use σ^2, s^2, or at times "var" to represent variance. The three labels will be used interchangeably throughout the book. It is important to note the units that correspond to the variance calculated. If the original data set units were dollars, then the variance would be in dollars squared.

This may seem strange. How can one compare dollars with dollars squared? This is the main difficulty with using the statistical measure of variance. The measure of dispersion used must be in the same units as the measure of central tendency. This difficulty is remedied easily and is detailed next.

Definition of Standard Deviation

The definition of *standard deviation* is simple:

$$\text{Standard deviation} = \sqrt{\text{Var}} = \sqrt{\sigma^2}$$

For the aforementioned example,

$$\text{Standard deviation} = \sigma = \sqrt{202} \approx 14.2$$

Since variance is in terms of squared units, taking the square root of the variance is all that must be done to get the measure of dispersion into the proper units. The Excel formula for standard deviation is STDEV(number1, number2, . . .).

Once again, standard statistical nomenclature labels standard deviation as σ. However, statisticians use σ, s, or at times SD to represent standard deviation. The three labels are used interchangeably throughout the book.

Standard deviation is the most common measure of dispersion. Many other industries and disciplines use standard deviation. For example,

- Insurance companies use SD in determining rates and coverages.

- Marketing researchers use SD to describe consumer preferences.

- Economists use SD to analyze variability in markets.

- Information systems analysts use SD to describe network traffic.

- Stockbrokers use SD in analyzing investments.

As a health care professional, you must think in terms of central tendency and dispersion. In using both measures, you will become a more effective and efficient problem solver. By using both measures you gain insight into the underlying patterns of the data sets. Combining the use of central tendency and dispersion gives you the ability to describe and analyze data sets much more fully and communicate that information to your client.

The following example illustrates this point.

Painting the Full Picture: A Waiting Room Example

Let's say your emergency room head nurse tells you that the average time for a patient to wait is around 30 minutes. Now, apart from being stunned by the low average, a student of health care operations and SCM may still be confused as to the makeup of the data set used to calculate the simple mean. This confusion is not uncommon. In fact, the confusion is justified because by using only the simple mean only half the story has been told.

For illustration, let's say the nurse explains that there are actually two different queues within the ER, one for adults and one for children (i.e., a separate pediatric ER area). The simple averages for these two queues are both 30 minutes.

TABLE 4.3 Emergency Room Waiting Time Information

	Waiting Time (minutes)			
	10	28	32	50
Adult ER	50	0	0	50
Pediatric ER	0	50	50	0

However, the nurse imparts the extra information contained in Table 4.3. From Table 4.3 it can be seen that out of 100 patients in the adult ER queue, 50 wait 10 minutes and 50 wait 50 minutes. In the pediatric ER, 50 patients wait 28 minutes while 50 patients wait 32 minutes.

On closer look at the two data sets, it is apparent that the simple averages are the same:

$$\text{Mean waiting time of adult ER queue} = (10 \times 50 + 50 \times 50)/100 = 30$$
$$\text{Mean waiting time of pediatric ER queue} = (28 \times 50 + 32 \times 50)/100 = 30$$

However, these two ER queues are very different from each other. The adult ER tends to be very spread out; half of the patients wait 10 minutes, while the other half wait 50 minutes. In contrast, the pediatric ER queue is very tightly packed around the mean of 30 minutes (i.e., no child waits much more than any other child).

Many individuals use words like *variation* or *variance in the data*. These individuals are not really referring to the statistical calculation of variance but are more likely talking about standard deviation. However, unless you are a statistician or around statisticians, rarely will you hear the common person use the term *standard deviation*.

With this in mind, health care professionals must remember what the statistical definitions of variance and standard deviation are, even while individual clients or colleagues may be using layman's terms such as variation or variance to actually describe the standard deviation of a data set.

Using Central Tendency and Dispersion

To become a more effective and efficient problem solver, a decision maker must use measures of central tendency and measures of dispersion to analyze and describe data sets.

This is readily apparent in the ER queue distribution data given in the preceding example. On the basis of mean alone, the two ER queues look identical. However, after seeing the dispersion of the data around the mean, it is obvious they are two different data sets. It is unnecessary to calculate a measure of dispersion such as the standard deviation, because the simple range calculation does a good job by itself.

Excel Tutorial on Using the Histogram Tool Function

The histogram tool in the data analysis section of Excel has the capability to create frequency distributions, histograms, cumulative frequency diagrams, and Pareto charts. The following section demonstrates the use of the Data Analysis menu to create graphs of these types.

Frequency Distributions

The first step in developing any of the aforementioned distributions, diagrams, or charts is to specify the classes or intervals for the distribution. The specification of the classes includes the number of classes, the width of the classes, and the beginning value for the first class. The histogram tool refers to classes as "bins."

If bins are not specified, the number of bins will be set approximately to the square root of the number of values in the data set. In addition, width will be determined as the difference between the largest data value and smallest data value divided by the number of values. Finally, the beginning value for the first class is set equal to the lowest data value. At first glance the output from the histogram tool may not be helpful.

Installing Excel's Data Analysis Add-In within Excel

Frequently, the data analysis menu item under tools will not be shown. If you cannot find the data analysis menu item, it means that the Analysis ToolPak has not been added into the Excel program. To add in the Analysis ToolPak, it is necessary to click on the File button in Excel 2010 and select the Excel Options window (a screen that resembles Figure 4.3 will appear). Within the Options window click on the Add-Ins menu and go to the Manage drop-down box at the bottom of the screen. Then select Excel Add-Ins from the menu and click on the Go button. This will prompt the Add-Ins menu to appear (see Figure 4.4).

FIGURE 4.3 Excel Options Window

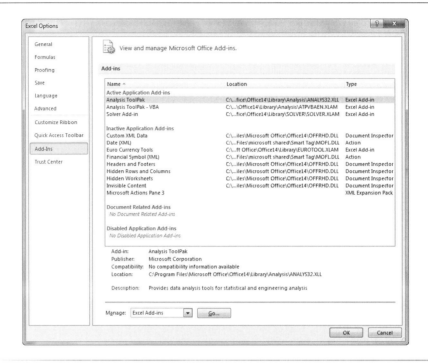

Two of the items in the Add-Ins window are Analysis ToolPak and Analysis ToolPak–VBA. It is necessary to check the box preceding both of these items for the data analysis options of Excel to be available. Once these have been checked, the Data Analysis option in the Analysis group under the Data tab will appear (see Figure 4.5).

When you click on the Data Analysis option, the Data Analysis window will open (refer to Figure 4.6). Shown in that figure is only a sampling of the 19 different analysis options available through the Analysis ToolPak. Selecting a specific analysis (e.g., Correlation) and clicking OK brings up an analysis window that will be tailored to the particular analysis requested. Specific analyses using the Analysis ToolPak are discussed as we move into the various categories of analysis available through this mechanism (e.g., correlation, ANOVA, regression, etc.).

Example: Using Excel's Data Analysis Add-In

The following example details the use of Excel's histogram tool. The steps in determining the number of classes/bins and the class width are discussed

FIGURE 4.4   Excel Add-Ins Choices within the Options Window

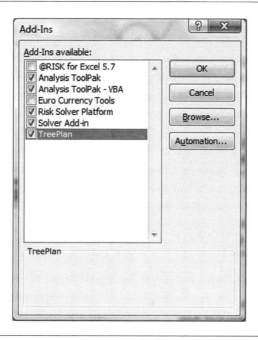

FIGURE 4.5   Excel Add-Ins Menu

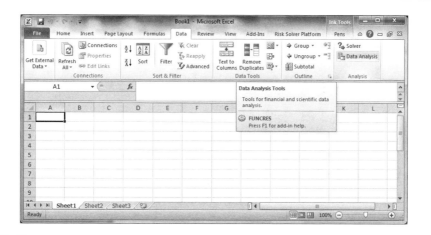

first, followed by an example using data from Table 4.4. Refer to the earlier section of this chapter for a tutorial on how to install Excel's Data Analysis add-in.

FIGURE 4.6 Data Analysis Window

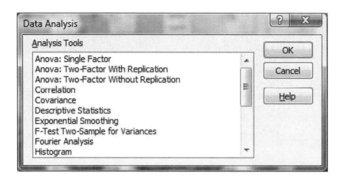

Steps for Determining Classes/Bins and Class Width   It is strongly suggested that you specify the classes/bins and class width for your data set. Follow this simple six-step process to determine the number of classes/bins and class width:

1. Identify the largest and smallest data points in your data set.

2. Round the smallest data point down to the nearest 10.

3. Round the largest data point up to the nearest 10.

4. Find the difference between these two rounded data points.

5. Divide this difference by numbers that are multiples of 2, 5, or 10, or an appropriate number of your choice that allows for easy analysis. The resultant integer will be the number of classes/bins.

6. The class width is equal to the number you divided by in step 5, and the number of classes/bins is the resultant integer from step 5.

As an example, given the information in Table 4.4, let's determine the appropriate number of classes/bins and class width:

> *Step 1:* Identify the largest and smallest data points in your data set. The smallest number in the data set = 27. The largest number in the data set = 89.

TABLE 4.4 Daily Census for Rehabilitation Center

Day	Rehabilitation Census	Day	Rehabilitation Census	Day	Rehabilitation Census	Day	Rehabilitation Census	Day	Rehabilitation Census
1	44	5	47	9	55	13	89	17	85
2	43	6	59	10	46	14	72	18	56
3	59	7	66	11	43	15	27	19	57
4	42	8	56	12	46	16	54	20	73

Step 2: Round the smallest data point down to the nearest 10. Round 27 down to 20.

Step 3: Round the largest data point up to the nearest 10. Round 89 up to 90.

Step 4: Find the difference between these two rounded data points. Difference of rounded data points = 90 − 20 = 70.

Step 5: For this example, 10 is chosen as the divisor. Divide the difference in step 4 by 10 (the resultant integer will be the number of classes/bins): 70 divided by 10 = 7.

Step 6: The class width is equal to 10, and the number of classes/bins is 7.

If the class width in step 6 is too large, too much data smoothing takes place (i.e., too few bins with too many data points). On the other hand, if the class width in step 6 is too small, too little aggregation occurs (i.e., too many bins with not enough points for data distinction). Now, using the answers developed in the six steps, let's illustrate how to create a frequency distribution, histogram, and Pareto chart with Excel's histogram tool.

Excel's Histogram Tool

Use the following 10 steps to create diagrams and charts with Excel's histogram tool.

1. Open Excel and a new Excel worksheet.

2. In cell A1 type Week and in cell B1 type Rehabilitation Census. Proceed to enter the numbers 1 through 20 in the column under the label Week (cells A2 through A21). In addition, enter the rehabilitation census data contained in Table 4.4 in the column under the label Rehabilitation Census (cells B2 through B21).

3. In cell C1, type Bin. Proceed to enter the values 20, 30, 40, 50, 60, 70, and 80 in the column under the label Bin (cells C2 through C8). Your Excel worksheet should resemble Figure 4.7.

4. Within Excel go to the Data Ribbon and select the Data Analysis menu from the Analysis tab. The Data Analysis dialogue box will then be

FIGURE 4.7   Excel Spreadsheet to Accompany Histogram Example

	A	B	C
		Rehabilitation	
1	Week	Census	Bin
2	1	44	20
3	2	43	30
4	3	59	40
5	4	42	50
6	5	47	60
7	6	59	70
8	7	66	80
9	8	56	
10	9	55	
11	10	46	
12	11	43	
13	12	46	
14	13	89	
15	14	72	
16	15	27	
17	16	54	
18	17	85	
19	18	56	
20	19	57	
21	20	73	

displayed. From this dialogue box, select Histogram and click on the command button labeled OK. The Histogram dialogue box will appear, and you now need to input your data (see Figure 4.8).

5. Move the cursor to the textbox to the right of the Input Range label and left mouse click. Enter the range for the data, including the label. This may be accomplished by typing $B$1:$B$21 or clicking on cell B1 and dragging to cell B21.

6. Move the cursor to the textbox to the right of the Bin Range label and left mouse click. Enter the range for the Bin Range, including the label. This

FIGURE 4.8 Histogram Dialogue Box

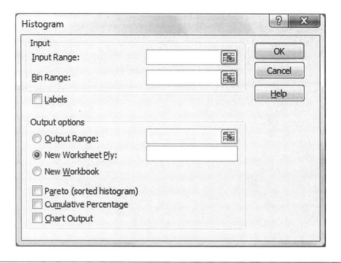

may be accomplished by typing $C$1:$C$8 or clicking on cell C1 and dragging to cell C8.

7. Move the cursor to the Labels checkbox and left mouse click to check the box. This informs the Histogram program that you have included labels with your data entries.

8. Move the cursor to where the Output options are and click on the appropriate output option. Generally, it is best to click on New Worksheet Ply. This option cuts down on the clutter of your main data sheet.

9. Sequentially, move the cursor to the last three check boxes labeled as Pareto (sorted histogram), Cumulative Percentage, and Chart Output and click to check the boxes labeled Cumulative Percentage and Chart Output (see Figure 4.9).

10. Click on the OK command button and Excel will compute and display output resembling Figure 4.10.

Figure 4.10 displays a histogram overlaid with a cumulative percentage diagram. The scale on the left depicts the frequency, and the scale on the right depicts the cumulative percentile. The data table in the upper left of

FIGURE 4.9   Histogram Dialogue Box with Specific Graphing Options Checked

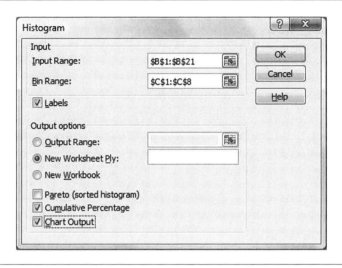

FIGURE 4.10   Histogram with Cumulative Percentage Overlay

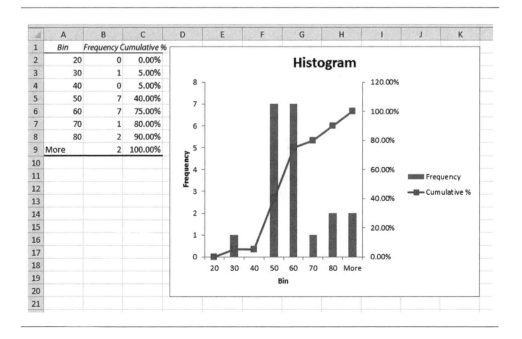

the spreadsheet displays the bin and frequency data (the "More" row appears automatically).

Expected Values

In this chapter, we have explored the concepts of central tendency and dispersion, and have concluded that decision makers need to investigate data sets with regard to both central tendency and dispersion to fully describe the situation facing them. Health care professionals will inevitably be confronted with data sets that contain random variables. Consequently, it is very important to describe random variables in terms of central tendency and dispersion.

The central tendency of a random variable is often referred to as the *expected value* of the probability distribution. Expected value is calculated by using the following formula (Equation 4.5):

$$E(x) = \sum_{i=1}^{n} x_i p(x_i) \tag{4.5}$$

Multiplying each random variable by its corresponding probability and then summing these products calculates the expected value. Let's take, for example, another average wait scenario. Table 4.5 displays the probability distribution for average wait times in an ER.

For the ER wait example, the expected wait time is computed as shown in Table 4.6. From Table 4.6, it is seen that the expected wait is 35 minutes.

Decision makers use the expected value calculation to compare different alternatives. The assumption that is made and will be used throughout this book

TABLE 4.5   ER Wait Times with Wait Time Distribution

Average Wait Time = x	p (Average Wait Time) = p(x)
5	0.05
15	0.07
25	0.18
35	0.40
45	0.20
55	0.05
65	0.03
75	0.02

TABLE 4.6   ER Wait Times with Expected Wait Time Calculated

Average Wait Time = x	p (Average Wait Time) = p(x)	x * p(x)
5	0.05	0.25
15	0.07	1.05
25	0.18	4.5
35	0.4	14
45	0.2	9
55	0.05	2.75
65	0.03	1.95
75	0.02	1.5
	Expected value – E(x) = 35	

is that decision makers wish to maximize expected value. Therefore, when comparing numerous alternatives, a decision maker will choose the alternative with the highest expected value.

Keep in mind that maximizing expected value is only one way to make decisions. It is a basic assumption that is made in decision theory, but it is not the only assumption one can apply to expected values. If a decision maker were dealing strictly with costs or (for our example) wait time, the assumption would be that the expected value of costs or wait times should be minimized. It would not be logical for a health care professional to wish to maximize expected costs or wait times.

When we use the assumption of maximizing or minimizing expected value, it is a single objective. Many problems in the real world do not have just one objective. On the contrary, the problems health care professionals face may actually have numerous objectives, and those objectives will more than likely conflict with each other.

Overall, multiple objective analysis is outside the scope of this text; the basic assumption followed here is maximization or minimization of a single objective, namely expected value.

HYPOTHESIS TESTING: ANALYZING THE DIFFERENCE
OF TWO MEANS

This section describes a procedure for hypothesis testing. This type of hypothesis testing examines differences between two independent groups, using numerical samples. Hypothesis testing is also referred to as analyzing the difference of two means or testing two means.

Introduction to Hypothesis Testing

Before the exact procedure for testing two means is described, a short discussion of standard deviation is in order. As was presented earlier in this chapter, standard deviation is one measure of dispersion. Coupled with the mean, the standard deviation describes what the data in the data set look like. Statisticians generally consider the totality of items or data being considered as a population. Therefore, it can be said that the mean and standard deviation of the data describe the shape of a population and the underlying population distribution.

There are many reasons why a health care professional would wish to compare two populations or distributions. They may wish to:

- Validate a claim.

- Discriminate between two data sets.

- Statistically prove a similarity or difference between data sets.

In essence, when a health care professional wishes to compare two population means, a comparison of the underlying distributions is appropriate. In comparing populations or underlying data distributions, a decision maker is attempting to make a claim or, in statistics language, test a hypothesis.

The Z-Test Statistic

The question at hand is how does one go about claiming two underlying distributions are the same or different from each other. A hypothesis could be established that states the following:

Population mean 1 = Population mean 2

The Z-test statistic is used to test this hypothesis. However, the difference between two population means is based on the difference between two sample means.

Before we detail the Z-test statistics, let's first represent the descriptive statistics of the two populations as in Table 4.7. The difference between the sample means, $\bar{x}_1 - \bar{x}_2$, is a test statistic that follows a standard normal distribution for samples that are large enough. The Z-statistic itself is as follows (Equation 4.6):

$$Z = \frac{(x_1 - x_2) - (\mu_1 - \mu_2)}{\sqrt{\frac{\sigma_1^2}{n_1} + \frac{\sigma_2^2}{n_2}}} \qquad (4.6)$$

However, rarely does a decision maker know the actual standard deviation of either of the populations. Usually the only information that is obtainable is the sample means, $\bar{x}_1$ and $\bar{x}_2$, and the sample standard deviations, s_1 and s_2.

Therefore, the next section discusses another test statistic, the t-test statistic, which allows us to use sample means and sample standard deviations to test for differences in two means.

The t-Test Statistic

The t-test statistic is similar to the Z-test statistic but uses information drawn from sample data. For the t-test statistic, the following assumptions are made:

- Samples are drawn randomly and independently from a normally distributed population.

- Population variances are equal, i.e., $\sigma_1^2 = \sigma_2^2$.

- A pooled-variance t-test will be used to determine significance.

These assumptions are necessary because of the lack of knowledge regarding the population standard deviations.

TABLE 4.7   Descriptive Statistics of Two Populations

Population 1	Population 2
μ_1 = mean of population 1	μ_2 = mean of population 2
σ_1 = standard deviation of population 1	σ_2 = standard deviation of population 2
n_1 = sample size of population 1	n_2 = sample size of population 2

The t-test can be performed as either a two-tailed or a one-tailed test. This text will concentrate on the two-tailed t-test. A two-tailed t-test is used to test whether population means are similar or different. A good rule of thumb to follow is:

Two-tailed t-tests use an equals sign in the null hypothesis.

They do so because the test is attempting to show merely a similarity or difference in the two means.

Four Components of a Hypothesis Test for Two Means

The t-test for hypothesis testing of two means, commonly referred to as the test of two means, is the most common method for comparing the means of two data sets.

The procedure for testing two means consists of four components:

1. Null hypothesis: H_0

2. Alternative hypothesis: H_a

3. Test statistics: t-statistic and t-critical value

4. Rejection/acceptance regions: rules of thumb to follow

The next sections detail each of the four t-test components and are followed by an application example.

The Null Hypothesis

The null hypothesis is the claim you are trying to make or prove. For the two-tailed t-test, it will consist of a statement similar to the following:

> H_0: the means are from the same sample population
>
> or
>
> H_0 : mean 1 = mean 2
>
> or
>
> H_0 : mean male salaries = mean female salaries

Standard statistical nomenclature assigns the moniker H_0 to the null hypothesis. The experimenter or decision maker is responsible for formulating and stating the null hypothesis. The null hypothesis is generally formulated and stated first.

The Alternative Hypothesis

The alternative hypothesis is the converse of the null hypothesis. For the two-tailed t-test it will consist of a statement similar to the following:

H_a: the means are from the same sample population

or

H_a : mean 1 $\neq$ mean 2

or

H_a : mean male salaries $\neq$ mean female salaries

Standard statistical nomenclature assigns the moniker H_a to the alternative hypothesis. The experimenter or decision maker is responsible for formulating and stating the alternative hypothesis. The alternative hypothesis is generally formulated and stated second.

The Test Statistics: t-Statistic and t-Critical Value

Two test statistics are needed to conduct a test of two means. These statistics are:

1. The t-statistic is calculated by using a pooled-variance t-test or Excel.
2. The t-critical value is a value based on a level of significance (usually 5 percent) and degrees of freedom (DoF) and obtained from a statistical t table or Excel.

t-Statistic   The t-statistic is calculated by using a pooled variance t-statistic (Equation 4.7). This statistic can be computed as follows:

$$t = \frac{(\bar{x}_1 - \bar{x}_2) - (\mu_1 - \mu_2)}{\sqrt{S_p^2 \left(\frac{1}{n_1} + \frac{1}{n_2}\right)}} \qquad (4.7)$$

where the pooled variance (Equation 4.8) is:

$$S_p^2 = \frac{(n_1 - 1)s_1^2 + (n_2 - 1)s_2^2}{(n_1 - 1) + (n_2 - 1)}$$

$S_p^2 =$ pooled variance

$S_1^2 =$ variance of sample 1 $\qquad\qquad$ (4.8)

$n_1 =$ size of sample 1

$n_2 =$ size of sample 2

The pooled variance t-test statistic follows a t-distribution with $n_1 + n_2 - 2$ degrees of freedom. The test gets the name *pooled variance* because the test statistic requires the pooling or combination of the sample variances.

The terms S_1^2 and S_2^2, in addition to n_1 and n_2, are combined, or pooled (see the pooled variance formula, Equation 4.8), to yield a variance estimate that is common to both populations under the assumption that the population variances are equal.

t-Critical Value   The t-critical value is a value based on a level of significance (usually 95 percent) and a number of degrees of freedom. The level of significance is also referred to as the alpha value.

Like the t-statistic, the number of degrees of freedom for the t-critical is based on $n_1 + n_2 - 2$. The actual t-critical value can be obtained from a statistical t table or from a commercial statistical software package such as Excel.

Rejection/Acceptance Regions: Rules of Thumb

After the t-statistic has been calculated and the t-critical value obtained, a decision can be made about rejecting or accepting the null hypothesis. A few simple rules of thumb exist for rejecting or accepting the null:

if :|t stat| > t crit, reject the null hypothesis H_0

or

if :|t stat| < t crit, accept the null hypothesis H_0

or

if|t stat| = t crit, investigate further

FIGURE 4.11   Reject/Accept Regions for Two-Tailed t-Tests

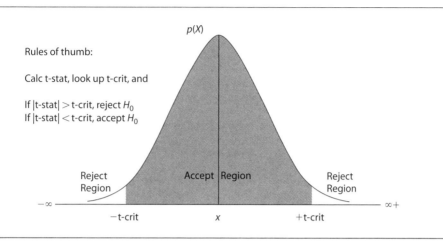

These rules of thumb instruct a decision maker for a given level of significance when the null hypothesis can be rejected or accepted. The rules of thumb for rejecting or accepting the null hypothesis can also be displayed as reject and accept reasons on a normal curve as in Figure 4.11.

Rules of thumb:

$$\text{Calc t-stat, look up t-crit, and}$$
$$\text{if} |\text{t-stat}| > \text{t-crit, Reject } H_0$$
$$\text{if} |\text{t-stat}| < \text{t-crit, Accept } H_0$$

t-Test Application Problem

This section presents a numerical example of the pooled variance t-test. Novine wishes to test a hypothesis. She works at a university that has two pharmacies, one on campus and one off campus. Novine wishes to compare the overall average purchase prices of the prescriptions that are filled by the two pharmacies.

She has collected receipts for the total dollar amounts of prescriptions from the two different pharmacies. Overall, the types and amounts of medicines that have been purchased are generally the same for both pharmacy locales and over time. Therefore, she believes the comparison can be made without too much bias.

TABLE 4.8   Novine's Average Prescription Data

On Campus Pharmacy			Off Campus Pharmacy		
$57.92	$50.35	$41.64	$77.89	$70.61	$104.97
$63.79	$76.22	$72.23	$83.99	$77.34	$89.18
$69.20	$38.57	$35.48	$52.61	$57.99	$35.04
$39.32	$45.90	$65.80	$30.82	$87.03	$86.96
$59.73	$60.17	$29.27	$103.28	$49.54	$85.66
$71.83	$30.29	$59.86	$39.92	$72.29	$57.58
$53.30	$52.36	$58.23	$70.16	$49.97	$31.38
$53.11	$33.19	$46.20	$29.42	$50.83	$44.62
$80.31	$75.84	$73.32	$65.79	$49.35	$51.13
$26.08	$37.59	$58.50	$60.76	$33.23	$96.12
$52.52	$53.98		$87.84	$77.47	$55.80
			$79.80	$49.44	

She has 32 receipts for the On Campus Pharmacy and 35 receipts for the Off Campus Pharmacy. The results are presented in Table 4.8.

Novine has heard rumors from students that the Off Campus Pharmacy charges higher prices than the On Campus Pharmacy even though the two locations by policy should not be differing on price. Therefore, Novine wishes to determine if there is a difference in the average prescription bills between the two populations of receipts. She understands that her data is just a sample of receipts but does have enough data to test. The null and alternative hypotheses are:

H_0: On Campus mean pharmacy receipts = Off Campus mean pharmacy receipts

$$H_0 : \mu_{\text{On Campus Pharmacy receipts}} = \mu_{\text{Off Campus Pharmacy receipts}}$$

$$H_0 : \mu_{\text{On Campus Pharmacy receipts}} - \mu_{\text{Off Campus Pharmacy receipts}} = 0$$

We will assume that the samples are taken from underlying normal distributions with equal variances. Therefore, a pooled variance t-test can be used to test the hypothesis. Novine chooses a significance level of 0.05 (a standard level in statistics), and the t-test statistic would follow a t-distribution with $n_1 + n_2 - 2$ degrees of freedom, or $32 + 35 - 2 = 65$. Referring to an F-distribution table, we find the critical value for the t-test is 1.997.

Table 4.9 displays the summary statistics for Novine's pharmacy t-test. The t-statistic is calculated as follows (Equation 4.9):

$$t = \frac{(\bar{x}_1 - \bar{x}_2) - (\mu_1 - \mu_2)}{\sqrt{S_p^2 \left(\frac{1}{n_1} + \frac{1}{n_2}\right)}} \tag{4.9}$$

where the pooled variance (Equation 4.10) is:

$$t = \frac{(\bar{x}_1 - \bar{x}_2) - (\mu_1 - \mu_2)}{\sqrt{S_p^2 \left(\frac{1}{n_1} + \frac{1}{n_2}\right)}} \tag{4.10}$$

and therefore the t-statistic (Equation 4.11) is:

$$t = \frac{(\bar{x}_1 - \bar{x}_2) - (\mu_1 - \mu_2)}{\sqrt{S_p^2 \left(\frac{1}{n_1} + \frac{1}{n_2}\right)}}$$

$$S_p^2 = \frac{(n_1 - 1)s_1^2 + (n_2 - 1)s_2^2}{(n_1 - 1) + (n_2 - 1)}$$

$$= 353.18 \tag{4.11}$$

$$t = \frac{53.82 - 64.17}{\sqrt{353.18 \left(\frac{1}{32} + \frac{1}{35}\right)}}$$

$$= -2.252$$

Using the rules of thumb for rejection/acceptance of the null hypothesis, we compare the t-statistic to the t-critical value and make recommendations, as follows:

TABLE 4.9 Summary Statistics for Novine's Pharmacy Receipts

	On Campus Pharmacy	Off Campus Pharmacy
Sample size	$n_1 = 32$	$n_2 = 35$
Sample mean	$x_1 = \$53.82$	$x_2 = \$64.17$
Sample variance	$S_1^2 = 227.79$	$S_2^2 = 467.51$

$$|t \text{ stat}| = 2.252 \text{ and } t \text{ crit} = 1.997$$

In turn,

$$|t \text{ stat}| > t \text{ crit}$$
$$2.252 > 1.997$$

Therefore,

The null hypothesis is rejected

or

Mean On Campus Pharmacy Receipts $\neq$ Mean Off Campus Pharmacy Receipts

Take note that a 0.05 level of significance is used and 65 degrees of freedom. This can be interpreted as follows: If the null hypothesis were true, there would be a 5 percent probability of obtaining a t-test statistic larger than 1.997 standard deviations from the center of the underlying distribution.

The null hypothesis is rejected because the t-test statistic falls into the reject region. Novine can conclude that the average pharmacy receipts at the On Campus Pharmacy and the Off Campus Pharmacy are not equal.

Items to Note Regarding Testing of Two Means

A number of assumptions were made regarding the test of two means presented here. The first assumption was that the samples were drawn from normally distributed populations. The second assumption was that the two samples had equal variance. The third assumption was the level of significance that was chosen. Departures from these assumptions must be investigated.

Overall, a good rule of thumb to use when testing means by a t-test is to have large sample sizes. Large in this sense means samples of at least 30, and the phrase "more is better" definitely does apply. Normality assumptions are met with much more ease if samples are large. If large enough samples are not available because of time, money, or other constraints, then other nonparametric tests such as the Wilcoxon rank sum test may be used to investigate the data.

If for some reason it cannot be determined that the two underlying populations have equal variances, a test for unequal variances—still a t-test—can be used. The test is similar to the pooled variance t-test and carries the name unpooled variance t-test.

Finally, a standard level of significance is 0.05, or an alpha level of 5 percent. Decision makers may deviate from this level, depending on their intuition or experimental design, but 5 percent is considered the statistical standard. Any commercially available data analysis software package (Excel's Data Analysis package, for example) will allow you to investigate changes to the underlying t-test assumptions. The next section presents Novine's t-test example using Excel's Data Analysis package.

Using Excel's Data Analysis Add-In for Testing Two Means

This section shows how to complete a t-test using Excel's Data Analysis add-in. A t-test assuming equal variances will be used here, but Excel does offer t-tests for paired samples and for data sets with unequal variances.

Steps for Using Excel's Data Analysis Add-In

The following steps should be followed if the raw data—not just summary statistics for the data—are available.

Step 1: Create a new spreadsheet in Excel and enter your raw data for the two samples (see Figure 4.12).

Step 2: Go to the Data tab and the Analysis group and choose Data Analysis (see Figure 4.13). *Note:* If the Data Analysis option does not appear in the Tools menu or the Data tab, refer to the section earlier in this chapter entitled "Installing Excel's Data Analysis Add-In within Excel."

Step 3: In the Data Analysis menu, scroll down until you locate the option "t-Test: Two-Sample Assuming Equal Variances," and click the OK button (see Figure 4.14).

Step 4: A dialogue box appears prompting you to enter information concerning your data sets (see Figure 4.15). *Note:* The t-test dialogue box in Figure 4.15 already has information entered according to the steps

FIGURE 4.12 Pharmacy Data in Excel

	A	B
	On Campus Pharmacy	Off Campus Pharmacy
1		
2	$57.92	$77.89
3	$63.79	$83.99
4	$69.20	$52.61
5	$39.32	$30.82
6	$59.73	$103.28
7	$71.83	$39.92
8	$53.30	$70.16
9	$53.11	$29.42
10	$80.31	$65.79
11	$26.08	$60.76
12	$52.52	$87.84
13	$50.35	$79.80
14	$76.22	$70.61
15	$38.57	$77.34
16	$45.90	$57.99
17	$60.17	$87.03
18	$30.29	$49.54
19	$52.36	$72.29
20	$33.19	$49.97
21	$75.84	$50.83
22	$37.59	$49.35
23	$53.98	$33.23
24	$41.64	$77.47
25	$72.23	$104.97
26	$35.48	$89.18
27	$65.80	$35.04
28	$29.27	$86.96
29	$59.86	$85.66
30	$58.23	$57.58
31	$46.20	$31.38
32	$73.32	$44.62
33	$58.50	$51.13
34		$96.12
35		$55.80
36		$49.44
37		

detailed in step 5. When the t-test dialogue box opens initially, the edit and check boxes will be empty except for the Alpha level.

Step 5: Follow this set of instructions for entering information in the t-test dialogue box:

- In the Variable 1 Range edit box, enter the range of the first data set.

- In the Variable 2 Range edit box, enter the range of the second data set.

- In the Hypothesized Mean Difference edit box, either enter 0 or leave it blank.

FIGURE 4.13 Tools Menu and Data Analysis Option in Excel

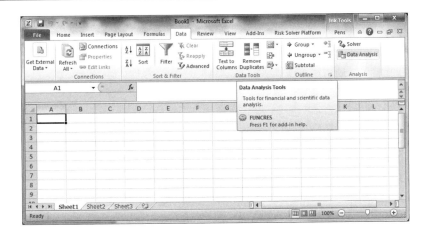

FIGURE 4.14 t-Test: Two-Sample Assuming Equal Variances Option in Excel

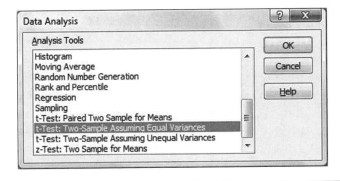

- Select the Labels check box if you have included headers or labels in your data set.

- In the Alpha edit box, enter the level of significance you have chosen (usually 5 percent, 0.05).

- Select the New Worksheet Ply option, and if desired enter an appropriate name of your choice.

FIGURE 4.15   t-Test Dialogue Box in Excel

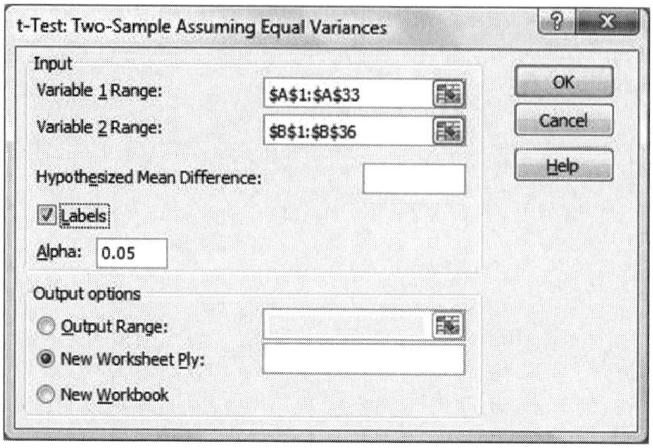

FIGURE 4.16   Data Analysis Output for t-Test

◇	A	B	C
1	t-Test: Two-Sample Assuming Equal Variances		
2			
3		On Campus Pharmacy	Off Campus Pharmacy
4	Mean	53.82	64.17
5	Variance	227.78	467.49
6	Observations	32.00	35.00
7	Pooled Variance	353.16	
8	Hypothesized Mean Difference	0.00	
9	df	65.00	
10	t Stat	−2.25	
11	P(T<=t) one-tail	0.01	
12	t Critical one-tail	1.67	
13	P(T<=t) two-tail	0.03	
14	t Critical two-tail	2.00	
15			

The resultant t-test dialogue box should now resemble Figure 4.15. Click the OK button and Excel will generate an output worksheet that resembles Figure 4.16.

Figure 4.16 displays the descriptive statistics, t-statistic, and t-critical values for the data set. The two most important pieces of information are located in cell B10 (the t-statistic) and cell B14 (the t-critical two-tailed value).

Other statistics of interest are in cells B4 and C4 (On Campus Pharmacy and Off Campus Pharmacy mean values) and in cells B5 and C5 (On Campus Pharmacy and Off Campus Pharmacy variance measurements). These additional statistics are important because they will assist us in further interpreting the test of two means.

Following the rule of thumb set down for testing of two means, we can see that $|$t stat$| = 2.252$ while t-critical two-tailed value $= 1.997$.

Therefore,

$$|\text{t-stat}| > \text{t-critical and the null hypothesis is rejected}$$

or:

$$\text{Mean receipts at the On Campus Pharmacy} \neq \text{mean receipts}$$
$$\text{at the Off Campus Pharmacy}$$

Comparing a t-statistic with a t-critical value is one way to determine whether to reject or accept a null hypothesis. The next section briefly discusses the interpretation of the t-test via p-values.

Interpreting t-Test Results via p-Values

Results from Figure 4.16 can also be interpreted by using what is called the p-value. Cell B13 contains the $p(T <= t)$ two-tailed value for the t-test. Alternatively, the p-value can be used to determine the reject/accept criteria. The p-value in cell B13 is 0.03. The p-value must be compared to the level of significance chosen earlier. The rule of thumb is as follows:

$$\text{If } p\text{-value} < \text{level of significance, reject the null hypothesis.}$$

or:

$$\text{If } p\text{-value} > \text{level of significance, accept the null hypothesis.}$$

In sum, the p-value for Novine's t-test is 0.03, which is less than the level of significance, 0.05. Therefore we reject the null hypothesis that average receipts from the On Campus Pharmacy and the Off Campus Pharmacy are equal. Note that this is the same conclusion gleaned from the t-statistic and t-critical analysis.

PARETO ANALYSIS

In the earlier section on histograms, we discussed relative frequency and cumulative percentage diagrams. Figure 4.10 displays a histogram overlaid with a cumulative percentage diagram. Although we chose not to display the data as a sorted histogram, we could have (see step 9 in the section labeled "Excel's Histogram Tool").

A sorted histogram is akin to a Pareto diagram when the histogram is sorted from highest frequency to lowest frequency. A sorted histogram is created by checking the Pareto (sorted histogram) check box in the Histogram menu of Excel's Data Analysis package (see Figure 4.9).

The principle is named after Italian economist Vilfredo Pareto, who observed that 80 percent of income in Italy went to 20 percent of the population. Later Pareto conducted surveys on a number of other countries and found that a similar distribution applied to income in those countries.

Pareto analysis could be characterized as an analytical technique in decision making that is used for the selection of a limited number of tasks that produce significant overall effect. The Pareto Principle, also known as the 80/20 rule, encompasses the notion that by doing 20 percent of the work you can generate 80 percent of the benefit of doing the whole job. Likewise, in terms of quality improvement, a large portion of problems (80 percent) are produced by a few key causes (20 percent). At times these two groups are also referred to as the vital few and the trivial many.

Pareto analysis can be applied to many health care operations and supply chain management (SCM) areas. For example:

- Eighty percent of delays or waiting by patients arise from 20 percent of the possible causes of the delays.

- Eighty percent of customer complaints arise from 20 percent of the health care services you provide.

- Twenty percent of your health care services account for 80 percent of your profit.

- Twenty percent of your customers make up 80 percent of your hospital's medical procedures.

- Twenty percent of a system's defects cause 80 percent of its problems.

The Pareto Principle has many applications in health care operations and SCM. It can be used as a guide for corrective action and to help decision makers take action to fix the problems that are causing the greatest number of defects first.

Creating and Interpreting Pareto Diagrams

When creating a Pareto diagram, use the same steps as for creating a histogram (see the earlier section labeled "Excel's Histogram Tool"). However, when you get to step 9, check the Pareto (sorted histogram) check box also. Figure 4.17 displays the histogram example developed earlier but now graphs the data in a sorted histogram (i.e., a Pareto diagram). A simple way to apply Pareto's rule is as follows:

- Draw a line at 80 percent on the *y*-axis parallel to the *x*-axis (see Figure 4.18).

- Drop the line at the point of intersection with the curve on the *x*-axis.

- The point on the *x*-axis separates the more important causes on the left from less important causes on the right.

For our rehabilitation example, Figure 4.18 illustrates that the 50- and 60-minute bins (approximately 40 minutes up to 59 minutes) account for around 70 percent (14/20) of the census values while the two bins make up about 25 percent (2/8) of the total bins.

The Pareto Principle's real value for a health care professional is that it reminds you to focus on the 20 percent of things that really matter. One could say, of the things you do during your workday, only 20 percent are really important. That 20 percent produces 80 percent of your results. Use the Pareto Principle to identify and focus on those things first, but don't totally ignore the remaining 80 percent, either. In other words, identify the low-hanging fruit first and go after it, but then turn your attention to the other 80 percent.

BOX-AND-WHISKER PLOTS

John W. Tukey is credited with the creation of the *box-and-whisker plot* in the mid-1970s. The box-and-whisker plot is many times referred to as a box plot, boxplot, or five-number summary. A typical box plot resembles Figure 4.19.

FIGURE 4.17 Pareto Diagram in Excel

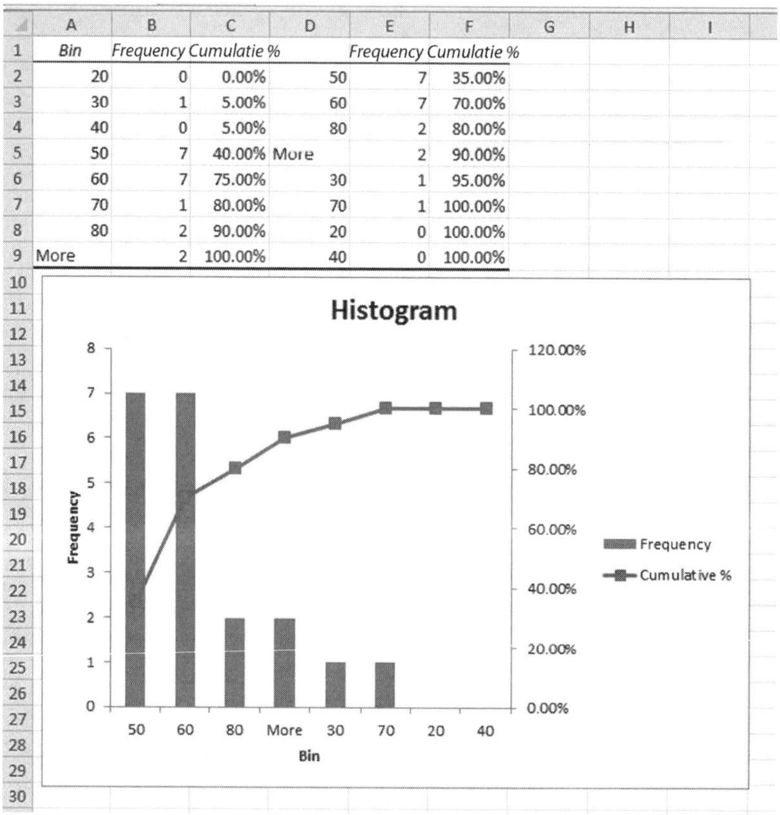

	A	B	C	D	E	F	G	H	I
1	*Bin*	*Frequency*	*Cumulatie %*		*Frequency*	*Cumulatie %*			
2	20	0	0.00%	50	7	35.00%			
3	30	1	5.00%	60	7	70.00%			
4	40	0	5.00%	80	2	80.00%			
5	50	7	40.00%	More	2	90.00%			
6	60	7	75.00%	30	1	95.00%			
7	70	1	80.00%	70	1	100.00%			
8	80	2	90.00%	20	0	100.00%			
9	More	2	100.00%	40	0	100.00%			
10									
11									

A box plot is a convenient way to graphically depict groups of numerical data through their five-number summaries:

1. Lower quartile (Q1)

2. Median (Q2)

3. Upper quartile (Q3)

4. Largest observation (sample maximum)

5. Smallest observation (sample minimum)

The box part of a box-and-whisker plot represents the interquartile range (IQR) that we discussed earlier in the chapter. In other words, the central 50

FIGURE 4.18   Pareto Diagram with 80 Percent Mark Displayed

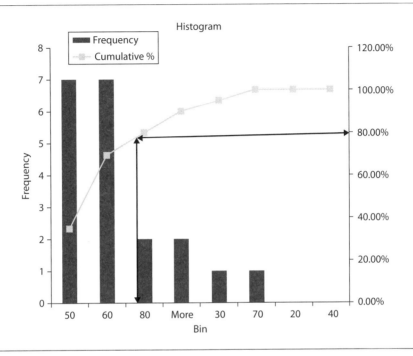

FIGURE 4.19   Basic Box Plot

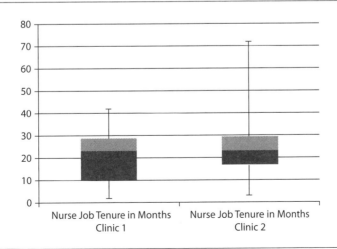

percent of the data is depicted by the box. The lower edge of the box plot is the first quartile or 25th percentile. The upper edge of the box plot is the third quartile or 75th percentile. The solid line inside the box is the median of the data. The whisker in a box plot represents the tails of the distribution. A box plot may also indicate which observations, if any, might be considered outliers.

The median line's location relative to the first and third quartiles indicates the amount of skewness or asymmetry in the data. If the distribution is symmetric, the median will be exactly in the middle. However, if the median is closer to Q3, the distribution is negatively skewed (or skewed to the left, meaning the left tail of the distribution is longer). Likewise, if the median is closer to Q1, the distribution is positively skewed to the right.

Box plots are nonparametric, meaning that they display differences between populations without making any assumptions about the underlying statistical distribution. The gaps between the different parts of the box help indicate the degree of dispersion (spread) and skewness in the data, and identify outliers. Box plots can be drawn either horizontally or vertically.

Box plots are very useful data visualization tools for depicting a number of different summary statistics and especially for graphically comparing multiple data sets. The next section illustrates how to create a box plot in Excel.

Creating a Box Plot

Box plots, or box-and-whisker diagrams, are used to look at statistical data, especially when there are multiple sets of data. Microsoft Excel does not offer an individual box plot template, but a normal line graph can be modified to create one.

It is important to have the five-number summary data arranged in a specific manner. Therefore, we will create a table of the results from five statistical functions that you have to run on each set of data. Figure 4.20 illustrates the data for the example and how to arrange the five-number summary data in an Excel spreadsheet.

The first quartile is listed first, followed by the median, the third quartile, the maximum, and finally the minimum. For the data set shown, use the Excel formulas in Table 4.10 to calculate the five summary numbers.

The five-number summary results must be modified since Excel doesn't have a box plot template built in. The box plot can be created in Excel by using a stacked column chart with three series. The first series is Q1, and within Excel the

FIGURE 4.20 Data for Box Plots

	A	B	C
		Nurse Job Tenure in	Nurse Job Tenure in
1		Months Clinic 1	Months Clinic 2
2		23	25
3		2	22
4		5	7
5		14	24
6		25	26
7		36	31
8		27	18
9		42	14
10		12	17
11		8	20
12		7	31
13		23	42
14		29	6
15		26	25
16		28	22
17		11	3
18		20	29
19		31	32
20		8	15
21		36	72
	Five-Number	Nurse Job Tenure in	Nurse Job Tenure in
22	Summary	Months Clinic 1	Months Clinic 2
23	1st Quartile	10.25	16.5
24	Median	23	23
25	3rd Quartile	28.25	29.5
26	Maximum	42	72
27	Minimum	2	3
	Modified Five-	Nurse Job Tenure in	Nurse Job Tenure in
28	Number Summary	Months Clinic 1	Months Clinic 2
29	1st Quartile	10.25	16.5
30	Median	12.75	6.5
31	3rd Quartile	5.25	6.5
32	Maximum	13.75	42.5
33	Minimum	8.25	13.5
24			

border and area properties are set to none so that the column is not visible in the chart (discussed in the step-by-step rules to follow). The second series is Median-Q1. The third series is Median-Q3. These two series stacked together make up the interquartile range. The area property is set to none for these two series to

TABLE 4.10 Excel Formulas for Box Plot

Formula Moniker	Cell	Formulas (Copy All Formulas to Column C)
First quartile, Q1	B23	=quartile(B2:B21, 1) or
		=percentile(B2:B21, 0.25)
Median, Q2	B24	=median(B2:B21) or
		=quartile(B2:B21, 2) or
		=percentile(B2:B21, 0.5)
Third quartile, Q3	B25	=quartile(B2:B21, 3) or
		=percentile(B2:B21, 0.75)
Maximum	B26	=max(B2:B21)
Minimum	B27	=min(B2:B21)
First quartile, Q1	B29	=quartile(B2:B21, 1) or
		=percentile(B2:B21, 0.25)
Modified median, Q2	B30	=B24-B23
Modified third quartile, Q3	B31	=B25-B24
Modified maximum	B32	=B26-B25
Modified minimum	B33	=B23-B27

create just the outline for the box plot. The whiskers are created using the modified minimum and maximum results.

Creating the Box Plot in Excel: Step-by-Step Instructions

This section contains step-by-step instructions on how to create a box plot in Excel.

1. Open the Excel file that contains the data you want to represent as a box plot (for our example, refer to Figure 4.20).

2. Set up the five-number summary as shown in Figure 4.20 using the formulas from Table 4.10. Use the headers, from top to bottom, listed in Figure 4.20 exactly as they appear (i.e., 1st Quartile first, followed by Median, etc.). Also include the modified five-number summary below the original five-number summary (cells A28 to C33).

3. Select cells B28 to C31 and click on the Insert tab in the ribbon. Next click on the Column menu and select the 2-D Stacked Column option (see Figure 4.21). Next, click on the Switch Row/Column in the Design tab. A figure that resembles Figure 4.22 should appear.

FIGURE 4.21   2-D Stacked Column Option

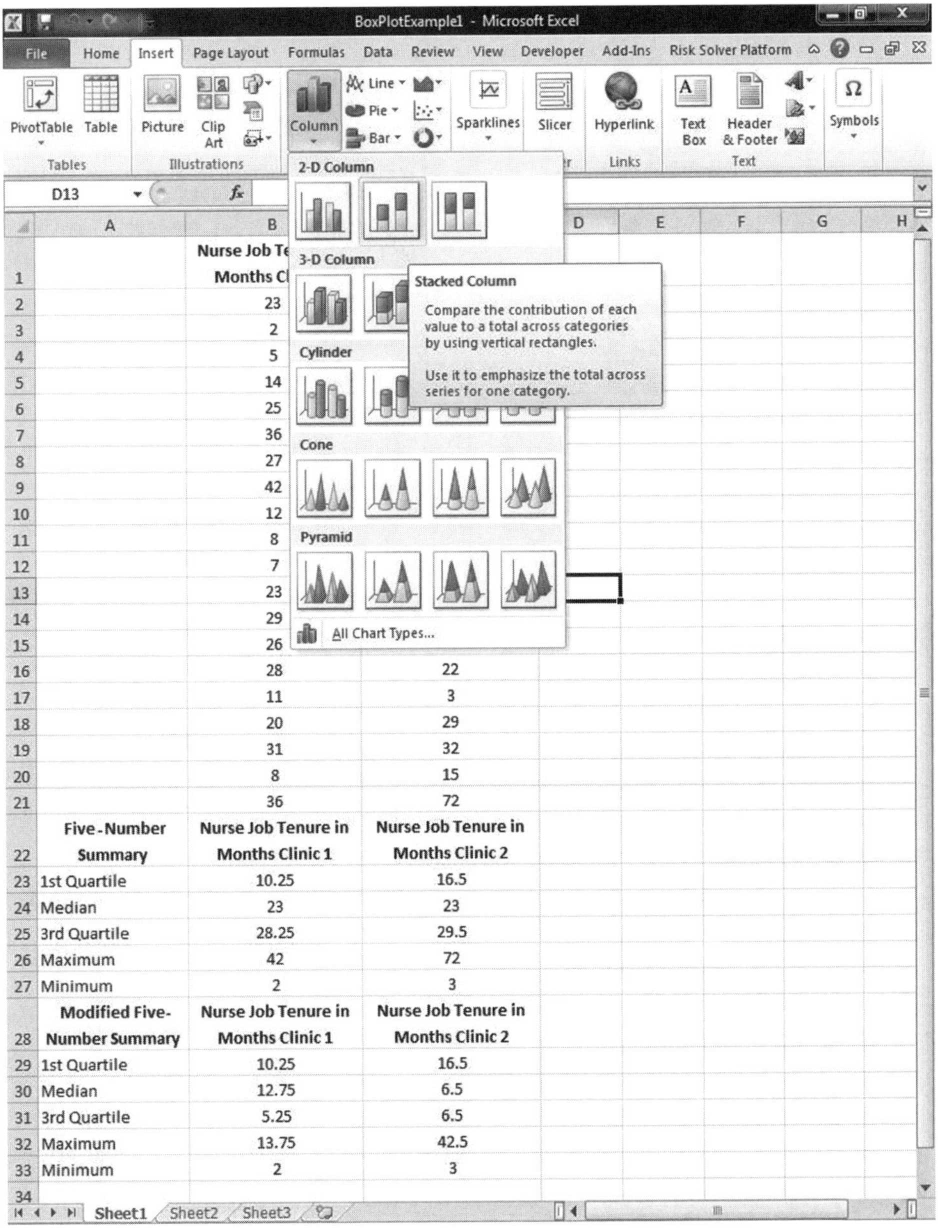

	A	B	C	D	E	F	G	H
1		Nurse Job Te... / Months Cl...						
2		23						
3		2						
4		5						
5		14						
6		25						
7		36						
8		27						
9		42						
10		12						
11		8						
12		7						
13		23						
14		29						
15		26						
16		28	22					
17		11	3					
18		20	29					
19		31	32					
20		8	15					
21		36	72					

	Five-Number Summary	Nurse Job Tenure in Months Clinic 1	Nurse Job Tenure in Months Clinic 2
22			
23	1st Quartile	10.25	16.5
24	Median	23	23
25	3rd Quartile	28.25	29.5
26	Maximum	42	72
27	Minimum	2	3
28	Modified Five-Number Summary	Nurse Job Tenure in Months Clinic 1	Nurse Job Tenure in Months Clinic 2
29	1st Quartile	10.25	16.5
30	Median	12.75	6.5
31	3rd Quartile	5.25	6.5
32	Maximum	13.75	42.5
33	Minimum	2	3
34			

FIGURE 4.22 Stacked Column Graph after Column Switch

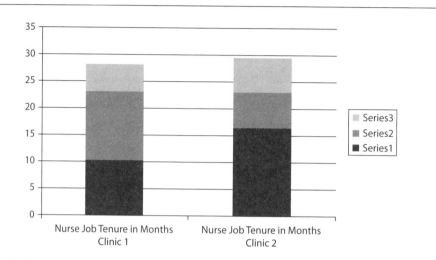

4. To add the whiskers, click on the Layout tab in the ribbon and then click on the Analysis menu. Within the Analysis menu select Error Bars and the More Error Bars Options option (see Figure 4.23).

5. A window resembling Figure 4.24 will open. In that window select Series 1 and click OK. A figure resembling Figure 4.25 will appear. This is the Format Error Bars menu. Inside this menu click on the Minus radio button and then click on the Custom radio button at the bottom of the figure and click on the Specify Value button.

6. A menu resembling Figure 4.26 will appear. Click in the Negative Error Value input area and on your data sheet highlight cells B33 to C33. Click OK and then click Close when Figure 4.25 appears.

7. Complete the instructions in steps 4 to 6 again, this time clicking on Series 3 in Figure 4.24. In turn, in Figure 4.25 (Format Error Bars menu) click on the Plus radio button, and then click on the Custom radio button, and finally click on Specify Value. When the Custom Error Bars menu (see Figure 4.26) appears, click in the Positive Error Value input area and on your data sheet highlight cells B32 to C32. Click OK and then click Close when Figure 4.25 appears.

8. At this point you will have a bar graph that resembles Figure 4.27. To make the bar graph depict a true box-and-whisker plot, the Series 1 bar must be

FIGURE 4.23   Error Bar Menus

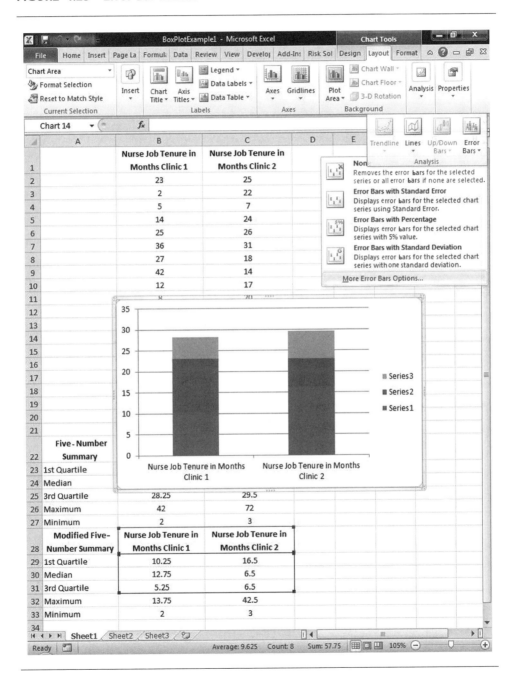

FIGURE 4.24   Input Window for Error Bar Input

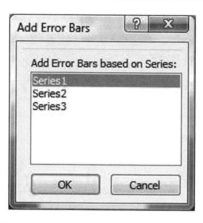

FIGURE 4.25   Format Error Bars Menu

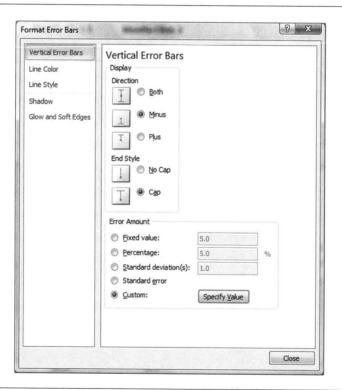

FIGURE 4.26   Special Value Input Menu

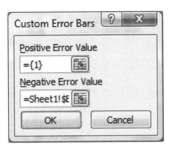

FIGURE 4.27   Box Plot Graph after Error Bar Formatting

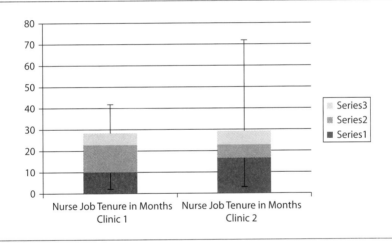

hidden. This is accomplished by right clicking on the Series 1 bar in Figure 4.27 and selecting the Format Data Series option.

Your box-and-whisker plot will then resemble Figure 4.28. There are many other formatting options that exist. We will allow users to make those choices on their own, but suggest that the legend be deleted and the median line be accentuated.

From Figure 4.28 it can be seen that the nurse job tenure for Clinic 1 and Clinic 2 tend to have the same median and third quartile point but differ on minimum, maximum, and first quartile. Overall, the data for Clinic 2 tend to be

FIGURE 4.28 Final Box Plot Graph

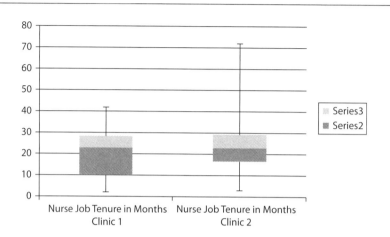

more tightly grouped (the difference between Q1 and Q3 is smaller than for Clinic 1) and the Clinic 2 nurses appear to be a more seasoned group than the Clinic 1 nurses (e.g., higher Q1 and higher maximum points). These facts may help a health care professional when making staffing choices or when interpreting variation in tasks performed.

Outliers

One issue with creating a box plot in Excel is how to show outliers—the points that fall outside of the range depicted by the box and whiskers and beyond the minimum or maximum. It is good practice that after the outliers are identified a table is created to indicate those outliers somewhere near the box-and-whisker plot.

Box Plot Variations

There are a number of subtle variations on box plots. However, the method to create those variations in Excel is cumbersome, so we won't describe them in detail, but we've included them here for your information.

Variable-Width Box Plot

It is common to represent the sample size by the width of the box plot when comparing samples with different sample sizes.

Notched Box Plot

At times decision makers wish to see the length of the confidence interval for the median. A notched box plot can be created to include the confidence interval for the median.

TORNADO DIAGRAMS AND SENSITIVITY ANALYSIS

Uncertainty exists in any planning process and subsequent operation. That uncertainty many times leads to added variability in an operation. This uncertainty and in turn variability is often the result of the combined effects of the uncertainty of the operations input variables. Some input variables may have large uncertainty yet have small effects on the operation because they are not heavily drawn on in the operation. Other input variables may contain low levels of uncertainty but influence the operation greatly.

These levels of impact on the operation are referred to as sensitivity: literally how sensitive an operation is to an input. Tornado diagrams are one method that allows a decision maker to determine the impact that each input variable has on the overall operation.

Single-Factor Sensitivity Analysis

A *tornado diagram* is made up of a set of single-factor sensitivity analyses combined in a single graph. The diagram can include all or a subset of the variables defined in a model. A tornado diagram visually displays the results of these single-factor sensitivity analyses. The uncertainty in the input associated with the widest bar has the maximum impact on the result, with each successive lower bar having a lesser impact.

Let's look at an example of a health care situation where a tornado diagram would assist a decision maker. Suppose that a medical team would like to test which inputs have the greatest influence on courses of action regarding staffing solutions. In our example, each input to the model (or, at least, each of the key inputs) could be changed by a specific amount. For each input change, the health care team might record the percentage impact on the model's main output.

The staffing solution has five input variables: hours of operation, number of physician's assistants (PAs) staffed, number of registered nurses (RNs) staffed, day

TABLE 4.11   Tornado Diagram Data Set

Variable	Impact on $ Cost	
	Minimum	Maximum
Hours of operation	$3	$47
# of PAs staffed	$4	$40
# of RNs staffed	$12	$29
Day of week	$19	$27
Demand for testing equipment	$21	$26

of week, and demand for testing equipment. The output the team is interested in is overall dollar cost for the plan. The team looked at the cost for each staffing solution based on changes (minimum and maximum values) in the five input variables. Table 4.11 contains the minimum and maximum cost numbers for each of the five variables.

Creating a Tornado Diagram in Excel

To create a tornado diagram for the data in Table 4.11, use the following steps:

1. First, select two series of data that show your maximum and minimum range for each sensitivity variable. Then choose from the Insert tab menu the Bar chart option and in turn choose the Clustered Bar option (see Figure 4.29).

2. A chart resembling Figure 4.30 will appear. Right click on the *x*-axis and choose the Format Axis option. The Format Axis menu, resembling Figure 4.31, will appear. In the Format Axis menu, go to the Vertical axis crosses option at the bottom of the menu. Click on the Axis value radio button and enter the midpoint of your data. For our example, the midpoint is 25. (*Note:* To estimate the midpoint, take the average of the variable that contains the largest minimum and maximum spread.)

3. Next, right click on any one of the individual bars in the graph and select the Format Data Series option. A screen resembling Figure 4.32 will appear, and in the Series Options menu move the slider bar from 0 percent overlapped to 100 percent overlapped. After this operation, your tornado diagram will begin to resemble a true tornado diagram.

FIGURE 4.29   Insert Tab and Bar Chart Option Menu

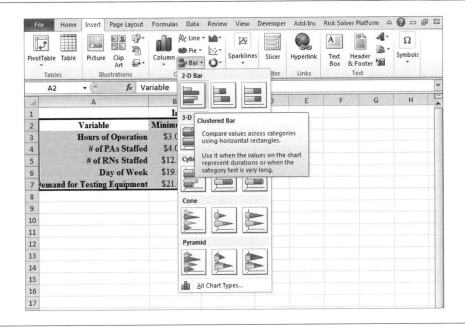

FIGURE 4.30   Preliminary Bar Chart for Tornado Diagram

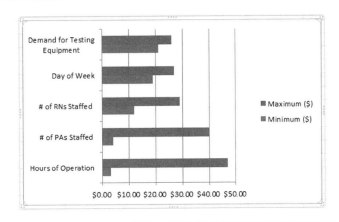

4. At this point you can format the tornado diagram in any manner you deem necessary. The last formatting we will discuss here is ordering the series from greatest impact to least impact. To accomplish this, right click on the *y*-axis

FIGURE 4.31 Format Axis Menu *x*-Axis

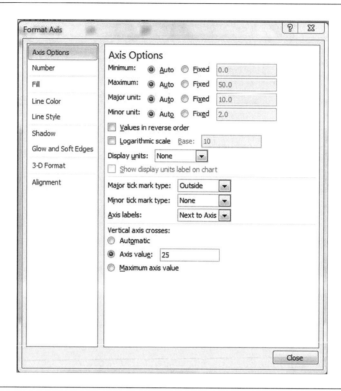

and choose Format Axis from the drop-down menu. A screen resembling Figure 4.33 will appear. In Figure 4.33, click on the Categories in reverse order button. This will reverse the *y*-axis categories, and the variable with the greatest impact will now be at the top of the graph.

Figure 4.34 displays the resulting tornado diagram for our example.

Interpretation of the Tornado Diagram

For Figure 4.34, a horizontal bar is generated for each variable being analyzed. Expected value is displayed on the *x*-axis, and each bar represents the range of expected values generated by changing the value of the related variable.

Thus, a wide/long bar indicates that the associated variable has a potentially large effect on the model's expected value. The bars are arranged with the widest

FIGURE 4.32   Format Data Series Option Screen

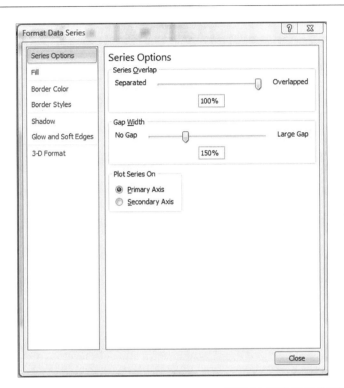

at the top and narrowest at the bottom, giving the graph a funnel-like appearance resembling a tornado. *Note:* We reversed the order of the variables to achieve this effect since the original tornado diagram was in a sense upside down.

The diagrams graphically display results of single-factor sensitivity analysis. The risk associated with the uncertainty in each of the variables that impact the outcome can be evaluated using the diagram. Single-factor analysis means that the effect on the outcome of each factor is measured, one at a time, while holding the others at their nominal (or base) values. Again, as has been mentioned before, the uncertainty in the parameter associated with the largest/longest bar, the one at the top of the chart, has the maximum impact on the result, with each successive lower bar having a lesser impact. This arrangement from largest/longest bars to smallest/narrowest bars is exactly why the result is called a tornado diagram (i.e., funnel from top to bottom).

FIGURE 4.33 Format Axis Menu *y*-Axis

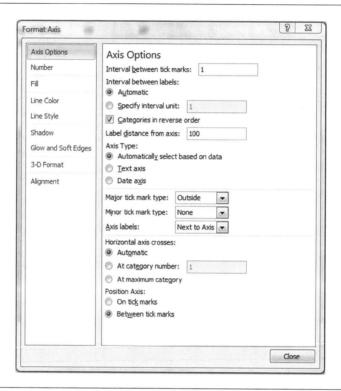

FIGURE 4.34 Tornado Diagram

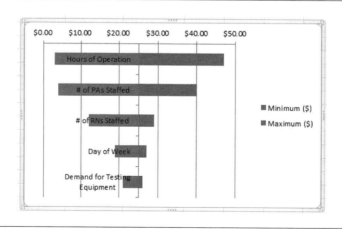

Disadvantages of Tornado Diagrams

Tornado diagrams are useful in demonstrating the impact that a fixed change in each parameter has on the main outcome. However, they tend to be not as useful in representing the confidence that a decision maker might have in the model's inputs. For example, the level of confidence in one particular parameter might be so low that it is entirely reasonable that the current input may be wrong by as much as 100 percent. This is seen in cases where no published data exist to support a particular model input or for new product introduction cases. A good health care example is the impact of a drug on a patient's long-term mortality, when only short-term trial data are available. However, some parameters (such as the price of an intervention) may be reasonably well known, and the user would have high confidence in that variable.

SUMMARY

The uses of data and statistical tools for health care operations improvement were presented in this chapter. The following areas were covered:

- Graphical methods of data description, specifically histograms.

- Measures of central tendency and dispersion.

- Use of Excel to construct histograms and calculate measures of central tendency and dispersion.

- Calculation and interpretation of expected values.

- Pareto analysis.

- Box-and-whisker plots.

- Tornado diagrams.

How to develop these concepts in Excel was also covered. The chapter should give a health care professional the tools needed to collect, analyze, and interpret data from health care operations and seek improvement where needed. For those looking for more resources pertaining to tools for data analysis, please refer to David 1962, Gonick & Smith 1993, Huff 1954, and Jaffe & Spirer 1987 for humorous views on the use of statistics. Peruse Gastwirth 1988, Hunt 2000,

McGervey 1989, and Peitetti et al. 1998 for data analysis pertaining to the health care field. In addition, for more traditional readings on statistics see Stigler 1986, Kruskal 1980, and Tukey 1977.

KEY TERMS

box-and-whisker plot	range
expected value	relative frequency diagrams
histograms	simple mean
interquartile range (IQR)	standard deviation
median	tornado diagram
Pareto analysis	variance

DISCUSSION QUESTIONS

1. In a specific hospital, if an employee is a direct care provider, then there is a 60 percent chance that he or she is from Asia. And if an employee is a supplemental service provider, then there is a 35 percent chance that he or she is from Asia. We also know that, at this hospital, 20 percent of employees are direct care providers and 80 percent of employees are supplemental service providers. What is the probability that an employee is a direct care provider given he or she is from Asia?

2. Given the following data set of patient ages: 21, 45, 34, 25, 61, 45, 6, 12, 49, 58, 38, 41, 9:

   a. Calculate the simple mean.

   b. Calculate the standard deviation.

   c. Calculate the median.

   d. Is the median equal to the mean? Why or why not?

3. The following data were collected from the American Medical Association regarding one group of doctors' attempts to pass their board certification:

% Grade	Letter Grade and Grade Points	% Grade	Letter Grade and Grade Points
94	A = 4.0	75	C = 2.0
81	B- = 2.7	77	C+ = 2.3
75	C = 3.0	65	D = 1.0
92	A- = 3.7	88	B+ = 3.3
51	F = 0.0	85	B = 3.0

Note: Standard grading scale is as follows: 94–100 = A, 90–93 = A-, 87–89 = B+, 84–86 = B, 80–83 = B-, 77–79 = C+, 74–76 = C, 70–73 = C-, 60–69 = D, all else F.

a. What is the mean % grade for the group?

b. What is the mean letter grade/grade points for the group?

c. What is the median % grade for the group?

d. What is the median letter grade/grade points for the group?

e. Are the mean and median % grades equal? Why or why not?

f. Are the mean and median letter grade/grade points equal? Why or why not?

4. The following data were collected regarding the number of patients admitted to a local emergency room each day for 18 days (patients per day, PPD).

PPD	PPD
23	22
24	26
16	24
26	21
22	20
21	26
26	25
17	24
15	14

a. What is the mean number of patients seen each day?

b. What is the standard deviation of the data set?

c. Construct a histogram for the data set using 2 PPD as your class width and starting with 14 as your lowest class.

5. The following data were collected regarding daily occupancy of a neonatal intensive care wing at a local hospital:

Occupancy					
99	12	94	21	11	88
88	2	89	18	97	5
10	5	10	87	100	10

a. What is the mean occupancy of the wing's data set?

b. What is the median occupancy of the wing's data set? Is there a difference or a similarity between the mean and the median? Explain the similarity or difference.

c. What is the standard deviation of the data set?

d. Construct a histogram for the occupancy data set using 5 as your class width and starting with 0 as your lowest class.

e. Relate the standard deviation you calculated in part c to your histogram in part d.

6. The following data were collected regarding the occupancy of two respective hospital departments:

Occupancy					
Critical Care			Intensive Care		
95	75	68	45	25	18
102	67	65	62	17	15
99	87	94	49	37	54
88	120	81	48	70	31
100	71	104	50	21	54

a. What are the means for the two departments?

b. What are the medians for the two departments? Is there a difference or a similarity between the mean and the median? Explain the similarity or difference.

c. What are the standard deviations for each of the departments?

d. Construct a histogram for each department using 5 as your class width, starting with 60 as your lowest class for the critical care department and 10 for the intensive care department.

e. Relate the standard deviation you calculated in part c to your histograms in part d.

7. For safety and health reasons, Perpetual Mercy Hospital is considering requiring all health care providers to wear latex gloves when interacting with patients. However, the board of directors is going to take a vote, and most of them have a latex allergy. The board of directors consists of 12 nonallergic and 18 allergic members, and 35 percent of the nonallergic members and 70 percent of the allergic members favor the glove policy.

a. Construct a probability tree for this problem.

b. Construct a probability table for this problem.

c. Determine the probability that a board of directors member who opposes the new policy is nonallergic.

8. The Mayon Clinic gets medical supplies delivered from two sources, Medex and ProMed. There is a probability of 60 percent that the order consists of medical supplies from Medex. According to the case, 20 percent of all medical supplies produced at Medex are defective and only 10 percent of the medical supplies from ProMed are defective.

a. Construct a probability tree for this problem.

b. Construct a probability table for this problem.

c. Find the probability that the medical supplies come from Medex and are defective.

d. Given that you have a defective medical supply, what is the probability that it came from ProMed?

9. One hundred male students attend medical school at Freeman University. Thirty of these students are from in-state undergraduate institutions and 70 went to out-of-state colleges for their bachelor's degrees. Students who attended in-state institutions as undergraduates have a 25 percent chance of passing their medical boards on the first attempt whereas those from out-of-state institutions have a 15 percent chance of passing their medical boards on the first attempt.

a. Construct a probability tree for this problem.

b. Construct a probability table for this problem.

c. What is the probability that a randomly selected Freeman University medical student will pass his medical boards on the first attempt?

d. Given a student passing his medical boards on the first attempt, what is the probability that he came from an in-state undergraduate school?

10. The standard heart rate for patients at a local hospital is normally distributed with a mean of 76 and a standard deviation of 9. What percentage of the patients will have a heart rate of 80 or greater?

11. The daily cost of a standard single hospital room in San Francisco is normally distributed with a mean of $800 a month and a standard deviation of $150. What is the probability that a patient will be assigned a standard single hospital room for $700 a month or less?

12. Akiko operates a private medical research facility in Japan. The clinic's monthly telephone bill is normally distributed with a mean of $67.69 and a standard deviation of $3. Akiko is considering a calling plan that has a great benefit for a customer who often uses international calling and whose phone bill is more than $75 per month; however, the plan also requires an extra basic fee for the service. What is the probability that Akiko's phone bill is going to be more than $75?

13. An ambulance is en route to the hospital. The time it takes to complete one emergency response call is normally distributed with a mean of 15 minutes and standard deviation of 7 minutes. What is the probability that it will take an ambulance more than 20 minutes to complete one emergency response call?

14. The following table gives the number of heart monitor failures experienced at a local hospital every week. It further shows the probability of each number of heart monitor failures. Determine the expected value of the number of heart monitor failures in a given week.

Number of Heart Monitor Failures (x_i)	Probability $p(x_i)$
1	0.15
2	0.10
3	0.25
4	0.30
5	0.20

a. Calculate the expected number of failures per week.

b. Find the standard deviation for the distribution.

c. If the hospital has one tech on duty at all times and one tech can fix two monitors a week, does the hospital need to staff more techs?

15. Matthew runs a small company that delivers medical supplies. Every week the company generates new revenue. The following table contains the past business records:

Revenue $\$(x_i)$	Probability $p(x_i)$
$2,000	0.30
$1,500	0.30
$1,000	0.20
$500	0.10
$0	0.10

a. Calculate the expected revenues for this week.

b. Find the standard deviation for the distribution.

REFERENCES

David, F. N. 1962. *Games, Gods, and Gambling.* New York: Hafner.

Gastwirth, J. L. 1988. *Statistical Reasoning in Law and Policy.* Vols. 1 and 2. San Diego: Academic Press.

Gonick, L., and W. Smith. 1993. *A Cartoon Guide to Statistics.* New York: HarperPerennial.

Huff, D. 1954. *How to Lie with Statistics.* New York: W.W. Norton.

Hunt, Dereck, et al. 2000. "User's Guides to the Medical Literature." *JAMA* 283, no. 14 (April 12).

Jaffe, A. J., and Herbert F. Spirer. 1987. *Misused Statistics: Straight Talk for Twisted Numbers.* New York: Marcel Dekker.

Kruskal, W. 1980. "The Significance of Fisher: A Review of *R. A. Fisher: The Life of a Scientist.*" *Journal of the American Statistical Association* 75, no. 372 (December): 1019–1030.

McGervey, J. D. 1989. *Probabilities in Every Day Life.* New York: Ivy.

Peitetti, R. D., et al. 1998. "Evaluation of a New Rapid Antigen Detection Kit for Group A Beta-Hemolytic Streptococci." *Pediatric Emergency Care* 14, no. 6 (December): 396–398.

Stigler, S. M. 1986. *The History of Statistical Measurement of Uncertainty before 1900.* Cambridge, MA: Harvard-Belknap.

Tukey, John W. 1977. *Exploratory Data Analysis.* Reading, MA: Addison-Wesley.

CHAPTER 5

PROBLEM SOLVING AND DECISION-MAKING TOOLS IN HEALTH CARE OPERATIONS

LEARNING OBJECTIVES

➠ Understand the components of decision analysis.

➠ Understand the types of decisions environments managers face.

➠ Understand how probability assessments impact the decision making process.

(Continued)

⪢ Conduct sensitivity analysis within the decision making process.

⪢ Develop decision trees to aid in the decision making process.

⪢ Use Excel to solve decision problems.

HEALTH CARE OPERATIONS AND SUPPLY CHAIN MANAGEMENT IN ACTION: HOW LEGAL DECISION MAKERS USE DECISION MODELS

Healthcare requires that decisions be made effectively and reliably and many times under extremely short notice. In turn, some of those decisions may be examined at a later date. This section describes one area pertaining to litigation costs.

Containing Litigation Costs

An increasing number of companies and their lawyers have turned to decision structures such as decision trees and influence diagrams to help them make better decisions in litigation management and settlement. The results have been lower transaction costs and better outcomes.

Litigators first identify the factual and legal uncertainties in a case—the issues—and then proceed, through fact discovery, legal research, and the use of experts, to cope with these uncertainties. Driving this costly process is the assumption that it will culminate in a trial, at which time a judge and jury will resolve the legal and factual issues.

The reality, though, is that more than 90 percent of all cases end up being resolved through settlement rather than trial (see Figure 5.1).

Decision trees can be enormously helpful in allocating resources before trial. They can effectively demonstrate the cost-effectiveness of forgoing the additional research or discovery, thereby saving the client time and money. Decision trees and influence diagrams make it possible to perform the analyses needed to

FIGURE 5.1   Decision Tree for Litigation Example

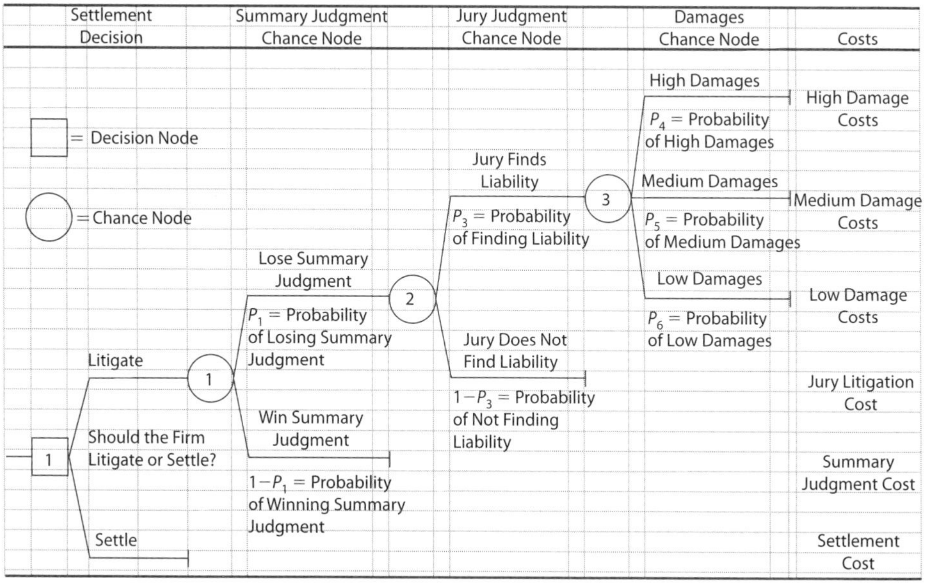

maximize opportunities for early settlement and reduced transaction costs while fully addressing the need to be prepared for trial.

Decision Analysis: Building the Structure for Solving the Problem

Health care professionals are faced with difficult problems and decisions each day. Many times the health care field offers multiple good alternatives with multiple associated outcomes or payoffs. In addition, those alternatives most likely are uncertain (i.e., the outcome has some probability of success or failure associated with it).

In Chapter 2, the importance of the financial aspects of health care operations was discussed to help assess the viability of alternatives. In Chapter 3, describing data sets in terms of central tendency and measures of dispersion was discussed to aid in comparing alternatives. Simple statistics, like mean, median, range, and standard deviation, were defined and described. However, a method to combine alternatives, outcomes/payoffs, and uncertainty is needed. Chapter 4 developed the framework for structuring decision making problems in a health care setting.

Importance and Relevance of Decision Analysis and Theory

The importance of health care managers' painting the full picture of data sets by using both measures of central tendency and measures of dispersion must also be developed. Managers do this by linking simple statistics with a mental and graphical picture of real-life data sets. This chapter builds up a framework to compare alternatives and set the stage for further analysis using probability and statistics to test differences in those alternatives.

FRAMING THE DECISION PROBLEM

A manager must think about building up an edifice and putting a structure, literally a framework, around decision-making problems. Health care managers must ask themselves an important question: "How do I make decisions and what is the process I go through?" Health care professionals make decisions all the time, and this book is not here to tell someone exactly how or what is the best way to make decisions. It would be folly to attempt to do this in one class or volume.

Take a moment and ask yourself the following question about decision making: "How do I make decisions and what is the process I go through as I choose one alternative over another?"

As a health care professional, you must develop your own decision-making process or rational methodology for solving problems. All of us understand that individuals make decisions all the time: we choose to come to class, to read the text, when and where to eat lunch, when to wake up, and when to go to bed.

The techniques individuals use to make these decisions obviously play an important role in everyday life. Decisions made regarding situations in medical staffing, vaccination choice, or even choice of college and career, for example, may also deal with a tremendous amount of uncertainty.

COMPONENTS OF A DECISION-MAKING PROBLEM

The next sections discuss one basic structure to build from. Bear in mind that it is simplistic and is just one way to structure a decision-making problem. With that said, the structure and subsequent framework are highly effective at communicating multiple alternatives, outcomes/payoffs, and uncertainty to other stakeholders.

Decision analysis problems generally have three distinct components:

1. States of nature

2. Decision alternatives

3. Outcomes

States of Nature

States of nature can be defined as events that may occur in the future. As health care professionals, we rarely have control over the states associated with a decision-making problem. In fact, the decision maker is generally uncertain about which state of nature will occur.

A good example of uncertain states of nature is the addition of medical equipment. The addition of the medical equipment will provide better services but as a health care professional you are uncertain about demand for the new machine. On one hand, demand for the equipment could be high and the equipment purchase will pay off. On the other hand, demand could be low for the equipment and in turn the equipment will not be fully utilized and purchase will not pay off.

However, as health care decision makers, we do have control over one item. The ultimate decision that is made is the purview of the decision maker. For the medical equipment example, the decision is to purchase or not purchase the equipment.

Decision Alternatives

Decision alternatives are the second component in a decision analysis problem. At times decisions are also referred to as alternatives. As stated earlier, the decision maker has ultimate control over the decision made or the alternative chosen.

For example, the decisions a health care decision maker could make regarding the medical equipment could be: purchase the equipment or do not purchase the equipment. These decisions must be made regardless of whether the demand for the equipment materializes in the future.

Purchasing medical equipment incurs certain consequences. Take, for example, the scenario that the equipment is purchased and demand for that equipment is high; thus the resources used to obtain the machine went to good use. In another scenario, if the demand is high but you have not purchased the equipment, an opportunity to service patients and make a return on the equipment is lost. These scenarios lead directly into the definition and discussion of outcomes.

Outcomes

The third component of a decision analysis problem is outcomes. An *outcome* is defined as the combination of a state and a decision. For our medical equipment example, we can choose to purchase the equipment or not purchase the equipment, coupled with demand for the equipment being either high or low. In this example, there really exist four possible outcomes. Table 5.1 lists the possible outcomes.

Outcomes versus Payoffs

It should be noted that outcomes are also referred to as *payoffs*. Pure decision analysts and economists generally refer to the combination of states and decisions as an outcome. However, managers tend to use the term *payoffs*.

Payoffs are typically expressed in monetary terms such as profits, revenues, or costs. One way to illustrate the outcomes from the medical equipment example being turned into payoffs is by equating purchasing the equipment and having low demand to the waste of hospital dollars and no payoff on the equipment.

TABLE 5.1   Possible Outcomes for Medical Equipment Example

Decision Alternative	State of Nature	Outcome
Purchase equipment.	Demand is high.	Equipment services patients, and hospital resources are effectively and efficiently used—win-win.
Purchase equipment.	Demand is low.	Equipment sits idle, and hospital resources are not used effectively or efficiently.
Do not purchase equipment.	Demand is high.	Patients are not serviced, and an opportunity is lost.
Do not purchase equipment.	Demand is low.	Patients are not serviced, but demand never materialized.

The term *payoff* is used because it directly links the combination of states and decisions to a monetary result. The authors will use the term *payoff* from this point on in the book.

Every decision problem has states, decisions, and outcomes/payoffs. Think about a recent decision you made and try to identify the states, decisions, and outcomes/payoffs associated with the problem. Were the states easy to describe? Were the outcomes/payoffs easily quantified?

PAYOFF TABLES

The layout of Table 5.1 allows the decision maker to see all the possible outcomes but does not organize the three components of a decision-making problem very well.

Traditional decision analysis uses what is called a *payoff table* to organize states, decision alternatives, and outcomes. Table 5.2 displays the payoff table for the medical equipment example.

The payoffs listed in Table 5.2 are situations rather than monetary amounts associated with the combination of a state and a decision alternative. However, one could quickly assign monetary amounts to the situations listed.

At times these monetary amounts may be negative, or considered costs. For example, the cost of not giving the medical care when the patient is healthy could initially be zero, whereas giving the medical care to a patient who is sick is the cost of the care.

As health care professionals you may be inclined to ask the question: "What is the probability of the demand being high?" This is a good question to ask, because the resulting answer to the question may help the decision maker choose a better course of action or save time and money.

TABLE 5.2 Payoff Table for Medical Equipment Example

	State of Nature	
Decision Alternative	**Demand Is High**	**Demand Is Low**
Purchase equipment.	Equipment services patients, and hospital resources are effectively and efficiently used.	Equipment sits idle, and hospital resources are not used effectively or efficiently.
Do not purchase equipment.	Patients are not serviced, and an opportunity is lost.	Patients are not serviced, but demand never materialized.

Health care professionals make numerous decisions each day. However, not all of those decisions are made by using probability assessments. Are there decisions you make each day without the use of probability assessments? How about where you are going for lunch?

The probability of a state occurring is not always readily available, and decision makers may have a difficult time assigning probabilities to events. Decision making without probability assessments is discussed next.

Health Care Operations and Supply Chain Management through the Ages: A Brief History of Decision Making

Historically, decision techniques have focused on outcome prediction, not decision process or technique. Take a look at the progression and remember that the way we make decisions today may come from decisions made in the past.

Soothsayers, Astrologers, and Fortune-Tellers

Elders were consulted for alternatives and probability of success.

Alexander the Great consulted oracles and fortune-tellers.

The Oracle at Delphi was famous and became hugely popular.

The Romans, the Babylonians, the Chinese, and the Use of Hard Data

Romans also had oracles but relied heavily on hard data—diviners called haruspices examined animal entrails to try to predict the future (we might say they used their gut feelings).

The Babylonians used the Talmud to deal with decisions on division of wealth; indirectly this document led to the understanding of cooperative games.

The Chinese developed the I Ching around 3000 BC. People consulted the I Ching for the prognosis of a given decision; an answer detailing potential risks and opportunities resulted.

The 1700s and 1800s

Benjamin Franklin is credited with the "balance sheet" approach to decision making.

William Playfair, in 1786, used the perspective ratios of height and width of graphs depicting government debt to imply skyrocketing national debt due to the British government's borrowing to support the various colonial wars of that century. Sound familiar?

In the late 1800s, the neoclassical revolution in economics elevated mathematical utility theory, and axiomatic methods of mathematics began to permeate decision theory; famous participants include Ramsey, de Finetti, Alt, and Frisch.

Modern Times

The 1960s and 1970s brought database systems and the cliché of "Let's crunch the numbers."

The 1990s introduced faster desktop and laptop computers and new software algorithms, and we began to see decision analysis tools available for our personal use.

And what does the new century bring? We'll let you decide.

DECISION-MAKING CRITERIA WITHOUT PROBABILITY ASSESSMENTS

Decision making that does not involve uncertainty is fairly simple. Without uncertainty, we tend to have limited choices (or just one choice) and simple outcomes. Many of life's basic choices are this simple, or the process used in making the choice is fundamentally an unconscious one, involuntary, or a learned response.

Decision makers use decision-making criteria when determining which alternatives to choose. When information regarding the probability of a state is limited or not available, decision makers use what are referred to as *nonprobabilistic criteria*. The following sections detail three of these criteria: the maximax, the maximin, and the minimax regret.

Spreadsheet Solution for Payoff Table Decision Problem

This section details the use of Excel spreadsheets to illustrate three nonprobabilistic criteria—a maximax, maximin, and minimax regret—and also demonstrates the Hurwicz decision criteron. A step-by-step creation of a graph to illustrate the three areas of sensitivity is developed.

Sarah's Magnetic Resonance Imaging Equipment Decision Problem

Sarah has a decision to make. She wishes to invest in one of three magnetic resonance imaging (MRI) machines offered in the market. Table 5.3 displays the three decision alternatives, the states of nature, the associated payoffs, and the probability of each state of nature occurring.

The payoffs are estimated percentage returns on the initial investment. One can take the information in Table 5.3 and input it into an Excel spreadsheet to obtain the results displayed in Figure 5.2.

Maximax Criterion

The *maximax criterion* is defined as the criterion where a decision maker selects the decision that will result in the best of the maximum payoffs. A decision maker who chooses to use this criterion is looking for the best of the best. It could be said

TABLE 5.3   Sarah's Equipment Payoff Table (Percent Return)

	States of Nature	
Equipment Type	High Demand	Low Demand
General Electric MRI machine	6%	4%
Fonar Upright MRI machine	20%	-8%
Philips Open MRI machine	12%	2%
Probability of states of nature	40%	60%

FIGURE 5.2   Excel Spreadsheet for Sarah's Equipment Payoff Table

	A	B	C
1	Sarah's Equipment Return Problem		
2	Payoff Table		
3		State of Nature	
4		High	Low
5	Equipment Type	Demand	Demand
6	GE MRI Machine	6%	4%
7			
8	Fonar Upright MRI Machine	20%	-8%
9			
10	Philips Open MRI Machine	12%	2%
11			

that a decision maker using maximax is optimistic (believes the best will always occur). It could also be said that the decision maker using maximax is willing to accept more risk.

Take a moment and think to yourself: "Do I know people who make decisions regularly using the maximax criterion?" Maybe you are the type of decision maker who uses the maximax criterion to make decisions. Can you think of professions that use this type of criterion? How about gamblers? High-risk derivatives or commodities traders?

A spreadsheet solution using the maximax decision criterion is shown in Figure 5.3. The payoff table with appropriate headings is placed in cells A4 through cell C10. The Excel formulas that provide the calculations and an optimal solution recommendation are:

> Cell D6 Compute the maximum payoff
> = MAX(B6:C6)

(Repeat formula for cells D8 and D10.)

> Cell E6 Determine which decision alternative is recommended
> = IF(D6 = MAX($D$6, $D$8, $D$10), A6, "")

(Repeat formula for cells E8 and E10.)

If the maximum payoff in cell D6 is equal to the best payoff in cells D6:D10, the MRI equipment's name will be displayed in E6; otherwise, this cell will be left

FIGURE 5.3 Excel Spreadsheet for Maximax Decision Criterion

	A	B	C	D	E
1	Sarah's Equipment Return Problem				
2	Payoff Table				
3		State of Nature			
4		High	Low	Maximum	Recommended
5	Equipment Type	Demand	Demand	Payoff	Decision
6	GE MRI Machine	6%	4%	6%	
7					
8	Fonar Upright MRI Machine	20%	-8%	20%	Fonar Upright MRI Machine
9					
10	Philips Open MRI Machine	12%	2%	12%	
11					

blank. As Figure 5.3 shows, the maximax criterion recommends the Fonar Upright MRI machine decision alternative with a best payoff of 20 percent.

Maximin Criterion

The *maximin criterion* is defined as the criterion where a decision maker selects the decision that will result in the maximum of the minimum payoffs. In other words, the decision maker is looking for the best of the worst. It could be said that a decision maker using maximin is pessimistic (believes the worst will always occur). A maximin decision maker could also be categorized as risk averse or not willing to accept more risk.

A spreadsheet solution using the maximin decision criterion is shown in Figure 5.4. The payoff table with appropriate headings is placed in cells A4 through C10. The Excel formulas that provide the calculations and optimal solution recommendation are:

Cell D6 Compute the minimum payoff
= MIN(B6:C6)

(Repeat formula for cells D8 and D10.)

Cell E6 Determine which decision alternative is recommended
= IF(D6 = MAX($D$6, $D$8, $D$10), A6, "")

(Repeat formula for cells E8 and E10.)

FIGURE 5.4 Excel Spreadsheet for Maximin Decision Criterion

	A	B	C	D	E
1	Sarah's Equipment Return Problem				
2	Payoff Table				
3		State of Nature			
4		High	Low	Minimum	Recommended
5	Equipment Type	Demand	Demand	Payoff	Decision
6	GE MRI Machine	6%	4%	4%	GE MRI Machine
7					
8	Fonar Upright MRI Machine	20%	–8%	–8%	
9					
10	Philips Open MRI Machine	12%	2%	2%	
11					

The only difference between the spreadsheets in Figures 5.3 and 5.4 is that the maximin criterion finds the minimum payoff in each decision alternative.

Notice that the formulas in E6, E8, and E10 remain the same. This is because Sarah is still looking for the maximum result in column D. With the appropriate changes, the spreadsheet in Figure 5.4 shows that the maximin criterion recommends the General Electric (GE) MRI machine decision alternative with the best minimum payoff value of 4 percent.

Take a moment and think to yourself: "Do I know people who make decisions regularly using the maximin criterion?" Maybe you are the type of decision maker who uses the maximin criterion to make decisions. Can you think of a group of people who use this type of criterion? How about those individuals who lived through the Great Depression in the United States?

Minimax Regret

The *minimax regret* criterion is defined as the criterion where a decision maker selects the decision that will result in the minimum regret. Before this criterion is detailed, the measure of regret must be defined.

Operations and Supply Chain Management Definition of Regret

Operations and supply chain management (SCM) managers define regret as the difference between the payoff from the best decision and all the other decision payoffs. Health care students must keep in mind that this is not the only discipline to define regret. Economics and marketing both have similar concepts of regret.

Economics Definition of Regret: Opportunity Cost

Economists use the words *opportunity cost* to define or refer to regret. *Opportunity cost* is the value of the next best alternative, or opportunity, that was given up by choosing the best alternative. For example, by choosing to spend your money on beer and pizzas you give up the opportunity to invest that money in a retirement account. Your opportunity cost is the choice you gave up.

Regret, as defined by operations and SCM, is akin to the concept of opportunity cost in economics. In operations and SCM, regret is the quantifiable amount a decision maker gives up to choose a different alternative.

Marketing Definition of Regret: Buyer's Remorse

The concept of regret is manifested in consumers by what marketers call *buyer's remorse*. Marketers describe the feeling consumers experience when they purchase an item and then feel as if they could have gotten a better deal on another item. At times this is also referred to as *postdecision doubt.*

Buyer's remorse can also manifest itself in consumers when they make a decision and then regret making that decision after the fact. Buyer's remorse occurs with some frequency in buying a home. Some home buyers have a sense of letdown after deciding to purchase a home.

Real estate brokers attribute this feeling to the fact that a home is a very large purchase, not in terms of just dollars but in the sense of status, ego, and commitment. A home buyer, after making the final decision, may look around and feel a sense of regret, believing that better deals existed and were missed.

Psychological Definition of Regret: Cognitive Dissonance

According to *cognitive dissonance* theory, there is a tendency for individuals to seek consistency among their beliefs and choices. Cognitive dissonance theory applies to all situations involving attitude formation and change. It is especially relevant to managers in the decision-making and problem-solving process.

Consider someone who is going to have an elective medical procedure completed but is very uncomfortable with hospitals. The patient believes that an expensive private clinic and private room should be comfortable. Cognitive dissonance exists, since the belief that an expensive private clinic and room should be a comfortable place is violated in that the person is really uncomfortable with any hospital.

In general, decision makers will alter their beliefs instead of removing the conflicting attitude or behavior. The patient will convince himself or herself that the expense of the room and private surgeon will make the trip to the hospital much better, thereby eliminating the conflict in beliefs. The problem arises when the patient comes to the conclusion that the expensive room and private clinic did not assuage the fear of hospitals in general.

The term *cognitive dissonance* has also been adopted by the marketing discipline. Many advertising campaigns attempt to eliminate cognitive dissonance or buyer's remorse by focusing on product strengths or developing new nonconflicting attitudes toward the product.

As a decision maker, have you ever felt regret? Have you ever thought about the opportunity costs of choosing one item over another? As a consumer, have you ever felt buyer's remorse? Should decision makers rely on minimizing regret as the criterion to make decisions or solve problems? Do you make choices based on minimizing regret, opportunity costs, or buyer's remorse?

Minimax Regret Criterion Process

A decision maker who chooses to use this criterion is looking to minimize the measure of regret. Regret has been defined as the difference between the payoff from the best decision and all the other decision payoffs. Therefore, the first step in the minimax regret criterion is to determine regret.

A spreadsheet solution using the minimax regret decision criterion is shown in Figure 5.5. The payoff table with appropriate headings is placed in cells A4 through C10. The Excel formulas that provide the calculations and optimal solution recommendation are:

Cell B16 Compute the amount of regret
= MAX($B$6, $B$8, $B$10) – B6

(Repeat formula for cells B18 and B20.)

FIGURE 5.5 Excel Spreadsheet for Minimax Regret Decision Criterion

	A	B	C	D	E
1	Sarah's Equipment Return Problem				
2	Payoff Table				
3		State of Nature			
4		High	Low		
5	Equipment Type	Demand	Demand		
6	GE MRI Machine	6%	4%		
7					
8	Fonar Upright MRI Machine	20%	-8%		
9					
10	Philips Open MRI Machine	12%	2%		
11					
12	Regret Table				
13		State of Nature			
14		High	Low	Maximum	Recommended
15	Equipment Type	Demand	Demand	Regret	Decision
16	GE MRI Machine	14%	0%	14%	
17					
18	Fonar Upright MRI Machine	0%	12%	12%	
19					
20	Philips Open MRI Machine	8%	2%	8%	Philips Open MRI Machine
21					

Cell C16 Compute the amount of regret
= MAX($C$6, $C$8, $C$10) – C6

(Repeat formula for cells C18 and C20.)

Cell D16 Compute the maximum regret
= MAX(B16:C18)

(Repeat formula for cells D18 and D20.)

Cell E16 Determine which decision alternative is recommended
= IF(D16 = MIN($D$16, $D$18, $D$20), A16, "")

In Figure 5.5, Sarah first calculates the amount of regret under each economic condition by subtracting each return figure from the largest figure in the appropriate economic condition. She then finds the maximum regret for each fund in column D. Continuing, she finds the minimum regret in the Maximum Regret column, and thus accomplishes the minimax regret decision. We can see from Figure 5.5 that the Philips Open MRI machine offers the least amount of regret.

Regret as a Measure of Risk

Measures of dispersion, such as range and standard deviation, are measures of risk. Regret can also be used as a means to define and quantify risk. The definition of regret has been established in the minimax regret example. Regret is usually presented in terms of units.

It is important to remember that regret is not something tangible. In the previous example, Sarah did not lose 8 percent by choosing the Philips Open MRI machine; she will experience the least amount of regret by choosing the Philips machine. As was detailed in the sections preceding the minimax regret example, regret can be thought of as an opportunity cost, or a feeling of buyer's remorse, or a psychological feeling of cognitive dissonance.

Regret is used as a measure of risk to give decision makers a sense of what the other alternatives have to offer. Sometimes regret is called upside or downside risk.

The concept of upside and downside risk will be detailed in the section "Sensitivity Analysis" later in this chapter.

DECISION-MAKING CRITERIA WITH PROBABILITY ASSESSMENTS

A more common occurrence in business decision modeling problems is decision making under uncertainty or decision making relying on probability assessments.

Equal Likelihood Criterion: Laplace and Simple Weighted Averages

Expected values are commonly referred to as *weighted averages*. In other words, each event has a weight or a probability assessment associated with it. The *equal likelihood criterion* also weights each state of nature. As the name implies, all events are weighted equally.

Have you ever used a weighted average before? More than likely you have. At times information on the likelihood of states is not available or time is limited to assess state probabilities, so in many cases a simple weighted average, or simple mean, is used. When managers use a simple mean, they are assigning equal probabilities to all states. When do you use a simple mean to calculate central tendency?

The equal likelihood criterion is also referred to as the Laplace criterion, named for the mathematician Pierre-Simon Laplace. By assigning equal weights to the events in the event space, the decision maker is assuming that the states of nature are also equally likely to occur. This approach is akin to summing the payoffs for each decision and dividing by the number of payoffs summed—in other words, taking a simple mean or an expected value where all the $p(x)$'s are equal. For Sarah's equipment example, we find the equal likelihood payoffs to be 5 percent for the GE MRI machine, 6 percent for the Fonar Upright machine, and 7 percent for the Philips Open machine; therefore the Philips Open machine is chosen.

Hurwicz Criterion

The *Hurwicz criterion* is said to be a compromise between the maximax criterion and the maximin criterion. The three criteria combined complete the entire spectrum of expected outcomes. The maximax criterion relays the best of the best outcomes, and the maximin criterion details the best of the worst outcomes, while the Hurwicz criterion covers every outcome in between.

The Hurwicz criterion uses a coefficient of optimism to weight the best and worst payoffs for each decision. This coefficient of optimism is referred to as *alpha* in standard decision analysis nomenclature. The idea of payoffs is not a new one. We weighted states of nature when we used the Laplace criterion.

The Hurwicz criterion is the same concept as expected value but referred to by a different name. The general equation for expected value is a weighted average or the sum of a set of unique probabilities (or weights) multiplied by the corresponding payoffs. The equal likelihood criterion is a specific case of the expected value where all the alphas, or weights, are equal. The difference in the Hurwicz criterion is that only the best and worst payoffs are used.

The payoff table with appropriate headings is placed in cells A3 through C12. The Excel formulas that provide the calculations and optimal solution recommendation are:

Cell D6 Compute the payoff
= MAX(B6,C6)*$B$12 + MIN(B6,C6)*$C$12

(Repeat formula for cells D8 and D10.)

Cell E6 Determine which decision alternative is recommended
= IF(D6 = MAX($D$6, $D$8, $D$10), A6, "")

(Repeat formula for cells E8 and E10.)

Given alpha equal to 0.4, Figure 5.6 displays, for the MRI machine example, the Hurwicz criterion. For example, in the equipment purchase scenario, the

FIGURE 5.6 Excel Spreadsheet for Hurwicz Criterion

	A	B	C	D	E
1	Sarah's Equipment Return Problem				
2	Hurwicz Decision Criteria: Alpha = 0.40				
3		State of Nature			
4		High	Low		Recommended
5	Equipment Type	Demand	Demand	Payoff	Decision
6	GE MRI Machine	6%	4%	4.8%	
7					
8	Fonar Upright MRI Machine	20%	-8%	3.2%	
9					
10	Philips Open MRI Machine	12%	2%	6.0%	Philips Open MRI Machine
11					
12	Probability of States	40%	60%		
13					

alpha of 0.4 would be applied to the high demand state. In this example, high demand and low demand are mutually exclusive events and, consequently, according to the rules of probability, the coefficient or weight applied to the bad economic conditions state is 1.0 – alpha, or 0.6. For situations with more than two states of nature, all the payoffs for each decision alternative are used in the maximum and minimum functions defined earlier (refer to cell D6 formulas).

In Figure 5.6, we first calculated the payoff by multiplying the return figures of each machine under both conditions against their appropriate probabilities of occurrence. Furthermore, if the maximum payoff in column D is equal to the best payoff of a piece of equipment, the equipment's name will appear in column E indicating that machine is the optimal recommended decision. In using the Hurwicz decision criterion, we can see that the Philips Open MRI machine offers the optimal payoff of 6.0 percent.

As a decision maker, ask yourself: "How do I assess probabilities of the occurrence of certain states?" Do you see the similarity when a manager guesses and applies the same probability to all states and uses the equal likelihood criterion? Can we apply the same principles of central tendency and dispersion to the Hurwicz criterion and decision-making processes?

Given Sarah's payoff table with probability assessments for all states of nature, the expected value of her decision alternatives can be calculated. The expected value calculation (Equation 5.1) is:

$$E(x) = \sum_{i=1}^{n} x_i p(x_i) \qquad (5.1)$$

For Sarah's MRI machine example problem, let's attach a probability of high demand (HD) happening as 0.6, and therefore the probability of low demand happening would be 0.4. The expected value of each decision alternative is then calculated as follows:

$$E(\text{GE MRI}) = 6\% \times 0.6 + 4\% \times 0.4 = 5.2\%$$
$$E(\text{Fonar MRI}) = 20\% \times 0.6 + (-8\%) \times 0.4 = 8.8\%$$
$$E(\text{Philips MRI}) = 12\% \times 0.6 + 2\% \times 0.4 = 8.0\%$$

Thus, according to the expected value criterion, Sarah would choose the Fonar MRI, since it garners the maximum expected value.

TABLE 5.4 Summary of Final Medical Equipment Example Choices

Decision Criterion	Maximax	Maximin	Minimax Regret	Equal Likelihood	Hurwicz Alpha = 0.40	Expected Value p(HD) = 0.60
Equipment to choose	Fonar Upright MRI	GE MRI	Philips Open MRI	Philips Open MRI	Philips Open MRI	Fonar Upright MRI

Summary of Decision Criteria Results

Table 5.4 displays the final medical equipment example decision choices for each decision criterion. It can be seen from Table 5.4 that no one equipment alternative dominates the decision criteria. Depending on the decision criterion, the Fonar, GE, or Philips MRI machine could be the best choice.

Strict dominance cannot be established for the medical equipment example. Dominance is the first area a manager should analyze in the decision-making process. The principle of dominance will be defined and discussed later in this chapter.

Faced with numerous optimal or good choices, how does a manager make the right choice? Is there a process that a person uses when faced with multiple conflicting good choices? Is there a set of standard analyses that a manager can follow that will assist in the decision-making process?

From these results, it seems that a manager has a dilemma. Unless a manager can assess the probability of the states exactly (i.e., predict the future) or has a very optimistic or pessimistic risk profile, there will be multiple optimal choices. In fact, there seem to be some interactions or trade-offs among the three choices. Decision makers might wonder if they could obtain additional information about the states of nature, say by employing an economist. It then would be useful to find out if that additional information might be of value. In fact, it is possible to find what is called the expected value of perfect information (EVPI).

EXPECTED VALUE OF PERFECT INFORMATION

Now let's suppose that Sarah has a good friend who is a prominent health care economist and who has given her some insight into the future state of MRI demand. Sarah's economist friend claims that he can tell with certainty whether the future economic conditions for MRIs will be high or low. This information would change Sarah's decision problem from one under uncertainty to one under certainty. This information would help her make a better choice and garner a better return.

However, Sarah's friend wants a cut of the action. Specifically, he wants a couple of percentage points of return for his efforts. In other words, if Sarah would garner an 8 percent return, 2 of those percentage points would go to Sarah's friend, leaving Sarah with a net 6 percent return. Is it worth it to Sarah to pay this fee? Is 2 percentage points fair, or what do you think it might be worth to Sarah? To answer these questions we need to calculate the expected value of perfect information (EVPI).

If Sarah's friend were able to determine which state of nature would occur, then they would know exactly what alternative to choose to maximize returns. Since the payoffs under this perfect information will increase, this knowledge has value. Therefore, we need to determine the value of this information. The expected value of perfect information (Equation 5.2) is defined as the difference between the payoff under certainty and the payoff under risk.

$$\text{EVPI} = \text{expected value under certainty} - \text{maximum expected value} \quad (5.2)$$

To find the EVPI, we must compute the expected value under certainty. The expected value under certainty is the expected return if the decision maker has perfect information before each decision has to be made.

In calculating this value, the decision maker chooses the best alternative for each state of nature and multiplies its payoff by the probability of occurrence of that state of nature. For Sarah's example, we will use 0.6 as the probability of good economic conditions (the same probabilities used to calculate expected value earlier), and expected value under certainty is then calculated as follows:

$$\text{Expected value under certainty} = 20\% \times 0.6 + 4\% \times 0.4 = 13.6\%$$

The 20 percent is the best payoff under high demand and the 4 percent is the best payoff under low demand. Therefore, the expected value of perfect information is, for the expected value under certainty and maximum expected value calculations:

$$\begin{aligned} \text{EVPI} &= \text{Expected value under certainty} - \text{Maximum expected value} \\ &= 13.6\% - 8.8\% = 4.8\% \end{aligned}$$

In other words, the most Sarah would be willing to pay for the perfect information is 4.8 percentage points.

If Sarah's friend is asking for 2 percentage points, then Sarah would come out ahead by at least 2.8 percentage points. So it appears that taking her friend's advice is worth it. This conclusion is based on the assumption that the probability of good economic conditions occurring will be 0.6. If the probability assessment of good economic conditions changes, then the expected value of information will change.

Confusion over Multiple Good Choices

Obtaining multiple conflicting good choices is often confusing to students of business decision modeling as well as to real-world managers. This confusion over choices is common when people are attempting to solve complex problems. Part of the confusion is linked to the belief that the decision analysis process will lead health care managers to one ultimate correct choice.

The decision analysis process should lead a decision maker to a set of good choices and subsequently produce a more robust picture of the entire problem. The tool to assist decision makers to produce a more robust picture is sensitivity analysis.

Three Areas of Sensitivity Analysis

The principles of dominance, trade-offs, and risks are commonly used in solving decision problems. If dominance cannot be established, multiple optimal choices arise. Multiple optimal choices lead to trade-offs between those choices and a need to analyze the risk involved with one choice compared to another. In sum, when faced with multiple optimal choices, managers must complete analysis with regard to three areas:

1. Dominance

2. Trade-offs

3. Risks

The principles of dominance, trade-off analysis, and risk analysis can be grouped together into a standard set of analyses. This standard set of analyses is referred to as *sensitivity analysis*. Sensitivity analysis and the three areas of analysis are detailed next.

Sensitivity Analysis Process

The sensitivity analysis process assists health care professionals faced with multiple conflicting good choices. Sensitivity analysis includes analysis in three areas: dominance, trade-offs, and risks. The three areas could be referred to as a three-step approach to building a more robust understanding of the decision-making problem. The three areas, or steps, are detailed next, followed by an application to the medical equipment payoff table example.

Step 1: Establish a Dominant Decision   Given that a decision maker wishes to maximize expected value, an alternative that always returns the highest expected value would be considered the dominant choice. However, in many problems there is not one dominant decision. In other words, the decision that maximizes expected value may change, depending on the decision maker's probability assessments of the states.

When strict dominance cannot be established, trade-offs among the alternatives will occur. Trade-off analysis is the second step of analyzing a decision problem.

Step 2: Examine the Trade-Offs between Dominant Decisions   If strict dominance cannot be established, trade-offs between the alternatives must exist. Trade-offs are akin to the break-even analysis detailed in Chapter 3. A trade-off is defined as the point where the expected value of two or more alternatives is equal. On the leading edge of this trade-off point one alternative dominates, while on the lagging edge of the trade-off point another alternative dominates.

In break-even analysis, the trade-off is the point where costs are equal to revenues. On the leading edge of the break-even point, costs dominate revenues (i.e., revenues are not covering fixed costs, resulting in losses). In turn, on the lagging edge of the break-even point, revenues dominate costs (i.e., revenues cover fixed costs, resulting in profits).

Trade-off analysis gives the decision maker a means to judge how much will be given up by choosing one alternative over another.

Step 3: Define and Quantify the Risk   The authors believe that, as health care professionals assess probabilities of states occurring, they are actually assessing a measure of risk.

Risk must be defined and then quantified for each decision-making problem. Risk can be defined in a number of different ways. Table 5.5 lists the ways in

TABLE 5.5 Definitions and Quantifications of Risk

Risk Measurement	Relation of Measurement	Definition of Measurement
Range	Larger ranges relate to higher relative risk	Difference of high versus low of a data set
Regret	Regret is not a monetary amount, but a feeling of loss	Buyer's remorse or opportunity costs (i.e., minimax regret criterion)
Standard deviation	Relatively higher standard deviations mean relatively higher risk	$SD^* = \sqrt{\dfrac{\sum (x - \mu)^2}{n - 1}}$ $SD^\dagger = \sqrt{\sum (x - E(x))^2 p(x)}$

*Use with raw data.
†Use when a probability distribution is given.

which this book has defined risk. A health care professional may employ all of these definitions and methods of quantification when making complex decisions.

Each method carries with it certain advantages and inadequacies. However, risk must be defined and quantified in order to fully analyze a decision-making problem.

Importance of Sensitivity Analysis

It is the decision maker's job, when solving complex problems, to complete the three steps of sensitivity analysis before coming to a conclusion. Some refer to sensitivity analysis as *"what if"* analysis or *scenario analysis*. These terms are synonymous with sensitivity analysis.

It is important to note that, while sensitivity analysis may be the most critical and meaningful aspect of the decision-making process, it often tends to be the most underutilized. It could be said that a problem is only half-solved if formal sensitivity analysis is not included. The next section details the three steps of sensitivity analysis with regard to the medical equipment purchase.

At times sensitivity analysis is referred to as "what if" analysis. In fact, the term "what if" analysis has become the standard nomenclature with the proliferation of the spreadsheet as a decision support tool. Have you ever conducted a "what if" or sensitivity analysis on a decision problem? We would bet you have, especially when final exam time rolls around.

Sensitivity Analysis: Sarah's Medical Equipment Example

Now that Sarah has computed the results of the maximax, maximin, minimax regret, and Hurwicz decision criteria, she is faced with a difficult decision because there is not one dominant decision.

This section details a sensitivity analysis, which offers Sarah a deeper understanding and will assist her in making a better decision on which MRI machine to invest in.

"What If" Analysis

Oftentimes sensitivity analysis is referred to as "what if" analysis. In other words, "What if something changes—does our recommended decision change?" Figure 5.7 shows an adequate method to analyze the outcomes for the expected value criterion. In addition, the information contained in Figure 5.7 can be graphed to reveal a much clearer picture of what is really happening as alpha changes.

Figure 5.7 uses different alphas ranging from 0.0 to 1.0 and shows the payoff potential for each. The following Excel commands produce the information in Figure 5.7.

FIGURE 5.7 Sensitivity Analysis Data Calculations

	A	B	C	D
1	Sarah's Equipment Return Problem			
2	Payoff Table			
3			State of Nature	
4		High	Low	
5	Equipment Type	Demand	Demand	
6	GE MRI Machine	6%	4%	
7				
8	Fonar Upright MRI Machine	20%	−8%	
9				
10	Philips Open MRI Machine	12%	2%	
11				
12	Expected Value Criterion			
13			Expected Payoff Value	
14	p(High Demand)	GE MRI	Fonar Upright MRI	Phillips Open MRI
15	0	4.00%	−8.00%	2.00%
16	0.1	4.20%	−5.20%	3.00%
17	0.2	4.40%	−2.40%	4.00%
18	0.3	4.60%	0.40%	5.00%
19	0.4	4.80%	3.20%	6.00%
20	0.5	5.00%	6.00%	7.00%
21	0.6	5.20%	8.80%	8.00%
22	0.7	5.40%	11.60%	9.00%
23	0.8	5.60%	14.40%	10.00%
24	0.9	5.80%	17.20%	11.00%
25	1	6.00%	20.00%	12.00%
26				

Cell B15 Compute the payoff figure for the GE MRI
= $B$6*A15 + $C$6*(1 – A15)

(Repeat formula for cells B16 through B25.)

Cell C15 Compute the payoff figure for the Fonar Upright MRI
= $B$8*A15 + $C$8*(1 – A15)

(Repeat formula for cells C16 through C25.)

Cell D15 Compute the payoff figure for the Philips Open MRI
= $B$10*A15 + $C$10*(1 – A15)

(Repeat formula for cells D16 through D25.)

Sarah has now computed all the possible combinations on the occurrence of the state of nature. Since she is more visual than mathematical, she decides to convert the tabular display into a graphical display. A detailed walk-through on creating a sensitivity graph in Excel is next.

How to Construct a Sensitivity Graph in Excel

This section is a step-by-step tutorial on converting tabular data into a graphical form. This should prove useful to any student who is unfamiliar with Excel. Figure 5.8 shows how to begin constructing a graph from the data in Figure 5.7. The eight steps are:

1. Highlight cells B14 through D25.

2. Click on the Insert tab on the Menu bar and select from the Charts group the Scatter option (see Figure 5.9).

3. Click on the option at the bottom of the Scatter pull-down menu, and select All Chart Types. A figure resembling Figure 5.10 will appear.

4. Choose X Y (Scatter) with straight lines and markers (the fourth icon in from the left); this will graph your table in a scatter plot format.

5. Click on the OK button, and the graph will appear within your spreadsheet as in Figure 5.8.

6. To format the graph's axes in Excel, position the cursor over the axis to format and right click. An options menu resembling Figure 5.11 will appear.

FIGURE 5.8   Final Chart Output in Excel

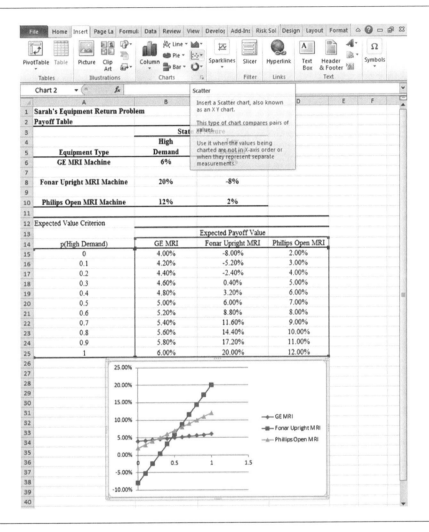

7. Click on the Format Axis option, and a screen resembling Figure 5.12 will appear. Use this menu to modify the axis options. Another method to accomplish this task is to click on the Layout tab and use the Axes group to complete modifications (see Figure 5.13).

8. To move the graph in Excel, right click anywhere on the graph itself. A menu resembling Figure 5.14 will appear. Click on the Move Chart option and a screen resembling Figure 5.15 will appear. From this menu, choose where you want the graph to be placed.

FIGURE 5.9   Scatter Chart Menu in Excel

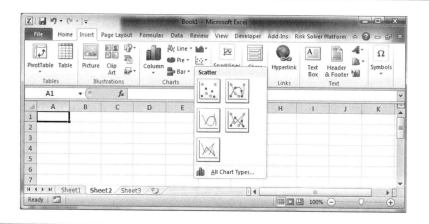

FIGURE 5.10   Insert Chart Menu in Excel

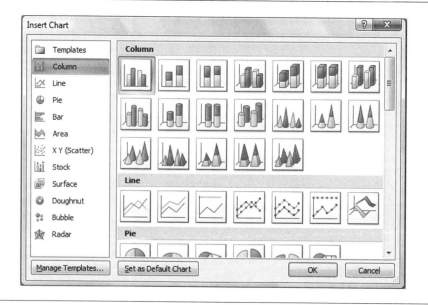

FIGURE 5.11   Format Axis Option after Right Click in Excel

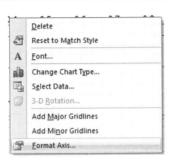

FIGURE 5.12   Format Axis Menu in Excel

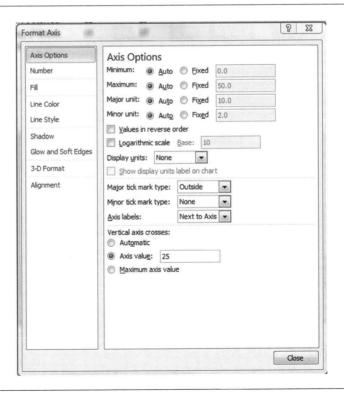

FIGURE 5.13   Layout Tab for Modifying Graphs in Excel

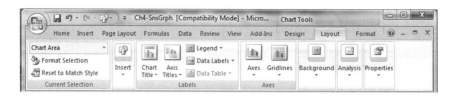

FIGURE 5.14   Move Chart Option for Modifying Graphs in Excel

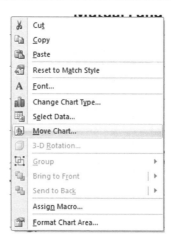

FIGURE 5.15   Move Chart Dialogue Box for Modifying Graphs in Excel

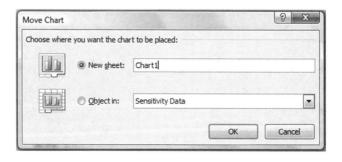

Analyzing the Sensitivity Graph

Figure 5.16 reveals some very interesting information about the medical equipment example. The sensitivity graph in itself illustrates the three areas of sensitivity analysis: dominance, trade-offs, and risk. Let's review the three steps of sensitivity analysis with regard to Figure 5.16.

Establish Dominance

The lines traced on the graph represent the dominant decisions for Sarah's medical equipment example. The graph is telling the decision maker the following:

- If your assessment of the probability of good economic conditions is less than about 25 percent, then the GE MRI is the best equipment alternative.

FIGURE 5.16   Excel Output for Medical Equipment Sensitivity Analysis

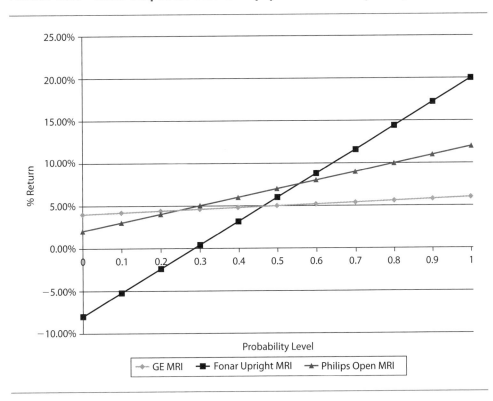

- If your assessment of the probability of good economic conditions is greater than about 25 percent but not greater than 55 percent, then the Philips Open MRI is the best equipment alternative.

If your assessment of the probability of good economic conditions is greater than about 55 percent, then the Fonar Upright MRI is the best equipment alternative.

Strict Dominance   Overall, a dominance structure has been established. However, this dominance is not strict dominance. Strict dominance is established when there is one decision that dominates in all situations. In the medical equipment example, there are three decision alternatives that dominate at different probability levels of high demand. Since strict dominance cannot be established, the decision problem will contain trade-offs between the conflicting choices.

Trade-Off Analysis

Let's assume a decision maker is clairvoyant and knows whether demand will be high. The decision, then, would be very simple. A decision maker with this clairvoyant edge would only look at the right-hand or left-hand side of the graph to make a decision. But as we all know, no one is clairvoyant. Therefore, the point at which the two dominant choices cross is very important.

The point at which the two dominant choices intersect is referred to as the *trade-off point*. The exact value of the trade-off point can be calculated, but is not of overall importance to the decision maker. The most important issue is the identification and acknowledgment of the trade-off point.

There are several trade-offs involved with the three medical equipment alternatives. It is Sarah's understanding that, should she yearn for a better return, she would have to take on more risk from the Fonar Upright MRI machine (represented by the steep slope of the line). Thus, in order for Sarah to make her decision, she should really think about her risk tolerance level.

Defining and Quantifying Risk

Risk must be defined and quantified when a decision maker is faced with trade-offs associated with numerous good alternatives. At the trade-off point, the alternatives look equally desirable. Subsequently, the risk associated with each of the alternatives may be the only way to differentiate the alternatives.

For the medical equipment example, risk is defined by using the measures of range and regret. Risk will not be defined by standard deviation, because of the small payoff sample size. Standard deviation will be used to define and quantify risk in Chapter 6, "Simulation."

Risk Defined and Quantified by Range

From Figure 5.16 it can be seen that the lines associated with the different equipment alternatives have different slopes. The Fonar Upright MRI machine tends to have a much steeper slope than the Philips or GE machines do. In this case, the slope of the line is related directly to range.

Range is defined as the difference between the highest value and the lowest value in the data set. Larger measurements of range mean the highest and lowest values in the data set are farther apart. As a line becomes steeper, the difference between the high and low values is greater. Hence, steeper slope, like larger values of range, translates into higher relative risk.

Table 5.6 contains the range calculations for the medical equipment example. From the table it can be seen that the Fonar Upright MRI machine has the highest range and could be considered to have the highest relative risk. Refer back to Figure 5.16 and relate the range measurements to the slope of each line.

If Sarah has assessed the probability of high demand to be around the trade-off point, 0.55, the range definition of risk could assist the decision-making process. A person who is optimistic or who is more risk tolerant may choose the Fonar Upright MRI machine because of the higher payoff in the best scenario. Conversely, a person who is less optimistic or less risk tolerant may choose one of the other two MRI alternatives.

TABLE 5.6   Range Calculations for the Medical Equipment Example

MRI Machine	Range
Fonar Upright	28
Philips Open	10
GE	2

Risk Defined and Quantified by Regret

If Sarah chooses to invest in the Philips Open MRI machine, the payoff received will be moderate compared to that from the Fonar Upright MRI machine but greater than the payoff from the GE MRI machine most of the time. Sarah could say she might have less regret by investing in the Philips Open MRI machine when comparing it to the highs and lows of the other MRI machines. In fact, it has been shown that the Philips Open MRI machine is the choice that minimizes regret. Table 5.7 contains the minimax regret calculations for the medical equipment example.

However, if Sarah chooses the Philips Open MRI machine in order to minimize regret, something is given up. Sarah may actually feel some measure of regret by choosing the Philips Open MRI machine. Specifically, she will lose the ability to receive higher payoffs from the Fonar Upright MRI machine or more stable payoffs from the GE MRI machine.

Risk-Return Trade-Off

A manager must analyze a problem with regard to measures of central tendency and dispersion in order to make an informed decision. In the words of decision analysis, a manager must analyze each decision problem with regard to return (i.e., expected values) and risk (i.e., range or regret). Only after analyzing the risk-return trade-offs can a decision be made.

Each of us must analyze complex decision problems in terms of return and risk. As health care professionals, we must integrate sensitivity analysis into the problem-solving process while developing critical reasoning and judgment skills with regard to the risk-return trade-off.

In sum, this book cannot tell decision makers exactly what decisions will be the best when they are faced with complex problems. It is a guide to assist in developing a rational methodology for solving problems. Overall, the book provides a process for becoming a more effective and efficient problem solver.

TABLE 5.7 Minimax Regret Calculations for the Medical Equipment Example

MRI Machine	Minimax Regret
Fonar Upright	12
Philips Open	8
GE	14

MODELING

A decision model can be defined as any quantitative or logical abstraction of reality that is created and used to help decision makers solve a problem. A model consists of states, decisions, payoffs, a structure to frame those decision components, and the definition and quantification of objectives the decision maker wishes to investigate.

Why Model?

A manager creates a model to assist in the decision-making process. Models assist in two ways. First, in building a model and structuring a decision problem, a decision maker can respond to increased levels of complexity that cannot be grasped or resolved by analyzing the individual pieces of a problem.

Second, a model, with computer support, can keep track of many details and rapidly perform all necessary computations and sensitivity analysis. This allows a decision maker to devote attention to judgments about the individual details and composite results produced by the model.

Five Main Reasons for Modeling

Five main reasons are detailed in this chapter. They encompass the major themes of modeling.

Necessity

Models are built from necessity. They are done when simpler approaches are not adequate. Models are not a goal in themselves even though they can be engaging and, at times, almost supplant the decision at hand in our attention. However, decision makers require the assistance that models can efficiently give. Learning to model requires adapting one's language in order to communicate the model and its results effectively.

Better Decisions

It could be said that a model has helped a decision maker if a better decision is reached. In general, the decision is better because the model has allowed a sensitivity analysis. Sensitivity analysis allows for the study of (1) the outcomes of interest as different assumptions are methodically varied, (2) the effect of uncertain factors on the surety of results, and (3) which assumptions affect the outcomes the most. The decision can include the interaction of influences over a much longer period of time so that the decision does not just respond to the most obvious short-term considerations.

Insight

A model gives the decision maker insight into a subject. The model allows a manager to explore the dominance of alternatives, the trade-offs among the factors that enter into those alternatives, and the risk associated with one alternative compared to another. Modeling equips a decision maker with the ability to break a problem into pieces and put it back together, offering insight along the way that otherwise might have been overlooked.

Intuition

Overall, complex systems behave nonintuitively. Modeling gives insight into these nonintuitive behaviors that come from time lags between actions and responses, from interactions, and from the dampening of one influence by another. The model provides intuition about the whole, starting with intuition about the parts.

The model tells you which uncertainties in your knowledge matter. In general, a decision maker may be working with an incomplete understanding and incomplete data. Some of this uncertainty may not affect the decision choice; however, the model analysis reveals which pieces of information are of the most importance. If time and money allow, a manager will know which areas to study more to improve the quality of the decision; in this way, intuition has been achieved.

Aid to Presentations

A model is an aid to the final presentation of the results. The presentation to the client uses the structure inherent in the model to explain those final results. The model illustrates the problem as compactly as possible. In general, clients need to see a physical structure in order to fully understand the problem and the alternatives presented.

Structuring Decision Problems

Earlier in this chapter the components of a decision problem were identified and defined. In addition, a simple structure, called a payoff table, was presented to aid in the decision-making process. As a health care professional, you will quickly find out that payoff tables, although straightforward and helpful, are inadequate for more complex problems.

Payoff tables are just one way to structure problems. What kind of structure is needed for these more complex problems? How should one proceed in modeling complex decision problems?

Take, for example, the medical equipment decision problem. A payoff table appeared to work well for Sarah's simple decision regarding MRI equipment choice. However, the payoff table framework soon becomes inadequate when additional variables are introduced. A review and refinement of the decision structure would be in order. The next section presents a structure, decision trees, that assists with more complicated decision problems.

DECISION TREES

A *decision tree* is a graphical representation of a decision problem. Decision trees are another method to structure a problem. The decision tree framework consists of nodes and branches.

Decision Nodes, Chance Nodes, and Decision Trees

A decision tree contains two types of nodes, decision nodes and chance nodes, as well as branches, defined as follows:

A *decision node*, represented by a square, denotes when a decision maker must make a choice or a decision.

A *chance node*, represented by a circle, denotes an event or state of nature that can occur in the future.

A *branch*, defined by a line, represents and links decision alternatives and/or states of nature.

In using a decision tree, a decision maker computes expected values at each chance node and makes a choice or decision on the basis of those expected values at decision nodes.

Decision trees provide a visual representation of the states, decisions, and outcomes of a sequential decision problem. Decision trees provide a framework for problems that payoff tables are unable to illustrate.

Building Decision Trees

To frame a problem by using a decision tree, the components of the problem must be identified and defined. Recall that the three components of any decision-making problem are states, decisions, and payoffs. Let's use Sarah's medical equipment problem example as the decision problem of interest. Figure 5.17 displays the payoff table for the medical equipment example.

From the information given in the payoff table, a decision tree can be built. First, let's relate the components of the decision problem to the graphical components of decision trees.

Obviously, the three decisions match up with the decision node component. A common starting place for most decision trees is a decision node. For the medical equipment payoff table, three decisions emanate from the initial decision node as decision branches.

At the end of each of the decision branches, a chance node is placed. From each chance node two branches depicting the two states—high demand and low

FIGURE 5.17   Payoff Table for Sarah's Medical Equipment Example

	A	B	C
1	Sarah's Equipment Return Problem		
2	Payoff Table		
3		State of Nature	
4		High	Low
5	Equipment Type	Demand	Demand
6	GE MRI Machine	6%	4%
7			
8	Fonar Upright MRI Machine	20%	-8%
9			
10	Philips Open MRI Machine	12%	2%
11			

demand—emerge. At the end of these chance branches the payoffs associated with each decision/state combination are listed. Figure 5.18 displays the corresponding decision tree.

For the medical equipment example, only one decision and one set of chance nodes are needed. The decision tree structure allows for any combination of decision and chance nodes. The next section briefly discusses the concept of folding back the tree. The application of decision trees to multiple sequential decision making will be detailed later in this chapter.

FIGURE 5.18   Decision Tree for Sarah's Medical Equipment Example

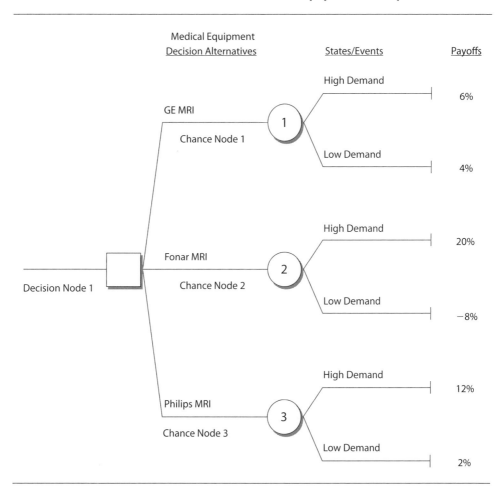

Folding Back the Tree: Calculating Expected Values

One goal of a decision tree is to calculate the expected value of the tree, or perform a process called *folding back the tree*. This process is based on a set of rules for decision trees. When analyzing a decision tree, a decision maker may encounter decision nodes or chance nodes.

Two rules govern decision trees regarding these nodes:

1. At a chance node, a decision maker computes an expected value based on the payoffs and probabilities given.

2. When faced with a decision node, a decision maker must make a decision. The criterion used to make the decision is to maximize the expected value of the various alternatives in question.

In other words, when a decision maker encounters a chance node, an expected value calculation is performed. Accordingly, at a decision node a decision maker makes a choice based on maximizing expected value.

In general, when faced with a decision tree, a decision analyst begins at the far right of the tree with the payoffs, at chance nodes calculates expected values, and at decision nodes chooses the decision that maximizes expected value. This process is followed until the decision analyst reaches the far left of the tree, a process that is referred to as folding back the tree.

Example of Folding Back a Decision Tree

Figure 5.19 displays the tree for the medical equipment example under the equal likelihood scenario. Expected values for the chance nodes are shown on the tree and will be calculated; in addition, a final recommendation is displayed on the tree at the final decision node.

According to the rules set down in the previous section, expected values are calculated at chance nodes 1, 2, and 3. The calculations are as follows:

$$\text{Chance node 1: } E(1) = 6\% \times 0.5 + 4\% \times 0.5 = 5\%$$
$$\text{Chance node 2: } E(2) = 20\% \times 0.5 + (-8\%) \times 0.5 = 6\%$$
$$\text{Chance node 3: } E(3) = 12\% \times 0.5 + 2\% \times 0.5 = 7\%$$

FIGURE 5.19 Decision Tree for Sarah's Medical Equipment Example under Equal Likelihood Scenario

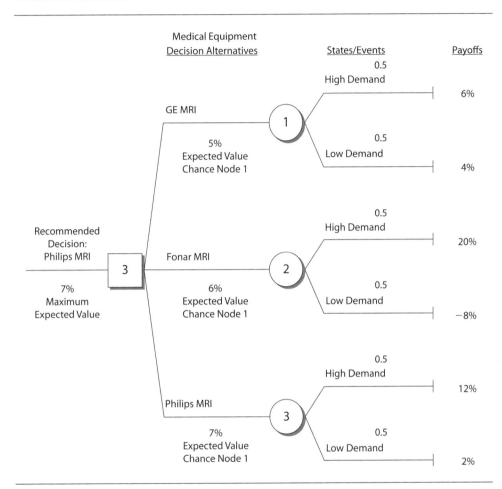

Subsequently, at the far-left decision node, the expected values are compared and the MRI machine with the highest expected value is chosen. Table 5.8 displays the three expected values and highlights the Philips Open MRI machine as the final recommendation made at the far-left decision node.

In summary, the process of folding back a decision tree consists of calculating expected values at chance nodes and making decisions at decision nodes based on maximizing expected values. Therefore, in the medical equipment example, when the decision maker's assessment of the occurrence of good economic conditions is 0.5, the Philips Open MRI machine will be the recommendation.

TABLE 5.8 Medical Equipment Decision Tree Expected Values

Equipment Alternative	Expected value, alpha = 0.5
GE MRI	5%
Fonar Upright MRI	6%
Philips Open MRI	**7%**

In sum, when a decision maker is confronted with a chance node, an expected value must be calculated; subsequently, when confronted with a decision node, the decision maker must make a choice based on maximizing expected value.

Multistage Decision Trees

In general, decision trees begin with a decision node. However, it is possible to begin a decision tree with a chance node. In addition, the decision tree structure allows for any number and combination of decision nodes and chance nodes.

For example, if Sarah wishes to make another decision after witnessing low demand, she may want to switch to the Fonar Upright MRI machine; the decision tree structure allows this very easily. In addition, Sarah knows that there is a chance of changes in Medicare payouts if she purchases the MRI equipment.

To accommodate these additional decisions and states, the original decision tree must be augmented. Figure 5.20 displays the modified decision tree including these added decisions and states.

From Figure 5.20 it is obvious that any order, combination, and/or number of decision and chance nodes is possible. This makes the decision tree framework very robust for structuring decision problems with multistage decisions and states.

Inadequacies of Decision Tree Structures

Although decision trees provide a more robust structure for framing decision problems, there may be times when a decision maker is faced with a problem that does not exactly fit the tree format. In fact, the basic tree format does not incorporate feedback well. In addition, the tree structure becomes large as the number of decision nodes and chance nodes grows. At times a simpler method may be appropriate. A method akin to a process flowchart is one way to assist decision makers.

FIGURE 5.20 Multistage Decision Tree Example

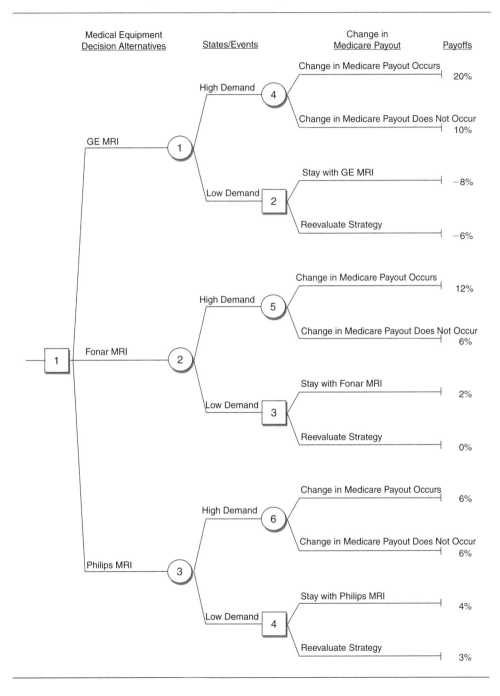

Using TreePlan to Develop Decision Trees in Excel

TreePlan is an add-in to Excel spreadsheets that greatly simplifies the process of constructing decision trees. Excel does have sufficient resources to develop decision trees without using an add-in software package like TreePlan, but that process is difficult and slow. This section describes and explains how to access, install, and use TreePlan in conjunction with Excel.

Loading and Accessing TreePlan

Since TreePlan is an add-in for Excel, the first step in using TreePlan is loading the software via Excel's Add-Ins menu. You must copy the Excel add-in file, TreePlan.xla, onto your hard disk drive. To add in TreePlan, it is necessary to click on the Office button and select the Options button at the bottom of the screen (see Figure 5.21).

This action brings up the Excel Options window; within this window click on the Add-Ins option on the left. A screen that resembles Figure 5.22 will

FIGURE 5.21 Excel Options Button

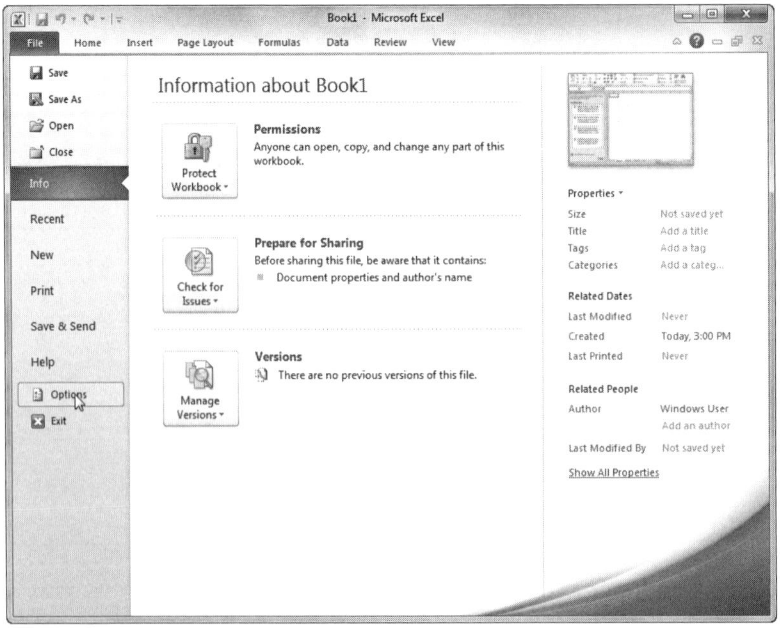

FIGURE 5.22 Excel Options Window

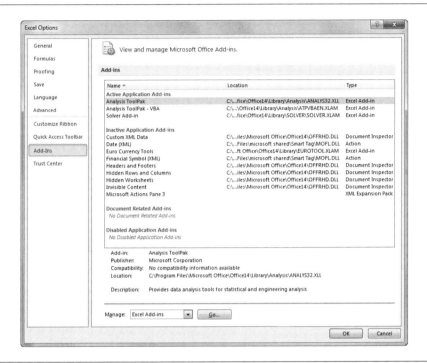

appear. In the Add-Ins menu go to the Manage drop-down box at the bottom of the screen, select Excel Add-Ins from the menu, and then click on the Go button. This will prompt the Add-Ins menu to appear (see Figure 5.23). TreePlan should be listed in the Add-Ins menu in Figure 5.22. If TreePlan does not appear in the Add-Ins menu, click browse in the Add-Ins menu (Figure 5.23), locate where you saved the TreePlan.xla file on your computer, and then click OK in the Browse menu. Click on the check box that is labeled TreePlan and then click OK. Once this has been completed, the TreePlan option in the Menu Commands group under the Add-Ins tab will appear (see Figure 5.24).

Creating an Initial Decision Tree in TreePlan

To use TreePlan, open Excel, choose the Tools menu, and click on Decision Tree . . . menu. The menu displayed should resemble Figure 5.25. TreePlan defines decision nodes in the same manner as this book, but refers to chance

FIGURE 5.23 Excel Add-Ins Menu

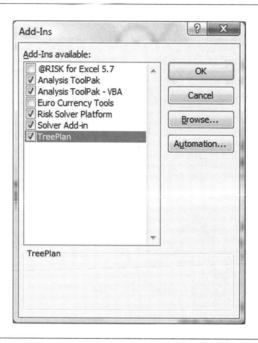

FIGURE 5.24 TreePlan Option in Add-Ins Tab

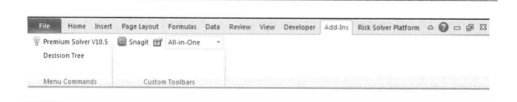

FIGURE 5.25 Initial TreePlan Menu

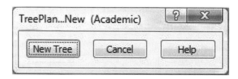

nodes as event nodes. The two terms will be used synonymously throughout the rest of the book.

Click the New Tree button, and a decision tree will appear in the active Excel worksheet. The decision tree generated should resemble Figure 5.26.

Adding to or Modifying a Decision Tree in TreePlan

Once the initial tree has been created in Excel, the user can modify it by adding branches, chance nodes, or additional decision nodes. Refer to Figure 5.27 for a visual display of the concept. *Note:* Regarding data input into TreePlan, do not type in cells that contain formulas, as this invalidates the tree and consequent tree calculations.

FIGURE 5.26   Initial Decision Tree

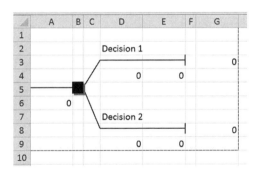

FIGURE 5.27   TreePlan Formula Example

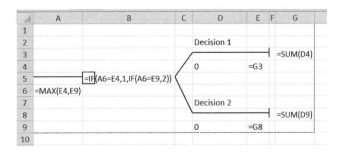

Adding Chance Nodes

1. To add a chance node in TreePlan, place the cursor at the end of a branch at the T intersection, or terminal node (see cell F3 in Figure 5.26).

2. After placing the cursor, click on the Tools menu and choose the Decision Tree option.

3. A dialogue box resembling Figure 5.28 will appear.

4. Choose the option you wish to perform. For example, in this case we wish to add an event node; therefore, click on the Change to event node button (not the Change to decision node button selected in Figure 5.28) and click OK.

5. The tree in your workbook should resemble Figure 5.29 after this procedure is finished.

Modifying Decision Nodes

1. To modify a decision node in TreePlan, place the cursor on the decision node you wish to modify.

2. Choose the Decision Tree option from the Tools menu. A menu resembling Figure 5.30 should appear.

3. From the menu in Figure 5.30, choose the instruction you wish to have TreePlan perform.

4. The same procedure can be used to modify chance nodes.

FIGURE 5.28 TreePlan Add/Change/Modify Dialogue Box

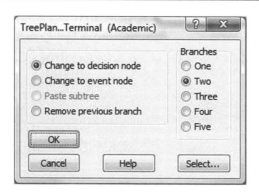

FIGURE 5.29 Decision Tree with Event Node Added

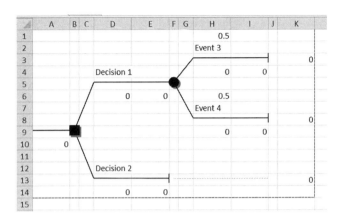

FIGURE 5.30 TreePlan Menu for Modifying an Existing Node

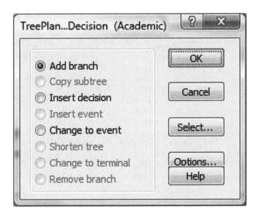

These commands for adding chance nodes and/or modifying decision nodes can be combined to create detailed sequential decision trees. A few items must be taken note of whenever you are developing a decision tree in TreePlan.

As a previous note cautions, *do not type in the cells* that contain formulas in TreePlan. Figure 5.31 displays a generic two-decision, two-state decision tree. Dashed boxes mark the cells where data should be entered and *italics* mark the cells where probabilities should be entered.

FIGURE 5.31 Example Tree Depicting Data Entry Areas

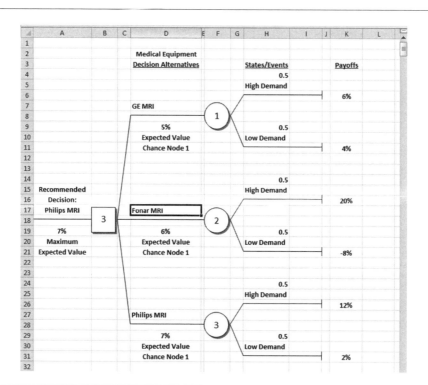

It is acceptable to enter data into any of the cells containing a probability (refer to the asterisked numbers in Figure 5.31 and corresponding cells H1, H6, H11, and H16). However, the user must keep in mind the rules of probability. *If the sum of the event probabilities does not add to 1.0, TreePlan will return an error.*

It is easier to go forward building a tree than to undo hastily made branches or nodes. Draw the tree on paper first and then proceed in TreePlan.

Health Care Operations and Supply Chain Management behind the Scenes: The Story of John von Neumann, the Father of Decision Analysis

John von Neumann (1903–1957), often considered to be the father of decision analysis, was a child prodigy born into a banking family in Budapest, Hungary. At the age of 6, von Neumann was able to divide eight-digit numbers in his head. From the age of 13 he showed a pronounced interest in mathematics, which was fostered by his teachers at the Lutheran High School of Budapest. After graduation from high school, von Neumann studied chemistry for two years in Berlin and for two years in Zurich, but spent much of his time with mathematicians, taking a PhD in mathematics at the University of Budapest not long after receiving his chemistry diploma at Zurich.

Mathematician, Economist, and Physicist

von Neumann lectured in Berlin from 1926 to 1929 and in Hamburg from 1929 to 1930. In 1930 he became a visiting lecturer at Princeton University, and was appointed a professor there in 1931. He became one of the original six mathematics professors in 1933 at the newly founded Institute for Advanced Study in Princeton, a position he kept for the remainder of his life.

von Neumann's brilliant work in mathematics also carried him into theoretical economics and technology as well as theoretical physics—areas where he was able to make vital contributions not only to science but also to the welfare of his adopted country. His work in quantum mechanics gave him a profound knowledge concerning the application of nuclear energy to military and peacetime uses, enabling him to occupy an important place in the scientific councils of the nation.

Developer of Atomic Bomb and Adviser to the Atomic Energy Commission

During World War II, he played a major role among the Los Alamos group of scientists who developed the atomic bomb. After the war he served on the advisory committee of the Atomic Energy Commission and on the commission itself from 1954 until his death.

SUMMARY

This chapter illustrates how decision analysis can be used to structure and analyze decisions involving numerous and conflicting alternatives. A rational methodology has been put forth for a health care professional to become a more effective and efficient problem solver. The goal of decision analysis is to identify the best alternative in the face of uncertain or risky future conditions.

Three types of criteria were presented for making decisions not based on probability assessments: the maximax, the maximin, and the minimax regret.

The concept of expected values and the Hurwicz criterion were linked with the issue of probability assessment and decision analysis. The chapter explored three areas of sensitivity analysis and presented the idea that the decision analysis framework and sensitivity analysis provide a manager with a rational method to compare and ultimately make a choice.

A completed decision tree expresses the structure of a formal model. Decision trees provide participants in the modeling process a means of communication. They also serve as the framework for expressing more specifically the exact nature of relationships.

Readers are encouraged to peruse the references listed at the end of the chapter for further information regarding the field of decision analysis. Classic readings include those by Miller 1956, Raiffa 1968, and von Neumann and Morgenstern 1944. More contemporary readings include those by Bazerman and Neale 1992, French 1986, Howard and Matheson 1983, Kahneman et al. 1982, and Keeney 1992.

KEY TERMS

buyer's remorse	maximax criterion
chance nodes	maximin criterion
cognitive dissonance	minimax regret
decision alternatives	opportunity cost
decision nodes	outcomes
decision trees	payoff tables
equal likelihood criterion	payoffs
Hurwicz criterion	states of nature

DISCUSSION QUESTIONS

1. Management at Washington Hospital Center is thinking about two investments. One is an MRI machine, which can make $100,000 in good economic conditions or $60,000 in bad economic conditions. Another is a CT scanner, which can make $150,000 in good economic conditions or

$10,000 in bad economic conditions. Thus the decision depends on the economic conditions. What is the probability of good economic conditions that equates the two investments?

a. Develop a payoff table for this situation.

b. Find the following:

   1. Maximax

   2. Maximin

   3. Equal likelihood

   4. Minimax regret

c. Create a sensitivity graph comparing the different alternatives as the probability of economic conditions changes.

2. Nathan is contemplating earning the Fellow of the American College of Healthcare Executives (FACHE) certification. He knows from experience that he can get a well-paying job with his current degree; the probability of getting a job with a salary of $40,000 per year is 75 percent and a job with a salary of $60,000 per year is 25 percent. However, if he chooses to earn the certification, his salary would likely increase; then the probability of getting a job with a salary of $80,000 per year is 75 percent and getting a job with a salary of $100,000 per year is 25 percent. Knowing that tuition cost and time spent on certification are not a concern for Nathan, should he find a job now or seek the certification?

   Find the better decision using the following:

a. Develop a payoff table for Nathan's situation.

b. Find the following:

   1. Maximax

   2. Maximin

   3. Equal likelihood

   4. Minimax regret

c. Create a sensitivity graph comparing the different alternatives as the probability of getting a job changes.

3. MedStar Health is expanding into Virginia. The firm must select one location where it can build a clinic to serve patients. The following table lists the expected profits for clinics in three locations and the expected probabilities of the two possible situations: high numbers of patients utilizing the clinic or low numbers of patients utilizing the clinic.

Location	High (0.75)	Low (0.25)
Alexandria	$1,500,000	$600,000
Woodbridge	$950,000	$900,000
Leesburg	$1,200,000	$200,000

Find the best decision using the following:

a. Develop a payoff table for this situation.

b. Find the following:

   1. Maximax

   2. Maximin

   3. Equal likelihood

   4. Minimax regret

c. Create a sensitivity graph comparing the different alternatives as the probability of numbers of patients changes.

4. Western Plastic Surgery Associates is planning on opening a cosmetic plastic surgery center in either Honolulu, San Francisco, or Seattle. There is a 60 percent chance that the demand for plastic surgery in the United States will increase in the near future, a 25 percent chance that the number will remain the same, and a 15 percent chance that the number will decrease. The developer estimates that the following profits would result from each decision given each set of economic conditions.

Location	Increase (0.60)	Same (0.25)	Decrease (0.15)
Honolulu	$1,102,000	$856,000	$502,000
San Francisco	$720,000	$640,000	$602,000
Seattle	$800,000	$702,000	$220,000

Find the best decision using the following:

a. Develop a payoff table for this situation.

b. Find the following:

1. Maximax

2. Maximin

3. Equal likelihood

4. Minimax regret

c. Can you create a sensitivity graph comparing the different alternatives as the probabilities of increase, same, and decrease change? Why or why not?

5. Genesis Medical Imaging is deciding whether to bid on a new contract to supply a local area hospital with a new MRI machine. Such bids are confidential and the lowest bid entered wins the contract. Genesis estimates it costs $1,000 to prepare for the bid and $900,000 for the MRI machine if it wins the contract. The following table shows the probabilities of Genesis winning the bid given the bids it submits.

Probability of Winning	Value of Bid
40%	$1,000,000
30%	$1,250,000
20%	$1,750,000
10%	$2,000,000

Set up a decision tree to find the bid that gives Genesis the highest chances of winning.

6. "If It Ain't Broke" Orthopedics is leasing a facility in Los Angeles for $20,000 per month. The partners are deciding on whether to buy a property and relocate the clinic or to continue leasing the current facility for another year and then relocate the clinic. They recently saw an advertisement for a new medical complex in Glendale at a price of $2,800,000. The current interest rate for a 20-year loan is 7 percent per annum. They believe there is a 40 percent chance that this interest rate will fall to 5 percent per annum in a year's time. They also believe that another facility they are interested in will still be available in a year at a discounted price of

$2,500,000. The partners have to decide whether to buy the new facility now or in a year. Interest payments will be made on the loan at the end of each year.

a. Develop a decision tree that will aid the owners in their leasing or purchasing decision.

b. Fold back the tree and find the expected value.

7. Victoria is currently a project manager for EPIC, an established integrated software company that services midsize to large health care organizations. Currently, her annual base salary is $150,000 per year. She also is eligible for a bonus at the end of the year, equaling 5 percent of all revenues if the company makes above $1,600,000 and 10 percent of all revenues if above $3 million. She is debating whether to leave this lucrative job to set up her own company. Although she has established client relationships, she believes only 65 percent of all existing clients will follow her in this new endeavor. Based on the previous year's performance, she believes there is a 25 percent chance the contracts would be worth $1,200,000, a 45 percent chance the contracts would be worth $2 million, and a 30 percent chance the contracts will be worth $3 million. She estimates that the total cost of operating her own company would be $700,000.

a. Develop a decision tree to help Victoria decide whether she should set up her own company.

b. Fold back the tree and find the expected value.

8. Fairfax Family Practice Center is considering whether to expand its practice to include an advanced on-site diagnostics center. The partners are considering whether to optimize existing space by purchasing and utilizing an extremity MRI machine or to expand the facility and add a full-body MRI at a significantly increased cost. The partners are trying to arrive at the most pragmatic decision to expand their business.

a. Identify the three components of the decision analysis.

b. Develop a table for each of the respective components.

9. Nathan has a friend who is a headhunter for several prestigious hospitals in the Northeast United States. This friend assures Nathan that she could find

placement with ample compensation if he were willing to compensate her for the service. The headhunter would like 10 percent of the portion of Nathan's salary that exceeds his expectation of $40,000 per year.

    a. Using the payoff table from question 2, determine the EVPI for the headhunter's services.

    b. Is the headhunter's offer fair?

10. Cognizant Consulting specializes in the expansion of medical firms. The consultants assert that they can determine whether demand for the medical facility's services will be high or low at each of the proposed locations. They have offered to provide their services to Washington Hospital Center for a $100,000 fee.

    a. Using the payoff table from question 3, determine the EVPI for the firm's services.

    b. Is the firm's offer fair?

11. Get Well Sooner, a local after-hours clinic, is losing money because it is unable to take advantage of the customer traffic at the clinic. Customers are spending inordinate amounts of time in the waiting room, while some of the clinic's rooms are left unfilled. The clinic has three doctors and nine rooms where patients are seen. Check-in is required and patients are given a 15-minute standard evaluation by one of the staff nurses before being seen by a doctor. Develop a flowchart outlining the steps to help the clinic reduce its waiting room times.

12. At emergency rooms in hospitals across the United States, waiting times are at an all-time high. Develop a flowchart that expedites patient care, which at the minimum includes patient check-in, insurance screening, triage, ambulatory care, waiting room availability, and doctor availability.

REFERENCES

Bazerman, Max, and Margaret Neale. 1992. *Negotiating Rationally.* New York: Free Press.

French, Simon. 1986. *Decision Theory: An Introduction to the Mathematics of Rationality.* London: Ellis Horwood, Ltd.

Howard, Ronald A., and James Matheson, eds. 1983. *The Principles and Applications of Decision Analysis.* 2 vols. Palo Alto, CA: Strategic Decisions Group.

Kahneman, Daniel, Paul Slovic, and Amos Tversky. 1982. *Judgment under Uncertainty: Heuristics and Biases.* Cambridge: Cambridge University Press.

Keeney, Ralph. 1992. *Value-Focused Thinking: A Path to Creative Decision Making.* Cambridge, MA: Harvard University Press.

Miller, G. A. 1956. "The Magical Number Seven Plus or Minus Two: Some Limits on Our Capacity for Processing Information." *Psychological Review* 63:81–97.

von Neumann, J., and O. Morgenstern. 1944. *Theory of Games and Economic Behaviour.* Princeton, NJ: Princeton University Press.

Raiffa, Howard. 1968. *Decision Analysis.* Reading, MA: Addison-Wesley.

CHAPTER 6

SIMULATION

INTRODUCTION

Simulation is a tool that utilizes a model of an existing or proposed system to determine the impacts that various parameters and changes to those parameters have on the system. These parameters may include the rate at which items arrive to the system, the rate at which items are serviced by the system, or the number of machines or workers in the system, among others. Simulation models are quite useful in that they can be employed for basic design, performance assessment, and process analysis (Pritsker 1974).

Over the past four decades, the field of computer simulation has grown immensely. Today there are over 50 commercially available computer simulation software packages in existence (Swain 2009), and they are capable of modeling systems from areas such as finance, pharmaceuticals, logistics, academics, health care, and air traffic control. While learning how to use a specific computer simulation software package is beyond the scope of this book, learning the basics of simulation design is not.

The sections that follow explain the concepts of process flows, probability distributions, random number generation, discrete-event simulation versus continuous simulation, Monte Carlo simulation, and queuing analysis, all in a health care context. An understanding of these concepts will enable a health care operations manager to determine appropriate times to apply simulation and will provide him or her with knowledge about the types of parameters and data required to create an accurate simulation model.

PROCESS FLOWS

In order to simulate a process, one must understand the steps of the process and how items flow through the system. *Process flows* can be used to map all kinds of health care systems, including the flow of patients through an operating room or emergency department (ED), the flow of blood work through a testing facility, or the flow of medication through a hospital. Critical measures for process flows include the input rate (i.e., the rate at which patients, samples, or prescriptions arrive to a system); the number of processors (i.e., the number of doctors, technicians, or nurses in the system); and the processing rate (i.e., the length of time needed to provide the required diagnoses, tasks, or services).

FIGURE 6.1 Process Flow at Low-Acuity Emergency Department

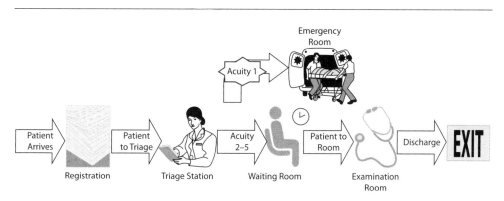

Icons are often used to diagram process flows. In Figure 6.1, the flow of patients through an emergency department is diagrammed. Although none of the critical measures are indicated in the diagram, they would be required for simulating the process. Since the primary purpose of the process flow diagram is to quickly give an audience an overview of the process's main steps, only these main steps are indicated in the diagram. When more detail is required, the diagram may be accompanied by explanatory verbiage.

In Figure 6.1, the diagram indicates that the basic steps for patients at this facility are arrival, registration, triage, going to a room, seeing a doctor, undergoing tests (possibly), and getting discharged. Those of us who have been to an emergency department recall a similar process for our visit. However, it is important to note that patients are often required to stay in the waiting area before or after triage and then may have to wait to see the doctor or to undergo testing. Depending on the purpose of a particular process flow diagram, it may become important to indicate waiting as a step in the process.

Additionally, it may be helpful to include a time line or some type of symbol to indicate the average length of time required from the first step of the process through process completion. When reducing total process time is the focus of a project, the time line is an easy way to clearly indicate the time saved via the new process.

PROBABILITY DISTRIBUTIONS

As mentioned, critical measures for simulating a process include the input rate (arrivals), the number of processors (servers), and the processing rate (service time). Typically, *probability distributions* are used to model the input rate and processing rate. As you may recall from statistics, probability distributions are functions that model long-term behavior. The two main categories of probability distributions are discrete and continuous. Distribution definitions included in the following pages are from Walpole and Myers (1989).

Before we examine some discrete and continuous probability distributions, it is important that we define the concept of a random variable. "A random variable is a function that associates a number with each point in an experiment's sample space" (Winston 2004, 715). Usually, random variables are denoted by boldface capital letters (such as **X**, **Y**, **Z**).

As an example, if we tossed a coin 50 times and recorded the number of heads that occurred and the number of tails that occurred, we could let the random variable **X** denote the number of heads resulting from our experiment and let the random variable **Y** denote the number of tails resulting from our experiment. Similarly, if we observed a health care facility for eight hours, we could let X_1 represent the number of patients arriving in the first hour, X_2 denote the number of patients arriving in the second hour, and so on. Or, more concisely, the random variable X_n could represent the number of patients arriving in the nth hour, for $n = 1$ to 8.

Random variables are used when defining both discrete and continuous probability distributions, as can be seen in the definitions given here. Discrete probability distributions include the uniform, binomial, multinomial, hypergeometric, negative binomial, geometric, and Poisson distributions. These distributions are employed when modeling systems whose arrival and servicing occur at discrete points in time, such as the arrival of patients to an emergency department. Of most interest when simulating health care systems and processes are the uniform, multinomial and Poisson distributions.

The assignment of nurses to cases may be modeled with a uniform random variable, assuming each nurse is equally likely to be assigned to a given case. The uniform distribution is described next (see Equation 6.1).

Uniform Distribution: If the random variable **X** assumes the values x_1, x_2, . . . , x_k, with equal probabilities, then the discrete uniform distribution is given by:

$$f(x;k) = \frac{1}{k}, x = x_1, x_2, \ldots, x_k \qquad (6.1)$$

When an experiment has more than two outcomes, the multinomial distribution is used to model the probability of occurrence of each of the distinct outcomes. In a health care setting, one may need to simulate responses to a drug regimen or results from a battery of tests. In order to simulate these situations, data regarding each possible outcome and the frequency of each outcome's occurrence would need to be available in order to correctly model the situation via a multinomial distribution. This distribution is described in Equation 6.2.

Multinomial Distribution: If a given trial can result in the k outcomes $E_1, E_2, \ldots, E_k$ with probabilities $p_1, p_2, \ldots, p_k$, then the probability distribution of the random variables $\mathbf{X}_1, \mathbf{X}_2, \ldots, \mathbf{X}_k$ representing the number of occurrences for $E_1, E_2, \ldots, E_k$ in n independent trials is:

$$f(x_1, x_2, \ldots, x_k; p_1, p_2, \ldots, p_k, n) = \left(\frac{n!}{x_1! \, x_2! \ldots x_k!} \right) p_1^{x_1} p_2^{x_2} \cdots p_k^{x_k} \quad (6.2)$$

with

$$\sum_{i=1}^{k} x_i = n \quad \text{and} \quad \sum_{i=1}^{k} p_i = 1$$

Factorial values (!) as above are calculated as follows: $n! = (n) * (n-1) * (n-2) * \ldots * (1)$

So, as an example, $6! = (6) * (5) * (4) * (3) * (2) * (1) = 720$.

The multinomial distribution plotted in Figure 6.2 is a special case of the multinomial. When $k = 2$, the multinomial distribution is the same as the binomial distribution because there are only two possible outcomes. Consider tossing a fair coin four times ($n = 4$); the two possible outcomes for each toss are heads and tails. If the coin is fair, then the probability of the coin landing heads up is the same as the coin landing tails up, so we say that $p_1 = p_2 = 0.50$. Figure 6.2 indicates the probability of obtaining a total of x heads in four tosses of a fair coin. The variable x can take on only the values of 0, 1, 2, 3, and 4, and the probability that x takes on each of these values is displayed at the top of each bar.

The Poisson distribution may be the most commonly used distribution when simulating processes. This distribution models the number of outcomes (e.g., arrivals, departures, occurrences) that happen during a given time interval or in a specified region of space. Required parameters include the average number of outcomes per unit of time or space (derived from given data) and the given time or space interval of

FIGURE 6.2   Graph of Multinomial Distribution

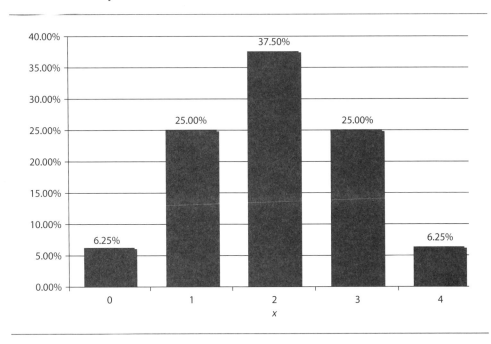

FIGURE 6.3   Graph of Poisson Distribution ($\lambda=5$)

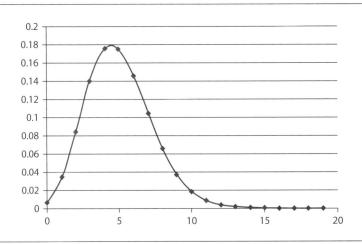

interest. In a health care setting, the arrival of patients at an emergency department is typically modeled using a Poisson distribution (see Equation 6.3 and Figure 6.3).

Poisson Distribution: The probability distribution of the Poisson random variable **X**, representing the number of outcomes occurring in a given time interval or specified region denoted by *t*, is given by:

$$p(x; \lambda t) = \frac{e^{-\lambda t}(\lambda t)^x}{x!},$$

x = 0, 1, 2, ..., *where* λ *is the average number of outcomes per unit time or region and*

$$e = 2.71828...$$

(6.3)

Continuous probability distributions include the normal, gamma, exponential, chi-squared, and Weibull distributions. These distributions are employed when the system to be modeled is a continuous system, such as the circulatory system of the human body. The continuous distributions most frequently encountered when simulating health care systems and processes are the exponential and normal distributions.

The exponential distribution is significant in simulation due to its ability to model processes and its relationship to the Poisson distribution. In health care, the time between arrivals of patients at an emergency department may be modeled using an exponential distribution, whereas the number of arrivals in a given time period may follow a Poisson distribution. If the parameter associated with the Poisson distribution is λ, as noted in Equation 6.3, then the parameter β associated with the exponential distribution is the reciprocal of λ, or $\beta = 1/\lambda$. The exponential distribution is modeled using Equation 6.4 and is shown graphically in Figure 6.4.

Exponential Distribution: The continuous random variable **X** has an exponential distribution, with parameter β, if its density function is given by:

$$f(x) = \begin{cases} \dfrac{1}{\beta} e^{-x/\beta}, & x > 0 \\ 0, & elsewhere \end{cases} \quad where \ \beta > 0. \qquad (6.4)$$

FIGURE 6.4 Graph of Exponential Distribution

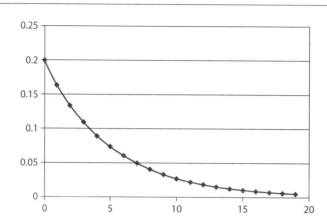

Theorem: Interarrival times are exponential with parameter λ if and only if the number of arrivals to occur in an interval of length t follows a Poisson distribution with parameter λt.

Computing Poisson and Exponential Probabilities in Excel

It is possible to use Microsoft Excel to determine probabilities for specific Poisson and exponential parameter settings (Winston 2004).

To calculate the probability that a Poisson random variable with a mean of MEAN is less than or equal to x, the syntax is:

$$=\text{POISSON}(x,\text{MEAN},\text{TRUE})$$

To calculate the probability that a Poisson random variable with a mean of MEAN is equal to x, the syntax is:

$$=\text{POISSON}(x,\text{MEAN},\text{FALSE})$$

To calculate the probability that a random variable with parameter λ assumes a value less than or equal to x, the syntax is:

$$=\text{EXPONDIST}(x,\text{LAMBDA},\text{TRUE})$$

FIGURE 6.5   Graph of Normal Distribution

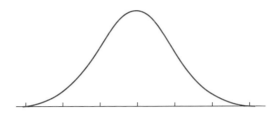

To determine the value of the density function for an exponential random variable with parameter λ, the syntax is:

$$=\text{EXPONDIST}(x,\text{LAMBDA},\text{FALSE})$$

See end-of-chapter question 4 for examples involving the application of these formulas.

"The most important continuous probability distribution in the entire field of statistics is the normal distribution" (Walpole and Myers 1989, 139). The graph of this distribution, known as the normal curve, is a bell-shaped curve that can be used to describe numerous events that occur in nature and in research (see Figure 6.5). The equation that describes the normal probability distribution depends on two parameters, the mean, μ, and the standard deviation, σ. In a health care setting, the length of time that it takes a technician to perform a specific test procedure or the number of patients seen at an emergency department each day may be modeled using a normal distribution (see Equation 6.5).

Normal Distribution: The density function of the normal random variable **X**, with mean μ and variance σ^2, is:

$$n(\text{x}; \mu, \sigma) = \frac{1}{\sqrt{2\pi}\sigma}e^{-\left(\frac{1}{2}\right)\left[\frac{x-\mu}{\sigma}\right]^2}, \; -\infty < x < \infty, \; where$$

$$\pi = 3.14159\ldots \quad and \quad e = 2.71828\ldots$$

(6.5)

Many commercially available software packages are able to determine which probability distribution best models a process's arrival or service rate if sufficient data are input into the simulation. Other times, the modeler may use data analysis tools such as Microsoft Excel or Minitab to determine appropriate probability distributions to employ. If the modeler elects to determine the probability distributions, he or she must ensure that the quantity and quality of the data are sufficient to do so.

RANDOM NUMBER GENERATION

Once it has been determined what probability distributions need to be utilized to model the arrival rate, service rate, and other probabilistic aspects of the simulation, then one must consider how to seed the streams from which the values of the probability distributions are retrieved. Random number generation has a long history (Hull and Dobell 1962). It is a topic covered in all simulation textbooks, sometimes taking up an entire chapter, and has been written about in countless journal publications.

The concept of *random number generation* centers around the fact that one must be able to reproduce the results of a simulation and one may also need to simulate a process for a long period of time, such as a week, a month, or even a year. To do this, the random number streams used for the probability distributions must be reproducible; however, one must ensure that the random numbers are not repeating themselves within a run and producing identical results for each time period of the simulation.

As an example, when simulating the flow of patients at an emergency department, one may determine that between 10:00 a.m. and 2:00 p.m., the patient arrival rate can be modeled by a Poisson distribution with a mean of 15. This does not mean that exactly 15 patients arrive each of those four hours. It means that when numerous data points are used, on average 15 patients per hour arrive at the facility between 10:00 a.m. and 2:00 p.m.

When simulating these arrivals, one would need to ensure that each larger period of the simulation (for example, a day at the emergency department) did not produce identical results for this four-hour period. That means, for example, each day should not show a total of 60 arrivals during each four-hour period for an average of 15 per hour (e.g., 17 arrivals in the first hour, 14 arrivals in the second hour, 12 arrivals in the third hour, and 17 arrivals in the fourth hour). Obviously, this behavior of identical arrivals each day is not representative of what actually happens at the emergency department, so the simulation must be designed to avoid such occurrences.

Law and Kelton (1991), in their text *Simulation Modeling and Analysis*, provide the following list of four properties that a good arithmetic random number generator should possess.

1. Numbers produced should appear to be distributed uniformly over the range [0,1] and not exhibit any correlation with each other.

2. The generator should be fast and not require significant amounts of storage.

3. A given stream of random numbers should be reproducible.

4. The generator should be able to produce several separate streams of random numbers.

Note that properties 3 and 4 are needed for purposes of reproducibility and for comparing simulation results, two critical aspects of any simulation study.

Today's computer simulation software packages come with their own random number generators. While it is not critical for health care operations managers to understand the intricacies of the code behind a package's generator, it is important for them to have confidence in the tool's ability to allow the reproducing of a stream (in order to simulate two scenarios with identical given conditions) and to know how many random numbers are needed so that the streams to be utilized can be selected in a manner that avoids overlapping that can occur when enough variates from one stream are generated that they cross over into a subsequent stream (Chance 1993).

In order to generate random numbers in Microsoft Excel, the RAND function should be employed. By default, the RAND function returns numbers from the interval [0,1)—that is, numbers greater than or equal to 0 but less than 1. If you need to generate numbers from a different interval, for example the interval [a,b), the following syntax should be used:

$$=RAND()*(b-a)+a$$

DISCRETE-EVENT VERSUS CONTINUOUS SIMULATION

Discrete-event simulation enables the modeling of a system as it changes over time and employs a representation in which the state of the system changes instantaneously at discrete points in time. Occurrences that alter the state of the system are called events. As an example, if we were to create a simulation of a hospital emergency department, a patient arrival, a nurse starting triage, and a patient departure arc all examples of events.

Most discrete-event simulation models employ the following components (Law and Kelton 1991, 10):

- *System state*—the collection of state variables necessary to describe the system at a particular time (i.e., number of doctors or nurses working in the ED, number of patients in the system, etc.).

- *Simulation clock*—a variable giving the current value of simulated time.

- *Event list*—a list containing the next time each type of event will occur (i.e., time of next patient arrival, time of next doctor to room event, etc.).

- *Statistical counters*—variables used for storing statistical information about system performance (i.e., utilization of doctors, nurses, or exam rooms).

- *Initialization routine*—a subprogram to initialize the simulation model at time zero.

- *Timing routine*—a subprogram that determines the next event from the event list and then advances the simulation clock to the time when that event is to occur.

- *Event routine*—a subprogram that updates the system state when a particular type of event occurs (there is one event routine for each event type).

- *Library routine*—a set of subprograms used to generate random observations from probability distributions that were determined as part of the simulation model.

- *Report generator*—a subprogram that computes estimates (from the statistical counters) of the desired measures of performance and produces a report when the simulation ends.

- *Main program*—a subprogram that invokes the timing routine to determine the next event and then transfers control to the corresponding event routine to update the system state appropriately.

Continuous simulation allows for the modeling over time of a system as it changes and utilizes a representation in which the state of the system changes continuously. "Typically, continuous simulation models involve differential equations that give relationships for the rates of change of the state variables with time" (Law and Kelton 1991, 109). From a health care perspective, modeling the cardiovascular system of a patient in order to help predict a drug's impact on blood flow would require a continuous simulation.

Most computer simulation software packages clearly indicate if they are intended for discrete-event simulation or continuous simulation. Some packages are capable of both types of simulation.

Figure 6.6 provides the basic steps of a discrete-event simulation of the process depicted in Figure 6.1. Typical flowchart notation is employed, with rectangular boxes indicating action, diamond-shaped boxes indicating a decision, and small circles signifying the start and finish of the process.

MONTE CARLO SIMULATION

"Monte Carlo simulation is a computerized mathematical technique that allows people to account for risk in quantitative analysis and decision making" (www .palisade.com). It has the advantage of being able to provide decision makers with a spectrum of possible outcomes along with the probability of each, based on a chosen action or decision.

The approach is named for a Monaco resort town renowned for its casinos (Monte Carlo) and was first utilized by scientists developing the atomic bomb. Over time, it has been applied in numerous arenas, including manufacturing, engineering, insurance, and finance.

Monte Carlo simulation provides a risk analysis. Uncertainties are modeled using appropriate probability distributions. Results are recalculated repeatedly, up to tens of thousands of times, producing a distribution of possible outcome values for each action or decision. Monte Carlo simulation provides a comprehensive picture of what might happen. "It tells you not only what could happen, but how likely it is to happen" (www.palisade.com).

Monte Carlo methods use random variables that are input by the user to determine the output distributions of an outcome variable or variables. Many health care decisions (e.g., total cost of patient care) contain variables that are actually functions of random variables (e.g., frequency of patient arrivals, length of stay). We might be interested in total cost of patient care and we know that patient length of stay is an input variable. We could use many different combinations of patient lengths of stay, generated in a random fashion, to create a distribution of possible values of total cost of patient care.

FIGURE 6.6   Discrete Simulation Flow for Process of Figure 6.1

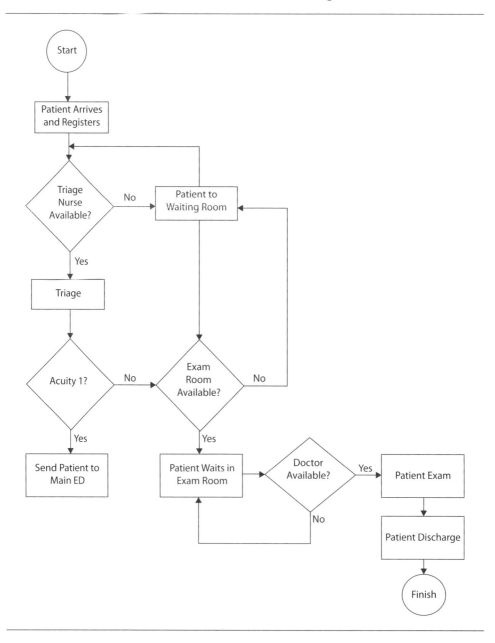

When applying Monte Carlo methods, it is possible to generate the random variables from many different types of probability distributions. For example, in many cases, arrivals in a service process (e.g., walk-in patients at a medical clinic) are characterized by a Poisson distribution. In all, Monte Carlo methods are used for analyzing risk but they are also very important statistically. The results of a Monte Carlo simulation give important insight into the statistical makeup of the inputs and outputs of the underlying model. In other words, it can provide information on what the variables of interest look like.

AGENT-BASED SIMULATION

Agent-based models allow for simulating the actions and interactions of autonomous agents (patients, teams of doctors, etc.) while attempting to assess each agent's effects on the system to which it belongs. Using agent-based simulation (ABS), the autonomous agents possess various attributes and behaviors that influence the way they interact with each other and the system environment. ABS allows an agent's behavior to depend on previous and current states of its environment, and this allows much more complex behaviors to be represented than with traditional simulation models (www.averill-law.com/simulation-training-agent .htm). Although the idea of agent-based modeling was developed in the late 1940s (Weaver 1948), its requirement of computationally intensive procedures prevented it from becoming widespread until the 1990s.

SIMULATION IN HEALTH CARE

Earlier, we described four types of *simulation (discrete-event, continuous, Monte Carlo, and agent-based)*. It is important for health care operations personnel to understand which type of simulation is best suited to solve the problem with which they are faced.

For example, discrete-event simulation would be appropriate to utilize for situations in which a process or patient flow needs to be modeled. The state of an emergency department changes at discrete points in time due to events such as patient arrivals, triage conducted on a patient, and lab work conducted on a patient. In contrast, as previously stated, continuous simulation would be applicable when modeling a system in which action is continuous, such as the human cardiovascular system.

Examples from the literature of health care applications of Monte Carlo simulation include its use to examine inequalities in access to emergency medical services (Mielczarek and Zabawa 2007) and also for determining risks for cancer patients undergoing radiation therapy (Stathakis, Li, and Ma 2007). Monte Carlo simulation is best suited for applications where determination of risks and their likely levels is the goal.

Agent-based simulation also has applications in health care. Currently, hospitals are under a lot of pressure to ensure that patients who are treated remain healthy and do not return, especially in a short period of time. Agent-based simulation could be utilized to model the behavior of various types of patients and their likelihood to return to the hospital in 30, 60, or 90 days or more.

QUEUING ANALYSIS

Queuing theory and analysis enable researchers and practitioners to determine statistics on the lines (queues) that form during various parts of a process. As customers arrive for some type of service, they may have to wait in line, depending on the number of servers present and the service time. Most queuing analysis formulas require the assumption that no more than one arrival can occur at a given instance. If this assumption is not required, then we say that bulk arrivals are permitted.

Arrivals

An additional assumption of queuing analysis is that the arrival of customers to the system is not affected by the number of customers presently in the system. We know this is not always the case. For example, if we enter a restaurant and see that there are currently 50 people waiting for a table, we may decide to leave and go elsewhere for dinner. When a customer arrives but fails to enter a system, this is known as balking.

In order to model the arrival of customers to a system, a probability distribution that models the time between successive arrivals is employed. Frequently, arrivals follow a Poisson distribution, meaning the interarrival times are exponentially distributed.

Service

After customers arrive and perhaps wait in line, they must undergo some type of service. We must also model the service time using a probability distribution.

Queuing analysis assumes that the service time is independent of the number of customers in the queue. In order to analyze a system, we must know the service time distribution, the number of servers, and whether the servers are in parallel or in series. For example, at a bank the servers are in parallel whereas on an assembly line the servers are in series.

Queue Disciplines

Most of the queuing examples we see in everyday life are first come, first served (FCFS). We wait in line and the person who is at the front of the line gets service before anyone behind him or her. There are some other queue disciplines that occur. These include last come, first served (LCFS), service in random order (SIRO), and a priority queuing discipline.

We may experience LCFS when riding an elevator, as the last person on is the first person off. SIRO is sometimes the manner in which phone calls to a call center are processed, although we hope that is not the case. Priority queuing discipline occurs at emergency departments on a daily basis, as the most severe cases are seen more quickly and ahead of many of those who have been waiting.

One other concept important to queuing analysis is the phenomenon known as jockeying. The term *jockeying* is used to describe the behavior of customers who move from one line to another in an attempt to receive service more quickly. We have all witnessed this at grocery stores.

Kendall-Lee Notation for Queuing Systems

In the 1950s, Kendall (1951) developed a set of standard notation to describe any queuing system. Specifically, this notation describes queuing systems where arrivals wait in a single queue and there are s identical servers working in parallel (as in a bank). The processing order is assumed to be FCFS.

Six characteristics are used to describe any queuing system. They are (Winston 2004):

1. The nature of the arrival process.

2. The nature of the service process.

3. The number of parallel servers.

4. The queue discipline.

5. The maximum number of customers permitted in the system.

6. The population size from which customers are drawn.

When describing a queuing system, typically abbreviations or identifiers for all six queue characteristics are given, separated by forward slashes. Possible identifiers for the characteristics include the following (Winston 2004):

Nature of Arrival Process

M	Interarrival times are independent and identically distributed (i.i.d.) random variables having an exponential distribution.
D	Interarrival times are i.i.d. and deterministic.
E_k	Interarrival times are i.i.d. Erlangs with shape parameter k.
GI	Interarrival times are i.i.d. and governed by some general distribution.

Nature of the Service Process

M	Service times are i.i.d. random variables having an exponential distribution.
D	Service times are i.i.d. and deterministic.
E_k	Service times are i.i.d. Erlangs with shape parameter k.
GI	Service times are i.i.d. and governed by some general distribution.

Queue Discipline

FCFS	First come, first served
LCFS	Last come, first served
SIRO	Service in random order
GD	General queue discipline

To illustrate this notation, consider an orthopedic clinic where the interarrival times are exponentially distributed, service times follow some general distribution, there are 12 doctors who see patients in an FCFS manner, and the total capacity of the clinic is 20 patients. Such a queuing system may be described using the notation M/G/12/FCFS/20/∞. In many instances, only the first three descriptors are used and the processing order is assumed to be FCFS.

Little's Formula

If we consider a system in two parts, its queue and its service, we can analyze numerous features of the system. Using available data, we can determine the average number of arrivals entering the system per unit of time (λ) and the average number of customers present in the queuing system (L). These two pieces of data can be used in Little's formula, $L = \lambda W$, to solve for W and to determine the average time a customer spends in the system (W).

Consider the following definitions:

L_q	Average number of customers waiting in line
L_s	Average number of customers in service
W_q	Average time a customer spends in line
W_s	Average time a customer spends in service

Little's formula can also be written as $L_q = \lambda W_q$ or $L_s = \lambda W_s$. It is important to note that Little's formula assumes that a steady-state distribution exists. We define π_j to be the steady-state probability that j customers will be present in the system. Assuming an arrival rate of λ and a service rate of μ, we define $\rho = \frac{\lambda}{\mu}$ as the traffic intensity of the system. For $\le \rho < 1$, we can calculate π_j using the formula $\pi_j = \rho^j(1 - \rho)$. If $\rho \ge 1$, then no steady-state distributions can exist.

Applications of Queuing Analysis

Queuing analysis plays an important role in many settings such as banks, amusement parks, sporting events, department of motor vehicles (DMV) offices, and doctors' offices. In the 1980s, queuing analysis enabled banks to determine that their customers would be better served by having one queue that fed the next available teller. Disney World and other amusement parks have implemented time savers such as Fast Pass in an effort to control line lengths and reduce wait times at the most popular rides. The number of these passes distributed and the times at which they are available are based on queuing analysis of the rides the passes serve.

In a health care setting, we are all familiar with having to wait for service at a doctor's office or at an emergency department. At a doctor's office, a lengthy patient wait may not be considered too important, particularly if the doctor is the only specialist in the community. However, lengthy waits at an emergency department (ED) may have extremely negative consequences. For this reason, hospitals are constantly looking for ways to reduce the waiting time in their EDs.

Queuing Analysis Example

This problem highlights some of the aspects of queuing covered in the preceding section, and also ties in several other concepts from the chapter. These include discrete (uniform) and continuous (normal) probability distribution functions and their use in Excel, as well as random number generation and the use of the RAND( ) function in Excel.

Scenario

New recruits at a military base must visit the medical lab and have their blood drawn by a phlebotomist (person who draws blood samples for medical testing). The interarrival times of recruits to the lab follow a uniform distribution with an upper bound of three minutes and a lower bound of one minute. The service times to have their blood drawn follow a normal distribution with a mean of two minutes and a standard deviation of 30 seconds.

Using Excel, we will demonstrate how to determine queuing and service statistics for the 300 recruits who visit the lab over a five-hour period. We will also calculate summary statistics such as average wait time, server utilization, and average number of recruits in line.

Modeling in Excel

Providing the distribution parameters (mean and variance) in cells in our spreadsheet allows for more flexibility. We can easily determine the effect of a change to the mean or variance of the interarrival or service times if they are stored in cells as opposed to being hard coded as numbers in the formulas we will utilize.

As can be seen from Figure 6.7, we have indicated the mean and variance of the interarrival times in cells B4 and B5 and the mean and variance of the service times in cells B8 and B9.

To create a table of data, we first label all of our columns (see row 13). The columns of data we will generate include patient ID, interarrival time, arrival time, service start time, wait time, service time, service completion time, time in system, and server idle time. The formula for each of these is provided in Table 6.1.

The formula for the patient ID (column B) is straightforward and should be dragged down until 300 patient IDs are created (to row 313). The formula for

FIGURE 6.7   Excel Screen Shot for Military Recruit Blood Work Example

	A	B	C	D	E	F	G	H	I	J
1	Military Recruit Bloodwork Example									
2										
3	Interarrival Times (Poisson)					SUMMARY STATS				
4	Mean	3				Number that wait		262		
5	STDEV	1				P(waiting)		0.87		
6						Avg. wait time		7.3747		
7	Service Time (Normal)					Max wait time		19.8037		
8	Mean	2				% time busy		0.9604		
9	STD DEV	0.5				Number waiting > 1		216		
10						Probability of Waiting >1 Minute		0.72		
11		Queuing Model				Average # in line		3.5337		
12										
13		Group	Inter. Time	Arrival Time	Serv. Start Time	Wait Time	Serv. Time	Compl. Time	Time in Sys.	Idle Time
14		1	1.5315	1.5315	1.5315	0.0000	2.3759	3.9074	2.3759	0.0000
15		2	2.3656	3.8971	3.9074	0.0103	1.4335	5.3409	1.4438	0.0000
16		3	2.7180	6.6151	6.6151	0.0000	1.5978	8.2129	1.5978	1.2742
17		4	2.8939	9.5090	9.5090	0.0000	1.8800	11.3889	1.8800	1.2961
18		5	2.3655	11.8745	11.8745	0.0000	2.8728	14.7473	2.8728	0.4856
19		6	2.6598	14.5343	14.7473	0.2130	1.7991	16.5464	2.0121	0.0000
20		7	2.3774	16.9117	16.9117	0.0000	2.0025	18.9142	2.0025	0.3654
21		8	2.2834	19.1951	19.1951	0.0000	1.8053	21.0004	1.8053	0.2809
22		9	1.7639	20.9590	21.0004	0.0413	2.3516	23.3519	2.3929	0.0000
23		10	1.7549	22.7139	23.3519	0.6380	2.0608	25.4128	2.6989	0.0000
24		11	1.6027	24.3167	25.4128	1.0961	2.1205	27.5333	3.2167	0.0000
25		12	2.6125	26.9291	27.5333	0.6042	2.2560	29.7893	2.8601	0.0000
26		13	2.5191	29.4483	29.7893	0.3410	1.7348	31.5240	2.0758	0.0000
27		14	2.2647	31.7129	31.7129	0.0000	2.1529	33.8659	2.1529	0.1889
28		15	1.8495	33.5624	33.8659	0.3035	1.3804	35.2462	1.6838	0.0000

TABLE 6.1   Excel Formulas for Queuing Example

Column	Row 14 Formula	Row 15 Formula
B—patientID	= 1	= B14+1
C—interarrival time	= $B$4+RAND()*($B$5–$B$4)	Same as row 14
D—arrival time	= 0+C14	= D14+C15
E—service start time	= D14	= IF(D15>H14, D15, H14)
F—wait time	= E14–D14	Same as row 14
G—service time	= ABS(NORMINV(RAND(), $B$8, $B$9))	Same as row 14
H—service completion	= E14+G14	Same as row 14
I—time in system	= H14–D14	Same as row 14
J—server idle time	= 0	= E15–H14

interarrival time (column C) contains three items that need explanation. First, as previously stated, the $ symbol in Excel is used to prevent the row ID or column ID from changing when a formula is copied to additional cells. Thus, cells B4 and B5 are used for all 300 rows of the data table since they are referenced using $B$4 and $B$5. Second, the RAND( ) function, as explained in the random number generation section earlier in the chapter, is used to return a random number that is from the interval [1,3).

The formula for arrival time (column D) is a sum of the previous patient's arrival time plus the current patient's interarrival time. This makes sense. In order to determine the service start time (column E), we must know if the server (phlebotomist) has finished with the previous patient. We use an IF statement to check to see if the current patient's arrival time is after the previous patient's service completion time. If it is, then we can start service on the current patient immediately. If it is not, we must wait until the previous patient completes service before starting service for the current patient.

The wait time (column F) is simply the difference between the time the patient arrived and the time he or she started service. The formula for service time (column G) includes two items that need explanation. First, the ABS function returns the absolute value of whatever is contained inside of the parentheses that follow it. NORMINV returns the inverse of the normal cumulative distribution for the specified mean and standard deviation.

The reason we must use NORMINV instead of NORMDIST is because the data needed are service times from a normal distribution. If we used NORM-DIST, it would return the probability of obtaining the service time resulting from the RAND( ) function in combination with the specified mean and standard deviation. In contrast, NORMINV returns the service time that occurs with RAND( ) probability, given our specified mean and standard deviation.

In order to calculate the service completion time (column H), we simply add the service time to the service start time. This is straightforward. Similarly, the straightforward calculation for time in system (column I) is the difference between the arrival time and the service completion time. Finally, to determine server idle time (column J), we examine the time between the service start of one patient and the service completion time of the previous patient. The server is idle only if this value is nonzero.

Summary Statistics

The reason for developing a queuing model in Excel is so that we can calculate summary statistics for our system and test varying scenarios by altering any problem-specific parameters. For this example, the formula for each statistic calculated is provided in Table 6.2.

The formula for number of patients who wait (cell G4) uses the COUNTIF function of Excel to determine which patients have a waiting time greater than 0.

TABLE 6.2   Excel Formulas for Summary Statistics

Statistic	Formula	Cell
Number of patients who wait	COUNTIF(F14:F313, ">0")	G4
Probability of waiting	G4/COUNT(B14:B313)	G5
Average wait time	AVERAGE(F14:F313)	G6
Maximum wait time	MAX(F14:F313)	G7
% of time server is busy	1-SUM(J14:J313)/H313	G8
Number waiting > 1 minute	COUNTIF(F14:F313, ">1")	G9
Probability of waiting > 1 minute	G9/COUNT(B14:B313)	G10
Average number of patients in line	G6*(B313/(H313)	G11

Similarly, the formula for the number of patients who wait more than one minute (cell G9) uses the same function and counts only patients whose wait time exceeds one minute.

The probability of waiting (cell G5) and the probability of waiting more than one minute (cell G9) are calculated very similarly. For cell G5, the numerator of the formula is simply the number of patients who wait and the denominator is the total number of patients. For cell G9, the numerator is the number of patients who wait more than one minute and the denominator is the total number of patients.

To calculate average wait time (cell G6) and maximum wait time (cell G7), use the Excel functions of AVERAGE and MAX, which you have probably used in other contexts. To determine the percentage of time the server (phlebotomist) is busy (cell G8), we simply determine the fraction of the time the server is idle (sum of idle time over total time system is operating) and subtract that fraction from 1.

To determine the average number of patients in line (cell G11) we must recall Little's formula, $L_q = \lambda W_q$. We know that W_q, the average wait time, has been calculated in cell G6. Recall that λ is the number of arrivals entering the system per unit of time. It can be determined by dividing the total number of patients who arrived (cell B313) by the total amount of system time (H313).

SUMMARY

In this chapter, we have examined a number of critical aspects of simulation. To begin, we discussed process flows and how understanding the flow of the process being modeled is critical to developing an accurate simulation. We looked at a number of discrete and continuous probability distributions to gain a better understanding of how to model system arrival and services times, and discussed random number generation in the context of simulation software and testing. Details of discrete-event simulation were provided, along with overviews of continuous, Monte Carlo, and agent-based simulation. Examples from health care were given to assist with determining appropriate application areas for each type of simulation.

The final section of the chapter focused on queuing analysis. It covered numerous critical definitions and introduced Little's formula and Kendall-Lee notation. To solidify understanding of both key queuing concepts and important Excel functions, a detailed example was provided, with Excel screen shots and explanations of all relevant formulas for both the queuing terms and the summary statistics.

KEY TERMS

probability distribution

process flow

queuing theory

random number generation

simulation (discrete-event, continuous, Monte Carlo, and agent-based)

DISCUSSION QUESTIONS

1. Create a process flow based on your observation of one of the following:

   a. Patients at the student health center on campus.

   b. Patients at a local ophthalmologist's office.

   c. Patients at a local hospital emergency department.

2. For each distribution listed, provide an example from your work that may be modeled using that distribution. You may not use any examples mentioned in this chapter.

   a. Multinomial distribution

   b. Poisson distribution

c. Exponential distribution

d. Normal distribution

3. Use Excel to create the following probability distributions. Graph your results using a scatter plot.

   a. Normal distribution

   b. Multinomial distribution

4. For the scenario that follows, solve by hand and then solve using the Excel functions POISSON and EXPONDIST.

   The time between arrival of patients to an urgent care center follows an exponential distribution with a mean of 30 minutes.

   a. What is the probability that exactly six patients will arrive in the next 90 minutes?

   b. What is the probability that at least two patients will arrive in the next 60 minutes?

   c. What is the probability that no patients will arrive in the next 60 minutes?

5. Provide the Excel code needed to generate a random number between [2,4]. In Excel, generate 100 random numbers in this interval. Count the number between [2,3) and the number between [3,4). Comment on the results of your count.

6. Conduct Internet research to determine three feasible alternative packages you might employ for discrete-event simulation. Rate the packages based on documented ease of use, cost, and ability to simulate health care scenarios.

7. Explain the differences between discrete-event simulation and Monte Carlo simulation. Provide an example of at least one situation from a health care arena when discrete-event simulation would be preferred and one when Monte Carlo simulation would be preferred.

8. Suppose we know that the average number of customers present in a queuing system is 10 and the average number of customers waiting in line is 4. Given that the average number of arrivals entering the system per hour is 20, determine the average time a customer spends in the system and the

average time a customer spends in line. Be sure to provide appropriate units for your answer.

9. Each Tuesday, the new residents at an inpatient rehabilitation clinic must visit the medication lab and have all of their existing medications inventoried when they arrive. The interarrival times of patients to the medication lab follow a uniform distribution with an upper bound of 45 minutes and a lower bound of 30 minutes. The service times to have their medication logged follow a normal distribution with a mean of 20 minutes and a standard deviation of 5 seconds.

Using Excel, determine queuing and service statistics for the 40 patients who visit the medication lab over a one-day period.

The columns of data you will need to generate include patient ID, interarrival time, arrival time, service start time, wait time, service time, service completion time, time in system, and server idle time.

10. Calculate the following summary statistics for question 9:

a. Number of patients who wait

b. Probability of waiting

c. Average wait time

d. Maximum wait time

e. Percentage of time server is busy

f. Number waiting > 1 minute

g. Probability of waiting > 1 minute

h. Average number of patients in line

REFERENCES

www.averill-law.com/simulation-training-agent.htm.

Chance, F. 1993. "On the Problem of Overlapping Pseudo-Random Number Streams: A Queuing Simulation Example." Technical Report No. 1055, School of Operations Research and Industrial Engineering, College of Engineering, Cornell University, Ithaca, New York.

Hull, T. E., and A. R. Dobell. 1962. "Random Number Generators." *SIAM Review* 4:230–254.

Kendall, D. 1951. "Some Problems in the Theory of Queues." *Journal of the Royal Statistical Society*, Series B, 13:151–185.

Law, A. M., and W. D. Kelton. 1991. *Simulation Modeling and Analysis.* 2nd ed. New York: McGraw-Hill.

Mielczarek, B., and J. Zabawa. 2007. "Monte Carlo Simulation Model to Study the Inequalities in Access to EMS Services." Proceedings of the 21st European Conference on Modeling and Simulation, Prague, Czech Republic.

www.palisade.com.

Pritsker, A. 1974. *The GASP IV Simulation Language.* New York: John Wiley & Sons.

Stathakis, S., J. Li, and C. Ma. 2007. "Monte Carlo Determination of Radiation-Induced Cancer Risks for Prostate Patients Undergoing Intensity-Modulated Radiation Therapy." *Journal of Applied Clinical Medical Physics* 8 (4): 14–27.

Swain, J. 2009. "Simulation Software Boldly Goes." *OR/MS Today* 36 (5).

Walpole, R., and R. Myers. 1989. *Probability and Statistics for Engineers and Scientists.* 4th ed. New York: Macmillan.

Weaver, Warren. 1948. "Science and Complexity." *American Scientist* 36:536–545.

Winston, W. 2004. *Operations Research Applications and Algorithms.* 4th ed. Belmont, CA: Thomson Learning.

CHAPTER 7

PROCESS IMPROVEMENT AND PATIENT FLOW

LEARNING OBJECTIVES

⟫ Identify the four steps of process mapping and draw a basic process map.

⟫ Understand how to create a value stream map and why it is useful.

⟫ Recognize the data required to set staffing levels.

⟫ Understand the concepts involved in workload management.

⟫ Comprehend the value of productivity analysis, especially as related to health care settings.

(Continued)

⟾ Recognize and understand common health care productivity measures.

⟾ Gain an awareness of steps that can be taken to improve productivity, particularly in health care settings.

INTRODUCTION

This chapter focuses on processes. In a health care setting, there are numerous processes that occur every day, many of which could be improved. The literature provides a seemingly endless list of research on the application of process mapping to health care (Koelling et al. 2005; Brown and Kros 2010; Cochran and Burdick 2011).

Processing mapping enables a health care manager to gain a better understanding of all steps in a process so that areas for improvement may be identified. This chapter explains the steps of process mapping and provides a basic process map for a hospital's room turnover process.

Value stream mapping has become a popular way for owners of a process to identify non-value-added steps in the process. By creating a *current state map* indicating areas for improvement, a *future state map* can be created that represents a streamlined process and removes as many non-value-added steps as possible. The chapter provides additional information about diagramming and utilizing value stream maps as well.

We also consider workload management issues in this chapter, and relate discussion of these issues to the critical topic of productivity analysis. We describe a number of productivity measures, and include an example from health care. Brief introductions to more complex productivity measures, such as data envelopment analysis and stochastic frontier analysis, are provided. The chapter closes with information on a number of health care productivity measures and a discussion of how to improve productivity and efficiency in health care settings.

PROCESS MAPPING

Process mapping is a technique used to analyze a process (Hunt 1996). The technique consist of four major steps:

1. Process identification
2. Information gathering
3. Interviewing and mapping
4. Analysis

The goal of the first step, process identification, is to acquire a full understanding of all the steps of a process. Instead of defining processes based on the company's understanding of itself and its processes, each process must be defined by the customers' understanding (Brown and Kros 2010). By thinking through experiences as a customer or patient, a reviewer is able to identify points in the process that can make or break success. These points serve as the focus of the process identification.

After process identification, information gathering begins. During this step the objectives, risks, fundamental controls, and measures of success for the process are identified, along with key process owners. It is important to correctly identify process owners, as they are the people who are most likely to be able to bring about change. Their buy-in and agreement throughout the process mapping activity are imperative.

The third step, interviewing and mapping, involves understanding the point of view of individuals in the process and designing actual maps. Worksheets may be helpful when gathering information such as process owners, trigger events (beginning and ending), inputs, outputs, objectives, risks, controls, and measures of success (Brown and Kros 2010).

The final step, analysis, actually occurs throughout the process mapping activity. Analysis involves determining what approaches and tools will make the process run more effectively and efficiently. Analysis may include identifying unnecessary steps in the process, removing redundant assignments, and investigating requirements that seem to have no reason for their existence. Process steps, assignments, and requirements should be analyzed in the context of the process map to ensure they support the objectives of the process.

One example from health care is the room turnover process (see Figure 7.1). In order for a hospital to improve its room turnover process, it must first identify and gain a full understanding of all of the steps of that process from a patient's point of view. Most often, when a bed is needed, it is because a patient at the emergency department has a condition that requires admission to the hospital. From a patient's perspective, someone needs to request a room and if none is ready, then a recently vacated room must be cleaned so the waiting patient can move into that room.

In information gathering, the objective for the patient is to get into the room as quickly as possible. Risks may include having to wait an excessively long time in the emergency department, being assigned to a room that was not cleaned properly, or being assigned to a room that is not on the proper floor based on the patient's diagnosis. For many hospitals, room turnover is controlled via a computerized bed tracking system that notifies the cleaning personnel when rooms are available for cleaning. A patient would measure success in terms of the waiting time and perhaps cleanliness of the room to which he or she is assigned. Although

FIGURE 7.1   Process Map for Room Turnover Process

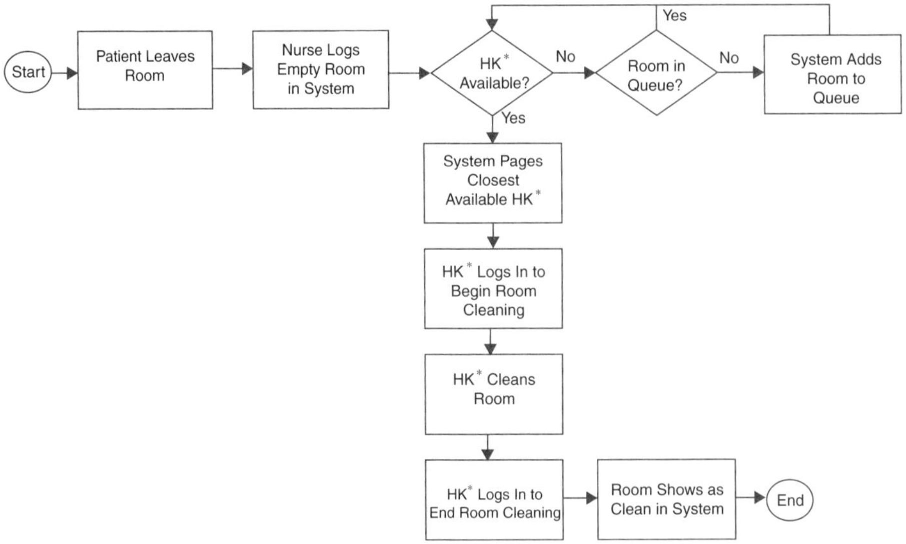

*HK—housekeeping.

process owners may vary from facility to facility, it is often nurses who must log the patient discharges that trigger the room turnover events via the bed tracking software. The managers of the cleaning personnel work to streamline the room turnover process, but must ensure that infection control remains a top priority.

The interviewing and mapping step for this example may entail speaking with floor nurses to determine how they know when to log an empty room into the system and what barriers exist for their performance of this task. Additional interviews with cleaning personnel or housekeeping (HK) and their management may shed light on other trigger events and existing measures of success.

As previously mentioned, the final step, analysis, involves determining what approaches and tools will make the process run more effectively and efficiently. If the first three steps of the process mapping activity have revealed process issues or inefficiencies, these should be resolved, removed, or reduced to the extent possible. The steps of the room turnover process, its task assignments, and its resource requirements should be analyzed to ensure they support the objectives of the process.

VALUE STREAM MAPPING

In a service industry such as health care, the value stream is all of the steps required to complete a service from beginning to end. *Value stream mapping* (VSM) is a tool to show work/materials and information flow using lead time, wait time, process time, and first-time quality as metrics (Haas and Torgerson 2010). VSM provides a visual analysis of the value stream and can lead to identification of problems and help focus attention in the most appropriate areas.

VSM involves sorting a process's activities into three categories: (1) those that create value as perceived by the customer, (2) those that create no value but are currently required and so cannot be eliminated, and (3) those actions that do not create value as perceived by the customer and can be eliminated immediately. Actions falling into category 3 are called *muda*. *Muda* is the Japanese word for waste, specifically any human activity that utilizes resources and creates no value (Womack and Jones 1996).

The process of VSM involves several levels of participants. Generally, these include members of a company's leadership team, workers who deal with service delivery on a daily basis, personnel from support areas, and a facilitator.

Examining the end-to-end flow of an outpatient radiology center patient (see Figure 7.2 and Figure 7.3) enables recognition of opportunities for improvement. This type of mapping process also facilitates an understanding of how support processes impact the delivery of care.

An additional benefit of mapping a patient's value stream is that the mapping process provides the opportunity for representatives from different functional organizations to gather as a group and see the care delivery system from a common point of view. It is very likely that this new perspective provides the additional benefits of improved communication and alignment of vision among the care providers (Wince 2007).

In order for the value stream mapping process to have a significant impact on the patient experience, the metrics of the various constituencies must be aligned as well. It has been suggested that the most effective way to do this is to translate all activities in the value stream to the common dimension of time (Wince 2007). In most health care settings, time is highly valued. Eliminating process steps that waste time and reducing the length of time that other required process steps take are two desirable results of the value stream mapping activity.

FIGURE 7.2 Current State Map

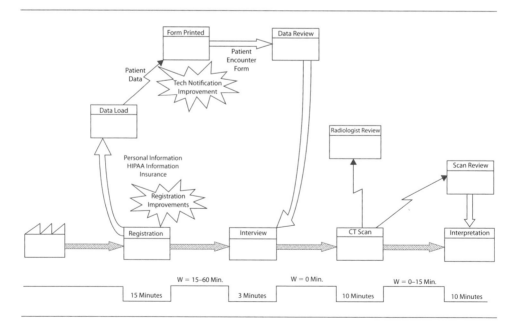

Value Stream Mapping Symbols

The symbols used for VSM are not standardized; however, some of the most common symbols are provided in Table 7.1. These have been adopted by numerous companies specializing in VSM.

Most of the symbols provided in Table 7.1 are explained by the brief meaning provided in the right-hand column. The only symbol that may require further explanation is the *kaizen* burst. In developing a current state map, as we will do in the following section, a *kaizen* burst can be used to highlight where improvement is needed and indicate steps of the process where *kaizen* events (see Chapter 10) may be essential in order to attain the desired future state map.

Current State Map

In order to develop a current state map, one must have a clear understanding of the process being mapped. This usually will require the VSM team to walk through the process to gain an understanding of its flow. There should be agreed-upon beginning and end points for the process being mapped.

FIGURE 7.3   Future State Map

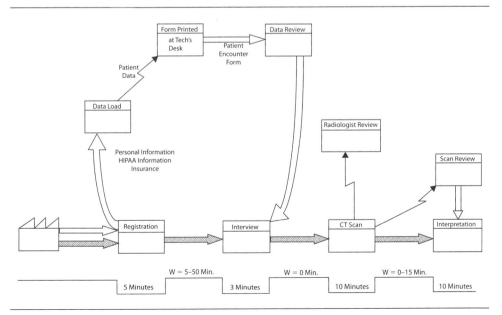

TABLE 7.1 Value Stream Mapping Symbols

Symbol	Symbol Meaning
	Customer or Supplier
	Process or Operation
	Shipment or Logistics
	Material Flow
	Information Flow
	Information Box
	Electronic Information
	Kaizen Burst

Some proponents of VSM recommend starting at the end of the process and mapping back to its start (http://lssacademy.com/2008/02/24/lets-create-a-current-state-value-stream-map/). Since the team will edit the current state map numerous times, it may work best to use a whiteboard and have one member of the team draw out the map as the other team members provide input. Another approach is to have each team member create a current state map, and then compare those and create a team map based on the individual maps. Last, some recommend having a portion of the team map the start of the process, a second subgroup map the middle of the process, and a third subgroup map the end of the process. The approach chosen will depend on the size of the team, the size of the process being mapped, the VSM experience of team members, and team preference.

Another recommendation when creating a current state map is to focus on the work or material flow first (http://lssacademy.com/2008/02/24/lets-create-a -current-state-value-stream-map/). Locate process and information boxes along the bottom portion of the map as shown in Figure 7.2. Information flow should then be added. Including a map of the information flow is critical for VSM. Without it, your resulting diagram will most likely be just a traditional process map (http:// lssacademy.com/2008/02/24/lets-create-a-current-state-value-stream-map/).

In order to be able to determine how much time in the process is value-added, a time line must be included in the current state map. This is typically inserted along the bottom of the map below the information boxes with times of process steps indicated along the time line (see Figure 7.2).

Although the list of symbols provided in Table 7.1 is not exhaustive by any means, it does provide a good starting point for developing a current state map. As can be seen in Figure 7.2, it is possible to develop a current state map using only the symbols of Table 7.1. Web resources may be consulted to investigate other widely accepted VSM symbols.

Figure 7.2 is a current state map for an outpatient radiology center. The process mapped is from an outpatient head, neck, and spine center that administers outpatient CT scans. Although many processes occur at the center, only the CT scan process is included in the current state map.

The current state map shows two *kaizen* bursts. The one near registration is included because currently all patients must complete all of their paperwork on-site. Often, patients do not realize that their place in line, so to speak, is not secured until their paperwork is completed and turned in to the workers at the registration area. When we examine the future state map in the following section, we will indicate what changes to registration may lead to reduced registration time. Another *kaizen* burst is located by the form printed step of the process. Changes to that step are also discussed in the section on the future state map.

Referring to the current state map of Figure 7.2, we see that, on average, a patient spends 78 minutes in the system. However, a patient may spend as much as 103 minutes in the system. Although registration is a necessary process, some of the time spent in the registration process is non-value-added. For the patient, all of the wait time is non-value-added. However, a small portion of the initial wait time that follows registration is necessary so that registration personnel can load relevant patient data into the system that generates the patient's encounter form.

We approximate that for an average time in the system of 78 minutes, about 28 minutes is value-added and 50 minutes is non-value-added. In our discussion of the future state map, we address how to reduce the non-value-added time patients must spend in the system.

Future State Map

The future state map is a picture of the desired flow of the material and information of the process under review. By using the current state map and its indicated value-added activities and non-value-added activities, the future state map can be created by removing non-value-added activities where possible, and improving communication or information flow where possible. The possible improvements indicated by the *kaizen* bursts in the current state map should be indicated in the future state map.

In health care, such improvements may center on opportunities to improve patient satisfaction. Specifically, there are many health care processes for which improvements could be made to the admittance and discharge procedures, the patient room readiness and cleanliness, physician availability, and the quality and timeliness of information given to the patient.

Additionally, there may be opportunities to improve employee satisfaction. Employees would prefer processes that reduce the time they spend searching for supplies and equipment, searching for a physician, searching for charts, or searching for the right information regarding a patient or procedure.

When developing a future state map, there are seven fundamental questions to consider (Locher 2008):

1. What does the customer/patient really need?

2. How often will we check our performance against customer/patient needs?

3. Which steps create value and which steps are wasted?

4. How can we flow work with fewer interruptions?

5. How do we control work between interruptions, and how will work be triggered and prioritized?

6. How will we level the workload and/or different activities?

7. What process improvements will be necessary?

In order to answer these questions, the VSM team must put themselves in a patient's shoes and see things from the patient's perspective. However, there will obviously be some aspects of medical care that a patient may not realize are value-added, so the VSM team must also use their knowledge of patient care. Although interruptions in general may not be good, interrupting a nurse who is about to administer the wrong medication or interrupting a doctor who cannot make a correct diagnosis without a needed test result would both be seen as needed interruptions.

Returning to the outpatient radiology center example of Figure 7.2, we can create a future state map using the information in the chart as well as possible impacts of the included *kaizen* bursts. The resulting future state map is provided in Figure 7.3.

Note that in the future state map, the registration time has been reduced from 15 minutes to 5 minutes. There are two actions that contribute to that reduction. First, the center will provide patients with the option of completing their paperwork prior to arrival by posting required documents online. This can be done at a minimal cost to the center and will allow patients to save waiting time at the center by bringing their completed forms with them and handing them to registration personnel upon arrival.

Additionally, signage and a colored piece of paper accompanying the registration forms will let patients know that they are not fully checked in until their paperwork is completed and turned in to registration personnel. This may increase the speed with which the forms are completed and submitted.

The other part of the process where waste can be eliminated is at the print form step. Currently, the form prints to a printer in a central location in the office of the registration personnel. This is not the same office used by the technician who must perform the CT scan. Under the current process, there is no indication given to the technician when to retrieve a document from the printer. The technician must check the printer periodically or rely on the registration staff to either call or drop off the printed form. A recommended change that would not be difficult or expensive to implement is to route the patient forms needed by the technician to his or her work area. This change would provide both a visual and an auditory cue for the technician to know the next patient is ready.

It is anticipated that if both of these waste-reducing actions are taken, then approximately 20 minutes could be cut from the non-value-added time a patient spends in the system. Ten minutes could be cut from the registration step and 10 from the initial wait to see the technician. This leads to a system with average time in the system of 58 minutes, with 28 minutes being value-added and 30 minutes non-value-added.

Value Stream Mapping Tools

There are a number of tools that can be utilized to assist with value stream mapping. Hines and Rich (1997) present seven of these tools. They are: (1) process activity mapping, (2) supply chain response matrix, (3) production variety funnel, (4) quality filter mapping, (5) demand amplification mapping, (6) decision point analysis, and (7) physical structure mapping. How each of these tools might be used is described very briefly in the following paragraphs. The interested reader is referred to Hines and Rich (1997) for further explanation.

Process activity mapping is described in the first section of this chapter. A supply chain response matrix attempts to show critical lead-time constraints for a specific process. Using a production variety funnel enables one to understand the complexities surrounding the operations of a company or its supply chain and can be useful when making decisions about inventory reduction. Quality filter mapping produces a map identifying where defects occur in the supply chain.

Demand amplification mapping can be utilized to demonstrate how demand changes along the supply chain. Decision point analysis provides a clearer understanding of where the decision point lies. That is, where in the supply chain do products start being made based on forecasted demand and not actual demand? Physical structure mapping aids in understanding the industry-level view of a supply chain.

USE OF MAPS AND CHARTS IN HEALTH CARE

The preceding sections provided details on process mapping and value stream mapping. In addition, most readers are familiar with flowcharts. It is important that health care operations personnel understand the differences among these approaches so that the most suitable approach can be selected for use in various situations.

Flowcharts are useful in many situations. Having their origin in computer programming, they allow one to depict the steps and decision points in a process.

Beginning and end points are indicated using ovals or circles. Steps are indicated using rectangular boxes, and decision points are indicated with diamonds. Arrows represent the flow through the process and may be used to indicate when the process contains subprocesses that are iterative in nature. There are numerous other shapes that may be employed in a flowchart, but the majority of those shapes are not required for basic process representation.

When first approaching a process flow problem, it may be a good idea to create a draft flowchart of the process and make sure that all personnel who contribute to the process agree on the draft. Often, it is not possible for one individual to create an initial draft flowchart that includes all steps, because one individual may lack familiarity with all process steps. Involving the contributing personnel will alleviate this problem and lead to an accurate draft flowchart.

As described earlier, process mapping involves several steps: process identification, information gathering, interviewing and mapping, and analysis. In some cases, the map designed as a part of the third step may include inputs and outputs. Other information that may be a part of a process map includes how, when, and where products or people move in the process; who the customers are; who the suppliers are; how information is recorded and shared; and how technology is applied (Endsley, Magill, and Godfrey 2006).

An Internet search of process mapping images reveals literally hundreds of process maps, a majority of which resemble flowcharts. The process map presented in Figure 7.1 could also be considered a flowchart of the room turnover process. Generally speaking, a flowchart is a tool that can be used to help depict a process. It may be used for process mapping, but the activity of process mapping involves other steps in addition to the mapping activity.

Value stream mapping (VSM) differs from process mapping in several ways. First, with VSM, one is trying to sort activities into three categories (see preceding section) in an effort to remove waste. Second, VSM looks at both material flow and information flow. In addition, VSM involves the use of a very specific set of symbols (see Table 7.1). If it is known ahead of time that an existing process involves a lot of non-value-added activities and the goal is to create a modified process that removes such activities to the extent possible, then the health care manager should employ VSM as a mapping tool and create both a current state map and a future state map. The literature is filled with examples of VSM applications. The interested reader is referred to Koelling et al. (2005) for an application of VSM to an emergency department.

STAFFING

In order to properly staff a service facility, one must first determine daily and hourly demand. It is important to note that demand may vary by day of week or month of year. For example, emergency departments often see a spike in demand on Mondays, as many who were sick or injured over the weekend wait until the start of the workweek to seek medical help. Similarly, Thanksgiving Day typically is a day of much lower demand at emergency departments and other medical facilities.

Most service facilities have standard service levels that are to be met, and these levels, combined with the forecasted demand, drive the *staffing* requirements. Figure 7.4 provides an example profile of nurse requirements for an emergency department with 24 beds. In the figure, the horizontal axis is the time of day beginning at 12 midnight and the vertical axis is the number of nurses assigned to work at that time of day. Each nurse works a 12-hour shift and is provided set times for breaks and meals. Due to the specialty nature of emergency department (ED) work, it is generally the case that nurses assigned to the ED work solely in the ED.

When care is taken in scheduling work shifts, the profile of the service supply can be made in such a way as to approximate demand. Work shift scheduling is a significant challenge for many service organizations, such as hospitals, that are faced with cyclic demand.

FIGURE 7.4   Staffing Profile

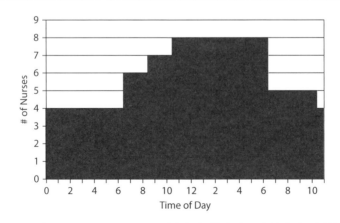

Work shift scheduling requires data to drive the process. The data are in the form of a forecast of demand by hour. This demand is translated into hourly staffing requirements. A schedule of shifts that matches the staffing requirements is then developed. As a final step, specific personnel are assigned to each shift.

In order to forecast demand by hour, historical data can be analyzed. Recall that demand may vary by hour of day, day of week, or month of year, so the historical data analyzed should cover a period of time long enough to recognize these types of fluctuations.

When scheduling shifts, it is important to note not only the quantity of workers needed, but also the type of workers needed for each shift. Even though many facilities cross-train their employees, it is often the case in health care that, based on qualifications and certifications, workers are not interchangeable. For example, at a hospital, nurses are permitted to perform the duties of nurse's aides, but nurse's aides are not permitted to perform the duties of a nurse.

Additionally, while it is critical to have an appropriate quantity of the right type of workers scheduled to work each shift, it is also important to make sure the skill mix and experience of those on duty are sufficient to cover all needs. For example, if your staff includes three nurses with 20-plus years of experience, it may be wise to assign one of them to each shift when scheduling nurses to work in the emergency department.

WORKLOAD MANAGEMENT

Workload management deals with the scheduling and utilization of resources in order to maintain efficiency of the service operations. Day-to-day workload management also involves distributing workloads, prioritizing activities, and managing unexpected events. Attention must be paid to the amount of work required at the present time and in the hours and days ahead so that decisions can be made regarding scheduling workers for overtime or early dismissal, if that is an option. Utilizing some workers to accomplish low-priority work (nonessential tasks), such as filing or taking inventory, may be an option if they are not kept busy by the current workload.

Managers must be aware that often workers become complacent during periods of low workloads and distracted during periods of excessive workloads. Maintaining a balance is critical.

Cross-training and specialization are other aspects to consider when it comes to workload management. In some situations, it may make sense to cross-train workers so that they can cover for each other and can spend their day performing a variety of tasks, not just one repetitive task. Having workers who are skilled at a wide range of tasks provides the company with more flexibility. Other situations may call for specialization, especially if there is much risk associated with a task being performed incorrectly or much cost associated with cross-training.

Another key aspect of workload management is the assignment of new customers or activities to workers. On a hospital floor with 24 beds and two nurses, typically the rooms are divided so that one nurse takes the patients in rooms 1 to 12 and the other nurse handles patients in rooms 13 to 24. Nurse managers will most likely try, to the extent possible, to ensure that difficult patients are divided evenly between the two sets of rooms.

There are a number of factors that influence workload management. These include but are not limited to activity, capacity, demand, and capabilities (Services for Australian Rural and Remote Allied Health, www.sarrahtraining.com). Activity is basically the work to be done, while capacity is the resources required to accomplish the activity. Demand includes all requests and referrals from various sources needing some or all of your company's services. Capabilities refer to the competencies necessary to perform the activities.

In the health care sector, case complexity plays a significant role in workload management decisions. As described in the report *Allied Health Professions: Workload Measurement and Management* (2006), case complexity includes consideration of comorbidities, social circumstances and emotional factors, complexity of interventions, identification and management of clinical risk, and factors relating to complex decision making. There is currently no standard method employed to ensure a balance of case complexity. As mentioned previously, nurse managers may try to divide the high-need patients, but oftentimes patients are assigned to a nurse prior to the complexity of their cases being ascertained.

Workload management can be simplified if demand management techniques are utilized. Using trend analysis, it is possible to predict demand for health care services, at least to some extent. Analyses of data on patient waiting times and planned admissions, as well as data on daily, weekly, and seasonal fluctuations, can be used to improve demand management and enhance workload management.

PRODUCTIVITY AND EFFICIENCY ANALYSIS

When investigating the performance of a manufacturing facility, often a *productivity analysis* is performed to determine throughput, machine utilization, worker utilization, cycle time, percent defects, and other relevant measures. When examining the performance of a service operation, efficiency analyses are utilized. Measures of interest may include customer satisfaction, average service time, and average wait time, among others.

To measure productivity, one must determine how well a given person, unit, or organization is converting inputs to outputs. In other words:

$$Productivity = \frac{Outputs}{Inputs}$$

Increasing productivity is a matter of making the ratio of outputs to inputs as large as possible.

Inputs are typically the people, resources, capital, energy, and other expenses used to run a business. Outputs vary based on the type of business being analyzed.

Work by Sumanth (1984) highlights a number of examples of *productivity measures*. The terminology they use makes it straightforward to see how their measures are applicable in both the production and service sectors. Four measures they provide are given in Equations 7.1 through 7.4 (Sumanth 1984):

$$Productivity = \frac{Output}{Labor} \qquad (7.1)$$

$$Productivity = \frac{Output}{Capital} \qquad (7.2)$$

$$Productivity = \frac{Output}{Materials} \qquad (7.3)$$

$$Productivity = \frac{Output}{Energy} \qquad (7.4)$$

These measures may be combined to create other productivity measures. When this is done, care must be taken to ensure that the units used are the same (e.g., dollars). If various units are used for measures that include multiple factors, then the measures may not make sense, unless they are used in conjunction with data envelopment analysis (DEA) or stochastic frontier analysis (SFA), both of which are discussed later in the chapter.

If we choose to combine all four of the measures listed, we would have a total measure as shown in Equation 7.5 (Sumanth 1984):

$$Productivity = \frac{Outputs}{Inputs} = \frac{goods/services\ produced}{resources\ used} \qquad (7.5)$$

Health Care Example

Consider an outpatient surgery center. It may elect to measure its daily productivity using the following measure:

$$Productivity = \frac{total\ number\ of\ patients\ seen}{total\ number\ of\ doctor\ hours\ worked} = \frac{18}{32} = 0.5625$$

This same measure could be used to determine the individual productivity of each of the doctors at the surgery center. For example, Dr. Smith's productivity on a specific day might be:

$$Productivity = \frac{number\ of\ patients\ seen}{number\ of\ doctor\ hours\ worked} = \frac{4}{8} = 0.50$$

and Dr. Wilson's productivity on that same day might be:

$$Productivity = \frac{number\ of\ patients\ seen}{number\ of\ doctor\ hours\ worked} = \frac{5}{8} = 0.625.$$

Based on this measure of productivity, we would conclude that on this day, Dr. Wilson was more productive than Dr. Smith. However, one must be careful when drawing conclusions about the results of productivity measure calculations. If multiple types of surgery are performed at the facility, it may not be possible to compare the productivity scores of several doctors. This is because not all types of surgeries take the same amount of time to perform, and not all types of surgeries cost the same amount.

Measuring Productivity and Efficiency

Measuring productivity or efficiency in health care settings is complicated by the various case mixes encountered, as well as the uncertainty regarding economies of scale that may or may not exist. The problem of measuring productivity in a health care setting is not new (Carr and Feldstein 1967; Neumann 1976). Work by Hollingsworth (2003) provides a summary and review of measures of health care efficiency.

According to Hollingsworth (2003), between 1983 and 2002, nearly 200 articles related to health care efficiency were published. Over half of these papers employ a method for measuring efficiency known as data envelopment analysis (DEA). Other approaches for measuring the efficiency of health care facilities are stochastic frontier analysis (SFA) and regression analysis (RA). Each of these methods is introduced next, and references are provided for the interested reader seeking additional detail.

Another measure commonly used in these papers is the Malmquist index. The Malmquist index is the mean of two indexes. It measures the change in efficiency from one time period to the next, and allows for a dissection of efficiency changes over time (Hollingsworth 2003).

Data Envelopment Analysis

Data envelopment analysis (DEA) is a mathematical programming technique that enables assessment of the relative performance of a set of like entities (e.g., banks, schools, hospitals). DEA measures how well the entities utilize their various inputs to produce outputs (Charnes, Cooper, and Rhodes 1978). Each entity in the group being analyzed is referred to as a decision-making unit (DMU).

Each DMU's performance is assessed relative to the best-performing DMU's performance using an efficiency measure that is the ratio of total outputs to total inputs. The best-performing DMU receives an efficiency rating of 1.00 or 100 percent. Other DMUs' efficiency scores vary between 0 and 100 percent. Once it has been determined which DMU is most efficient at converting inputs to outputs, further investigation may shed light on what characteristics of that DMU make it the top performer. When possible, those characteristics could be implemented or emulated by the other DMUs in an effort to improve their efficiency. Further details on DEA may be found in Ramanathan (2003).

Stochastic Frontier Analysis

A second popular approach to evaluate the efficiency of health care organizations is stochastic frontier analysis (SFA). Unlike DEA, which estimates a deterministic frontier, SFA allows for the separation of statistical noise from inefficiency by decomposing the error term into two parts. With SFA, the error for firm i is given by $\varepsilon_i = v_i + u_i$, where v_i is statistical noise and u_i consists of positive departures from the cost frontier and represents cost inefficiency (Rosko and Mutter 2008).

According to Berger and Humphrey (1997), SFA has at least two very important applications: (1) informing government policy on the impacts of deregulation, mergers, and so forth on industry inefficiency, and (2) improving managerial performance through the identification of best and worst practices. SFA allows an analyst to calculate a theoretical best-practices frontier and locate firms with respect to that frontier in order to objectively determine best practices (Charnes et al. 1978). This differs from DEA, where the frontier is based on actual firms. Further details on SFA may be found in Kumbhakar and Knox Lovell (2000).

Regression Analysis

The one approach to measuring health care facilities' efficiency with which you may be familiar is regression analysis (RA). Regression analysis may be used to help explain how the value of a dependent variable changes when any one of the independent variables is allowed to vary while the values of other independent variables remain fixed. Details on regression analysis are provided in Chapter 14.

COMMON HEALTH CARE PRODUCTIVITY AND EFFICIENCY MEASURES

For at least the past five decades, productivity measures in health care have been a topic of conversation and research. The work of Carr and Feldstein (1967) was the first comprehensive empirical investigation of hospital services. Later work by Neumann (1976) indicated that the productivity of a specific department within a hospital could be measured using cost and production functions, but it was not possible to aggregate these individual measures in order to evaluate an entire facility.

Today many facilities evaluate themselves against benchmarks established by health care bodies such as the American Case Management Association (ACMA) or the departments of social and health services (DSHS) that operate in each state. Many of these bodies establish and report on standards related to staffing and caseload, productivity, and outcome measures. For hospital workers such as nurses, this may translate into patient-to-nurse ratios, average times to distribute medication to patients, and length of stay (LOS) measures.

As described in the previous section, data envelopment analysis, stochastic frontier analysis, and regression analysis are techniques that enable hospitals and other health care facilities to evaluate their efficiency. In order to utilize these techniques, there must be data available on the system inputs (number of patients, number of care providers, size of facility, etc.) and on the system outputs (average length of stay, average patient waiting time, etc.). Table 7.2 provides sample outputs for various types of health care facilities. While these outputs may be viewed as measures themselves, they are often used in conjunction with DEA, SFA, or RA in order to determine the efficiency of a unit, department, or facility.

IMPROVING PRODUCTIVITY AND EFFICIENCY

Many of the analysis tools and operations management topics covered in this text can be linked to the goal of improving productivity and efficiency in a health care setting.

Understanding your company's supply chain and how to ensure that it operates efficiently and effectively (see Chapter 1) may help enable the establishment or modification of supply chain strategies to increase overall efficiency. Also, careful collection of financial data accompanied by determination of relevant financial ratios and metrics (see Chapter 2) can help indicate areas where efficiency improvement is possible. An understanding of the time value of money (see Chapter 2) is necessary when making decisions regarding the acquisition of the additional resources that are needed to improve efficiency.

Understanding decision analysis methods, decision support tools, and sensitivity analysis (see Chapter 4) enables a health care operations manager to make data-driven decisions that can lead to a break from business as usual when business as usual has become inefficient. Use of statistical tools to analyze relevant data (see Chapter 5) combined with simulation (see Chapter 6) to better understand the process being analyzed can lead to operational improvement.

For example, a box-and-whiskers plot may indicate that a current process has an acceptable mean but is highly variable. Development of a simulation of the process may offer insights into the causes of the high variance so that the process can be modified and its variance reduced.

A better understanding of patient flow, the focus of this chapter, has obvious ramifications for improving efficiency. Value stream mapping activities can highlight process steps that are non-value-added and detract from service delivery efficiency. Patient flow may also be inefficient due to a facility's design (see Chapter 8). Design alternatives that consider aisle width, service groupings, and closeness relationships can reduce bottlenecks and transportation time.

TABLE 7.2 Examples of Health Care Productivity and Efficiency Measures by Facility Type

Facility Type	Productivity and Efficiency Measures
Hospital emergency department	Length of stay (LOS), left without treatment (LWOT), patient wait time
Inpatient rehab center	LOS, worked hours per patient days, functional independence measure
Outpatient surgery center	On-time first cuts, patient throughput, cancellation rates
Long-term care facility	Billing errors per unit time, medication errors per unit time, patient satisfaction
Dialysis clinic	Machine turnover time, machine downtime, machine repair time
Hospital pharmacy	Dispensing errors per unit time, stock-outs, delivery time
Ophthalmologist office	Patient wait time, doctor idle time, billing errors per unit time
Low-acuity emergency department	LWOT, patient wait time, patient time to room
Hospital neonatal intensive care unit	Infection control measures in place, LOS, hospital-acquired infections
Doc-in-a-box	LWOT, patient throughput, patient wait time
Hospital operating room	On-time first cuts, retained surgical instruments
Blood donation center	Donations per unit time, no-shows, donor wait time

In health care, perhaps more than in other service industries, quality of service (see Chapter 9) and quality control and improvement (see Chapter 10) are critical. Poor quality may lead to a longer than necessary length of stay, the acquisition of hospital-borne infections, or even unnecessary fatalities. All of these consequences have a negative impact on a facility's costs, and thus directly impact productivity measures.

Reducing waste is synonymous with improving efficiency. Understanding and implementing lean concepts (see Chapter 11) leads to the reduction or even elimination of waste and enables health care processes to run more efficiently.

Acquiring needed resources at the last minute can be a costly endeavor. For this reason, a good understanding of basic forecasting concepts and techniques (see Chapter 12) is needed by health care operations managers to help them ensure that appropriate numbers of resources, such as beds and care providers, are available. Forecasting can also lead to better demand management and result in improved workload management, a side effect of which may be higher worker productivity.

Oftentimes, process improvement projects undertaken at health care facilities consume much more time, money, and resources than planned. A health care operations manager who is able to apply best practices in project management (see Chapter 13) can provide project oversight and guidance to enable the projects to finish on time and on budget, thus improving overall efficiency.

In order for a health care facility to operate efficiently, there must be sufficient qualified staff. Proper scheduling and capacity management (see Chapter 14) can help improve efficiency by ensuring that patients are not having to wait excessively long for the resources their care requires.

Application of best practices in inventory management (see Chapter 15) will minimize the possibility of stock-outs and ensure that sufficient quantities of vital supplies are on hand when needed. This will help improve efficiency by making sure care providers are not having to search or wait for the resources required to provide care. Maintaining proper levels of inventory will also ensure that inventory costs are controlled.

SUMMARY

In this chapter, we have examined process improvement and patient flow and learned about approaches and tools that will enable us to positively impact hospital performance. We defined process mapping in the context of the room turnover process and value stream mapping using an example from an MRI outpatient center. We briefly introduced some value stream mapping tools and pointed the reader toward additional details. We highlighted the similarities, differences, and features of flowcharts, process maps, and value stream maps, and provided examples from health care to emphasize which tool is most appropriate for various situations.

Staffing and workload management were explained using examples from health care. An overview of productivity and efficiency analysis was given, followed by information on the application of productivity measures in health care. More sophisticated approaches to efficiency analysis, such as data envelopment analysis and stochastic frontier analysis, were introduced, along with regression analysis. The chapter concluded with a look at productivity and efficiency analysis in health care and a description of how the entire content of this book contributes to the goal of improving productivity and efficiency in health care, with reference to how each chapter addresses this. A minicase is included to demonstrate chapter concepts.

KEY TERMS

current state map

future state map

process mapping

productivity analysis

productivity measures

staffing

value stream mapping

workload management

DISCUSSION QUESTIONS

1. For a basic process with which you are familiar from your current work or a previous work experience, carry out the four steps of process mapping (process identification, information gathering, interviewing and mapping, analysis). It will take considerable time to perform these steps correctly.

2. Draw a basic process map for the process investigated in question 1.

3. Using either the same process from question 1 or a different process with which you are familiar, develop a current state map using value stream mapping (VSM) approaches examined in the chapter.

4. Using the current state map developed in question 3, create a future state map using VSM approaches detailed in the chapter.

5. Describe staffing needs at your current work or a previous work experience. How are/were staffing decisions made? If you were in charge of staffing, what would you do differently? Why?

6. Explain why workload management is important for safe, effective, and efficient delivery of health care.

7. For a health care setting in which you have worked, provide a list of valid measures of productivity. What approach would you take to analyze productivity in that setting (i.e., how would you gather the data needed for the measures you have listed)?

8. One productivity measure at an emergency department is patient wait time to see a physician. What approaches might be effective at improving patient wait time? Describe how you would approach the problem of improving patient wait time at an emergency department.

MINICASE: IMPROVING PROCESS FLOW TO IMPROVE SERVICE-LEVEL PERFORMANCE STATISTICS

A local low-acuity emergency department wants to improve its patient flow. The facility has as its goal that 85 percent or more of the arriving patients will be seen by a doctor in 60 minutes or less. Currently, the facility is not meeting that goal.

An initial, high-level process map has been developed (see Figure 7.5), along with some observations from an outside team of analysts. Your task is to determine what else may be done to help this facility better understand the reasons it has been unable to meet its service-level goal. Specifically, explain in detail how each of the eight approaches listed might help this facility in determining where it should focus its change efforts if it wants to meet its current service-level goal.

FIGURE 7.5 Process Flow at Low-Acuity Emergency Department

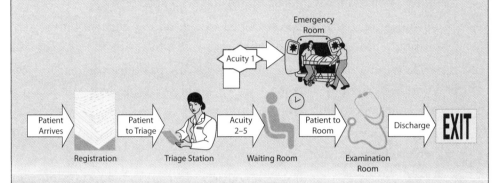

Observations

1. Time spent at registration is consistently less than five minutes.

2. Time spent in triage is consistently less than five minutes.

3. Time spent in the waiting room is highly variable (five minutes to 100 minutes) and depends on the patient's acuity (more severe patients are seen more quickly).

4. Time spent in exam room is highly variable (10 minutes to 100 minutes) and depends on availability of doctor and extent of testing required.

5. Time spent at discharge is consistently less than five minutes.

6. The facility operates 15 hours a day, seven days a week.

7. The facility has 10 patient exam rooms, two full-time doctors, one part-time doctor, two nurses, and one triage nurse.

8. All patient diagnoses must be entered into a computer system by the doctor at the conclusion of a patient's exam.

Approaches to Consider

• Process mapping (for subprocesses).

• Value stream mapping.

- Staffing and workload management

- Productivity analysis.

- Analysis of data for key emergency department productivity measures.

REFERENCES

Allied Health Professions: Workload Measurement and Management. 2006. Edinburgh: Scottish Executive Publications.

Berger, A., and D. Humphrey. 1997. "Efficiency of Financial Institutions: International Survey and Directions for Future Research." *European Journal of Operational Research* 98:175–212.

Brown, E., and J. Kros. 2010. "Improving Room Turnaround Time at a Regional Hospital." *Quality Management in Health Care* 19 (1): 90–102.

Carr, J., and P. Feldstein. 1967. "The Relationship of Cost to Hospital Size." *Inquiry* (June): 45–46.

Charnes, A., W. W. Cooper, and E. Rhodes. 1978. "Measuring the Efficiency of Decision Making Units." *European Journal of Operational Research* 2:429–444.

Cochran, J., and T. Burdick. 2011. "The Impact of the Door-to-Doc Emergency Department Patient Flow Model." *Proceedings of the 2011 Industrial Engineering Research Conference*, T. Doolen and E. Van Aken, eds. Reno, Nevada.

Endsley, S., M. Magill, and M. Godfrey. 2006. "Creating a Lean Practice." *Family Practice Management* 13 (4): 34–38.

Haas, R., and C. Torgerson. 2010. "Value Stream Mapping a Patient Care Unit." Tutorial posted at Society for Health Systems website, www.shsweb.org.

Hines, P., and N. Rich. 1997. "The Seven Value Stream Mapping Tools." *International Journal of Operations and Production Management* 17 (1): 46–64.

Hollingsworth, B. 2003. "Non-Parametric and Parametric Applications Measuring Efficiency in Health Care." *Health Care Management Science* 6:203–218.

Hunt, V. D. 1996. *Process Mapping: How to Reengineer Your Business Processes.* New York: John Wiley & Sons.

Koelling, C. P., D. Eitel, S. Mahapatra, K. Messner, and L. Grove. 2005. "Value Stream Mapping the Emergency Department." Society for Health Systems Annual Conference.

Kumbhakar, S., and C. A. Knox Lovell. 2000. *Stochastic Frontier Analysis.* New York: Cambridge University Press.

Locher, D. 2008. *Value Stream Mapping for Lean Development: A How-To Guide for Streamlining Time to Market.* New York: Taylor & Francis.

http://lssacademy.com/2008/02/24/lets-create-a-current-state-value-stream-map/.

Neumann, B. 1976. "Hospital Productivity: An Evaluation of Proposed Measurement Methods." *Public Productivity Review* 1 (5): 23–36.

Ramanathan, R. 2003. *An Introduction to Data Envelopment Analysis.* Thousand Oaks, CA: Sage Publications.

Rosko, M. D., and R. L. Mutter. 2008. "Stochastic Frontier Analysis of Hospital Inefficiency." *Medical Care Research and Review* 65 (2): 131–166.

Services for Australian Rural and Remote Allied Health, www.sarrahtraining.com.

Sumanth, D. 1984. *Productivity Engineering and Management: Productivity Measurement, Evaluation, Planning, and Improvement in Manufacturing and Service Organizations.* New York: McGraw-Hill.

Wince, R. 2007. "Improvement in Healthcare Is Possible—Just 'Be the Ball.'" *Patient Safety and Quality Healthcare.*

Womack, J., and D. Jones. 1996. *Lean Thinking.* New York: Simon & Schuster.

CHAPTER 8

FACILITY LAYOUT

LEARNING OBJECTIVES

➠ Understand various layout considerations affecting health care operations.

➠ Develop and apply Muther diagrams in the proper context.

➠ Understand how to properly evaluate different types of layouts, particularly those utilized in health care settings.

➠ Apply concepts for optimal facility layout and design.

INTRODUCTION

For purposes of this chapter, *facility layout* will be considered in the context of health care facilities. Layout at production facilities takes many factors into consideration that will not be discussed here. The interested reader is referred to Tompkins et al. (2003).

In health care facilities, a number of layout considerations factor into the design of the building. Details on the considerations are provided in the opening section of this chapter. This is followed by an overview of different types of layouts. Muther diagrams are introduced and their usefulness is highlighted in an example involving a health care facility.

The chapter describes the impact that design can have on workload management and evaluates different types of layouts. In order to choose among various designs, one must be able to model the situation and employ optimization techniques, so we include a section that provides basics of optimization. A common tool for linear optimization is Solver, an add-in to Excel; we therefore provide a small health care example utilizing Solver. The chapter closes with a section on optimal facility layout and design.

LAYOUT CONSIDERATIONS

Depending on the type of facility being constructed, there are numerous layout considerations that will influence the design. Some basic considerations for all facility layouts are discussed here, with examples from health care.

Flow is a major consideration when designing facilities. The patients at any health care facility need to be able to flow easily through the facility, and unnecessary travel should be avoided whenever possible. Depending on the types of patients that frequent a facility, flow considerations may be dealt with differently. For example, a facility whose primary patients are obese, immobile, or elderly may choose a flow pattern that requires little movement by the patients (i.e., check-in and then go straight to exam room). Other facilities, in an attempt to break up patients' wait into multiple short waits, may have patients check in, wait in one area, get temperature and blood pressure taken, wait in another area, get blood work done, and then proceed to the exam room (or some similar flow pattern).

In health care facilities, halls should be designed and located in a manner that promotes effective flow. Halls that are too narrow may result in safety issues during times of high traffic, whereas halls that are too wide may be difficult to keep clean and result in wasted space. In some hospitals, two sets of halls are built to allow employees to use one set and hospital visitors to use the other set.

Another layout consideration is how much space is required to conduct the activities that will occur in a given area. There are federal regulations and other guidelines that must be followed, but there are also practical reasons to consider space. The comfort and privacy of the patients must be a priority. The setting, or ambient conditions, will also be important. For example, the noise level, lighting, and temperature of an area can impact patient satisfaction as well as employee morale.

Other design aspects to consider include adequate waiting facilities, easily maintained surveillance, lack of clutter, and clear exit and entry points (www .ateneonline.it/chase2e/studenti/tn/6184–7_tn05.pdf). All of these features contribute to patient safety and security.

When making design changes to an existing facility or part of a facility, it is important to make sure the new design utilizes space and labor efficiently, eliminates bottlenecks, and reduces process and service time. A good design will also allow for visual control of activities, improve communications, and provide flexibility to adapt to changing conditions (www.cbpa.ewu.edu/~pnemetzmills /OMch5/OMFAC.html).

There are always multiple objectives to accomplish when designing a health care facility. Often, some of these objectives are in conflict with others. Consider a unit at a hospital that has 20 patient rooms and is rectangular in shape (see Figure 8.1). When deciding how to design the storage area(s) for the medication needed on the unit, two alternatives seem promising. The first, shown in Figure 8.2a, places a large, secure dispensary cabinet in the center of the patient

FIGURE 8.1 Hospital Unit

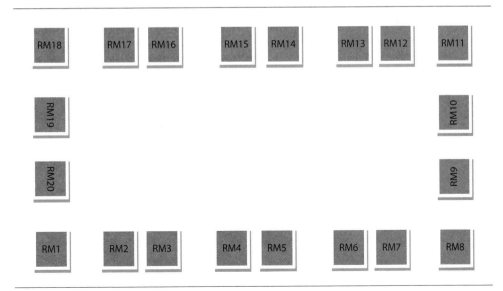

FIGURE 8.2a   Centralized Medication Storage

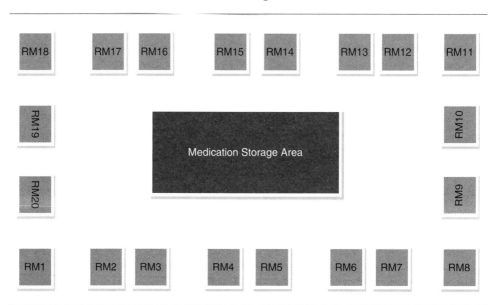

room area. All nurses can access the medication delivered from the pharmacy and distribute it to their patients on the unit. The second design alternative, shown in Figure 8.2b, provides for small medication cabinets between each set of two rooms, with a nurse having access to the cabinets for his or her patients only. Which design do you think is better?

The question of which design is better is somewhat tricky. Is the objective to minimize the walking the nurses must do to deliver all medications? If so, then the design of Figure 8.2b is preferred. But if that design is implemented, the pharmacy workers will now have to make 12 stops at the unit instead of one stop, which increases their workload and the time it takes them to deliver medications.

Design optimization cannot be looked at in isolation. The impacts of design decisions must be evaluated from a system perspective. More discussion of design optimization is included in the sections that follow.

Evidenced-Based Health Care Architecture

Work by Ulrich (2006) provides important information on the link between the architecture of health care facilities and health-related outcomes. Key findings of Ulrich are summarized in this section.

FIGURE 8.2b Decentralized Medication Storage

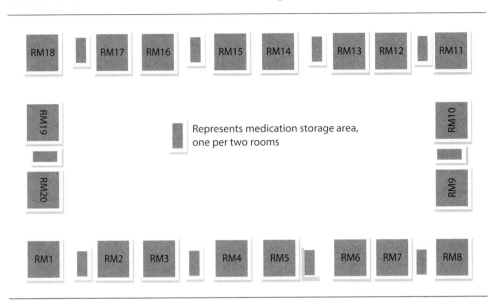

Research now indicates that good design of a health care facility's physical environment leads to better clinical outcomes, increased safety, and reduced stress for both patients and care providers. In many hospitals, high noise levels have a detrimental effect on patients and employees and can lead to sleep loss, high blood pressure, elevated heart rates, reduced recovery rates for myocardial infarction, and lower oxygen saturation in neonatal intensive care patients. The fatigue and job strain experienced by staff working in noisy environments can increase the risk of error.

Additionally, research supports the supposition that proper design of health care facilities can lead to a reduction in the incidence of transmission of infections. Evidence indicates single-bed rooms are advantageous in that they are easier to clean, offer less chance of both airborne and contact transmission of infection, and enable isolation of patients at their time of admission, when perhaps some existing infections have not yet been diagnosed. Infection control can also be improved by locating sinks and hand sanitizers in plain view of staff and in their work paths so that additional walking is not required in order to wash their hands.

Finally, there is increasing evidence supporting the idea that higher daylight exposure in patients' rooms reduces depression and pain. This realization highlights the significance of building orientation. Design plans that include buildings

TABLE 8.1 Types of Facility Layouts

Name	Description	Example
Process-oriented layout	For low-volume, high-variety production	Hospital emergency department
Product-oriented layout	Maximizes utilization in repetitive or continuous production	Pharmaceutical manufacturing
Fixed-position layout	For layout of large, stationary projects	Children's hospital
Retail layout	For allocating shelf space in response to customers' desires	Hospital gift shop
Office layout	For information movement among office workers and their equipment	Health insurance office
Warehouse layout	For addressing trade-offs between space and material handling	Surgical supplies distributor

that block sun exposure to rooms in other buildings are not optimal. When possible, the view from patient rooms should include nature or pleasant views, as research findings indicate such views reduce patient stress and pain.

TYPES OF LAYOUTS

There are a number of types of layouts to consider when designing a facility, area, or department. Some of the most common types of layouts are given in Table 8.1, along with their descriptions and an example of each (Heizer and Render 2004). More detail is provided in the subsections that follow.

Process-Oriented Layout

What we often see in health care settings is a *process-oriented layout*. It allows for flexibility in locating equipment and labor. One disadvantage of this layout is that it tends to have queues or bottlenecks that form due to difficulties in scheduling the required resources and changing setups (Heizer and Render 2004). Process-oriented layout is covered in more detail in the final section of this chapter.

Product-Oriented Layout

Repetitive production, such as the production of adult diapers, and continuous production, such as the production of pharmaceutical products, utilize *product-oriented layouts*. Fabrication lines and assembly lines are two types of product-oriented layouts (Ulrich 2006). Components are built on a fabrication line and then combined on an assembly line. One problem with this type of layout is that it is often difficult to balance the production line so that work flows smoothly, and at the same time produce the required level of output.

Fixed-Position Layout

A fixed-position layout allows the project to remain in one place and the resources, such as workers and equipment, to come to that place to work. As an example, a new children's hospital under construction would have a fixed-position layout. Problems faced with this layout include limited space within which to work, the need for a variety of materials as the project develops, and the dynamic nature of materials requirements (Heizer and Render 2004).

Retail Layout

The key to a retail layout is making sure the customers are exposed to the maximum number of products. Research indicates a sales increase as customers' exposure to products increases. There are a number of well-established guidelines to help with retail store arrangement. These include the recommendation to make sure high-impulse and high-margin items are located in prominent locations.

Office Layout

Information flow is a key component when designing an office layout. It is critical to group workers, their assigned working space, and their equipment in a way that provides both comfort and safety, and allows for efficient flow of information (Heizer and Render 2004). The section on Muther diagrams that follows can be helpful when designing an office layout.

Warehouse Layout

When designing a warehouse, it is important to seek a balance between warehouse costs (i.e., for the space) and handling costs (i.e., how high you stack things). Obviously, there are advantages to utilizing all of the space in a warehouse.

However, there is a cost associated with the use of space above reaching level, as material-handling equipment will be required to retrieve inventory stored up high. The location of shipping and receiving docks is also a critical component for warehouse layout design.

MUTHER DIAGRAMS

Flow, as mentioned before, may be measured in quantitative or qualitative terms. For quantitative measurement, a from-to chart can be employed to indicate the volume of goods (or number of patients) moved between departments or areas. For qualitative measurement, closeness relationships values introduced by Muther (1973) can be used to measure flows (Tompkins et al. 2003). When accompanied by information on the importance of each relationship and the reasons for the established closeness value, this information can be presented in a *Muther diagram* (see Figure 8.3).

A Muther diagram may be constructed in five steps in the following manner (Tompkins et al. 2003):

1. List all departments down the left-hand side of the diagram.

2. Interview or survey employees from each department listed and each department's manager in order to gather data on how each department views its relationships with the other departments.

FIGURE 8.3 Muther Diagram for Health Care Example

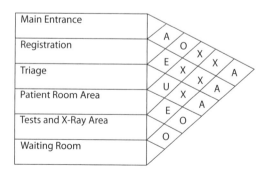

TABLE 8.2   Reasons for Closeness Rating

Code	Reason
1	High frequency of use
2	Medium frequency of use
3	Low frequency of use
4	High information flow
5	Medium information flow
6	Low information flow

TABLE 8.3   Importance of Relationship

Value	Closeness
A	Absolutely necessary
E	Especially important
I	Important
O	Ordinary importance
U	Unimportant
X	Undesirable

3. Define criteria for assigning closeness relationships and record the criteria as the reasons for relationship values on the diagram (see Table 8.2).

4. Determine the appropriate relationship value (see Table 8.3) and the justifying reason for that value for all pairs of departments.

5. Allow those employees and managers who were interviewed or surveyed during the development of the diagram to have an opportunity to evaluate and discuss changes to the diagram.

In the process for developing a Muther diagram, the inclusion of step 3 is optional. Numerous Muther diagrams you will find in the literature, such as Figure 8.3, include only the importance ratings (Table 8.3) and do not provide ratings for the reasons for closeness (Table 8.2).

Health Care Example

Consider a low-acuity emergency department (ED). In Figure 8.3, a Muther diagram is provided for a low-acuity ED. The six work areas considered are the main entrance, registration, triage, patient room area, tests and x-ray area, and the waiting room.

From the diagram, we can tell the following:

- It is absolutely necessary that the waiting room be located near triage, registration, and the main entrance. It is also absolutely necessary that the main entrance be located near registration.

- It is especially important to locate registration near triage, and the tests and x-ray area near the patient room area.

- It is of ordinary importance to locate registration near the main entrance, and the waiting room near the tests and x-ray area as well as near the patient room area.

- It is unimportant to locate triage near the patient room area.

- It is undesirable to have the tests and x-ray area located near triage, registration, or the main entrance. It is also undesirable to have the patient room area located near the main entrance or registration.

WORKLOAD MANAGEMENT

In manufacturing, assembly line balancing attempts to assign operations to workstations along an assembly line in a manner that minimizes cycle time or minimizes the number of workstations. The health care arena provides only a few situations in which application of assembly line balancing techniques is appropriate (Dowling and Cotner 1988).

Workload management, covered in Chapter 7, is related to facility layout and design. The time it takes to complete an activity may be directly impacted by the facility's design and layout. For example, health care facilities that are somewhat horizontal (i.e., fewer floors spread out over more space) must allow more travel time for workers. In those types of facilities, getting to an area where work needs to be done is not simply a matter of getting on a nearby elevator and pressing the button for the correct floor.

Additionally, as highlighted in the previous section on Muther diagrams, locating various departments, offices, and equipment correctly can reduce worker and patient travel time. This can positively impact workload management by reducing activity time and increasing capacity.

EVALUATING DIFFERENT TYPES OF LAYOUTS

Design evaluation measures have been around for more than half a century (Gantz and Petit 1953). Work by Konz (1985) indicates three main categories of measures relevant to facility design. These are resource utilization ratios, management control ratios, and operating efficiency ratios. These measures have documented limitations and deficiencies (Konz 1985).

More recently, Lin and Sharp (1999) developed three independent criterion groups for the facility layout evaluation problem. These groups are the cost criterion group, the flow criterion group, and the environment criterion group. Table 8.4 lists most of the cost, flow, and environment criteria Lin and Sharp considered. Those that would not relate to health care settings are omitted from the table.

In order to demonstrate how quantitative measures can be established and applied to evaluate different layouts, we will review the aisles criterion described by Lin and Sharp (1999), using their notation, formulas, and explanations for clarity.

In the table, the aisle is used to evaluate how effectively an aisle arrangement supports the flow of materials and personnel. There are two types of aisles to consider. There are the aisles that are developed based on building construction needs. These aisles are a part of the permanent building features. There are also aisles formed based on implementation of the layout plan. These aisles are considered movable building features. This criterion only considers major aisles, which must have identifiable widths and lengths.

TABLE 8.4 Design Evaluation Criteria

Cost Criterion Group	Flow Criterion Group	Environment Criterion Group
Initial cost	Clearness	Community environment
Annual operation and maintenance cost	Space sufficiency and utilization	Human-related safety
Future salvage value	Aisles	Worker-related comfort
Inventory holding cost	Distance and volume density	Property-related security
	Robustness of equipment capacity	Access for maintenance
	Building expansion	

TABLE 8.5 Impact Analysis of Aisle Arrangement

Objectives
Serve the areas adjacent to the aisles.
Handle the traffic without wasting space.
Lead to the areas needing access.
Provide alternative routes to an area.
Avoid congestion or blind corners.
Support the basic regularity of aisles and work areas.

In many cases, designers do not get to decide on aisle width, as that specification must be based on industry standards. Therefore, aisle length is how we will indicate the space occupied by an aisle system. For the design comparisons we will make, we will assume the aisles allow two-way traffic.

To develop an index that can quantify and allow for comparison of various aisle designs, Lin and Sharp (1999) consider six main objectives of an aisle system. These are listed in Table 8.5.

From the table, six issues worthy of investigation are discussed (Lin and Sharp 1999):

1. *Area served by the aisle.* The measure (total area served by whole aisle system)/ (total aisle length) is adopted for this issue.

2. *Ease of access.* Access from one department to another should have the following characteristics:

   • There is a connecting channel between every pair of departments.

   • No department is large compared to the others.

   • No department has a shape that is too long and thin.

3. *Alternative routes.* One may consider estimating the average number of possible routes that a part or patient can use in a facility; however, this is not easily measured.

4. *Intersection.* The differences among types of intersections are not considered here, but the quantity (sum of the number of intersections) is utilized.

5. *Department shape.* This is measured based on the three characteristics in issue 2.

6. *Straight aisles.* Two measures for straightness of an aisle are used:

   1. Number of turning points/length of ideal straight aisle.

   2. Actual aisle length/length of ideal straight aisle.

From the list, Lin and Sharp (1999) determined that the three measures most capable of providing insight into the aisle design are:

1. Total area served by whole aisle system/total aisle length.

2. Department shape ratio.

3. Sum of the number of intersections.

To simplify our example analysis, we will use only total aisle length and total number of intersections. We will compare the three design alternatives from Lin and Sharp (1999) that are given in Figure 8.4. Table 8.6 summarizes the aisle length and number of intersection values for these three designs.

Using these quantifiable measures for design evaluation, we would need to talk to the principal decision makers and determine answers to questions such as:

- Are fewer intersections preferable (for safety reasons)?

- Are higher numbers of intersections preferable (for access reasons)?

- Which of these two measures carries more weight with the decision makers?

The reader is referred to Chapter 5 for additional information on decision analysis tools.

FIGURE 8.4 Alternative Designs for Evaluation

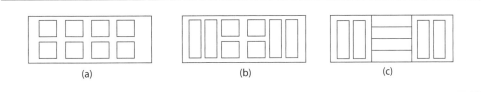

TABLE 8.6   Design Alternative Metrics

Alternative	Aisle Length	Number of Intersections
a	$3 \times 5 + 5 \times 3 = 30$	$4 \times 2 + 8 \times 3 + 3 \times 4 = 44$
b	$2 \times 5 + 7 \times 3 + 2.5 = 33.5$	$4 \times 2 + 12 \times 3 + 4 = 48$
c	$6 \times 3 + 2 \times 5 + 2.5 \times 3 = 35.5$	$4 \times 2 + 14 \times 3 = 50$

BASICS OF OPTIMIZATION

In order to understand what is required to optimize facility layout and design, we must first understand optimization. *Optimization* requires the modeler to determine an objective to be optimized, and the modeler must be able to express this objective in terms of the problem's variables, referred to as decision variables.

Depending on the problem being solved, the objective may be to minimize cost, minimize time, maximize revenue, or maximize throughput, among other things. The objective is defined in terms of a function of the decision variables. In addition to an objective function and decision variables, an optimization problem must include all relevant constraints. The constraints are also defined in terms of the decision variables. Let us consider a small example.

Let s_1 be the number of major surgeries scheduled for an operating room in a week and s_2 be the number of minor surgeries scheduled in the same operating room in a week. Thus, s_1 and s_2 are the decision variables for this problem. We will assume that each major surgery brings a profit of $2,000 to the facility and each minor surgery brings a profit of $800 to the facility. We will also assume that each major surgery takes four hours and consumes 15 total hours of labor, while each minor surgery takes 0.5 hours and consumes 10 total hours of labor. Finally, we will assume the facility has only one operating room, which is available 40 hours per week, and the facility has a total of 410 labor hours a week that can be devoted to surgeries.

From this description, we can formulate our optimization problem as shown in Equations 8.1 through 8.4:

$$\textit{maximize } z = 200s_1 + 800s_2 \quad \text{(objective function)} \qquad (8.1)$$

$$\textit{subject to}: 4s_1 + 0.5s_2 \leq 40 \quad \text{(operating room constraint)} \qquad (8.2)$$

$$15s_1 + 10s_2 \leq 410 \quad \text{(labor constraint)} \tag{8.3}$$

$$s_1, s_2 \geq 0 \quad \text{(non-negativity constraint)} \tag{8.4}$$

Note that in this formulation, Equation 8.4 is utilized to indicate that both of the decision variables can take on only nonnegative values.

Since the formulation requires only two decision variables, the problem can be solved graphically. Let the horizontal axis represent values for the decision variable s_1 and the vertical axis represent values for the decision variable s_2. Figure 8.5 indicates the feasible region for the linear programming problem. The feasible region is defined as the region in which all constraints are satisfied. In the figure, the feasible region is the shaded area.

FIGURE 8.5   Graphical Solution to Health Care Example

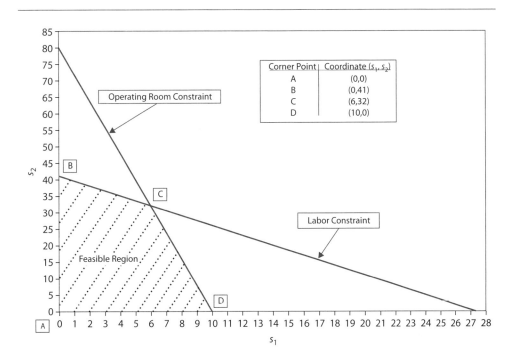

The mathematics of linear programming dictates that the optimal solution to such a problem, if an optimal solution exists, will lie at one of the corner points of the feasible region (Murty 1983). For Figure 8.5, we note that the four corner points are given by A = (0,0), B = (0,41), C = (6,32), and D = (10,0). By substituting these values for s_1 and s_2 into the objective function, we can determine that the optimal solution is point C, with $s_1 = 6$ and $s_2 = 32$. This can be interpreted to mean that the facility should perform 6 major surgeries and 32 minor surgeries per week and its weekly profit will be $37,600.

The formulation (Equations 8.1 to 8.4) may be referred to as a linear programming problem because the objective function and constraints are linear in terms of the decision variables. Linear programming problems are the most basic type of optimization problem, and the key to formulating them correctly is to ensure that the decision variables, constraints, and objective function are properly defined. Once formulated, many linear programming problems can be solved using the tool Solver, an add-in to Excel. For complex linear programming problems (i.e., those with more than 200 decision variables and more than 100 constraints), numerous other software options are available (*OR/MS Today* 2011).

A closer examination of the formulation reveals that it is actually an integer programming problem. Integer programming problems are linear programming problems whose decision variables are restricted to integers. Since we know it is impossible to perform a partial surgery, our decision variables s_1 and s_2 must be integers. The problem is referred to as a pure integer programming problem since all decision variables are restricted to integers. A mixed-integer programming problem includes some integer variables and some noninteger (or real-valued) variables.

Other types of optimization problems include nonlinear programming problems, multi-objective optimization problems, and combinatorial optimization problems, among others. The interested reader is referred to (Nocedal and Wright 1999).

OPTIMIZATION USING EXCEL SOLVER

For the small operating room example just given, it was possible to create a graphical representation of the situation and determine the optimal solution by hand. For problems involving more than two variables, the graphical approach is not feasible. In the example that follows, we expand the operating room example to include elective surgeries (s_3) and include an additional constraint related to the maximum number of elective surgeries that may occur each week (s_3 constraint). Using the Excel add-in Solver, we can determine optimal values for the decision variables s_1, s_2, and s_3. We will also add the constraint that all decision variables must be integers, since as previously discussed, we cannot perform partial surgeries.

For this example, consider a particular operating room. Let s_1 be the number of major surgeries scheduled in a week, s_2 be the number of minor surgeries scheduled in a week, and s_3 be the number of elective surgeries scheduled in a week. As before, we will assume that each major surgery brings a profit of $2,000 to the facility and each minor surgery brings a profit of $800 to the facility. Additionally, we will also assume that each elective surgery brings a profit of $1,500 to the facility. Each major surgery takes four hours and consumes 15 total hours of labor, each minor surgery takes 0.5 hours and consumes 10 total hours of labor, and each elective surgery takes 2 hours and consumes 12 total hours of labor. Finally, we will assume the facility has only one operating room, which is available 40 hours per week, and the facility has a total of 410 labor hours a week that can be devoted to surgeries.

Our problem formulation becomes (Equations 8.5 to 8.10):

$$maximize \ z = 2000s_1 + 800s_2 + 1500s_3 \quad \text{(objective function)} \quad (8.5)$$

$$subject \ to: \quad 4s_1 + 0.5s_2 + 2s_3 \leq 40 \quad \text{(operating room constraint)} \quad (8.6)$$

$$15s_1 + 10s_2 + 12s_3 \leq 410 \ \text{(labor constraint)} \quad (8.7)$$

$$s_3 \leq 4 \quad \text{(elective surgery constraint)} \quad (8.8)$$

$$s_1, s_2, s_3 \geq 0 \quad \text{(non-negativity constraint)} \quad (8.9)$$

$$s_1, s_2, s_3 \ \text{integer} \quad \text{(integer constraint)} \quad (8.10)$$

FIGURE 8.6   Excel Formulation for Health Care Example

	A	B	C	D	E	F
1	decision variables	s1	s2	s3	z=objective Function	
2		0	0	0	0	
3						
4						RHS
5	opearing room constraint	4	0.5	2	0	40
6	labor constraint	15	10	12	0	410
7	elective surgery constraint	0	0	1	0	4
8						

In order to utilize Solver, we must set up the formulation (Equations 8.5 to 8.10) in Excel. There are many ways to do this, one of which is indicated in Figure 8.6.

In Figure 8.6, values of 0 are entered for the three decision variables initially into cells B2, C2, and D2. The formula for the objective function z (see Equation 8.5), provided in cell E2 of the figure, is $=2000*B2 + 800*C2 + 1500*D2$. The values in the cell block B5 to D7 are the coefficients for each constraint and are taken directly from Equations 8.6 through 8.8. The values in cells F5 to F7 are the right-hand side (RHS) values of the constraints, and are also taken from Equations 8.6 through 8.8. The values in cells E5 to E7 show as zeros in Figure 8.6, but each of those three cells contains a formula based on the equation each constraint represents.

The formula for cell E5 is $=B5*\$B\$2 + C5*\$C\$2 + D5*\$D\$2$. By providing the constraint coefficients in cells B5 to D7, we are able to have more flexibility in our problem solving. If one of the coefficients changes, we simply change it and the formula for cell E5 is still correct. Also, by using the $ symbol when referring to cells B2, C2, and D2, we are able to drag the formula for cell E5 down to cells E6 and E7. When we do this, the coefficients (B5, C5, D5) change as needed, but the variables (B2, C2, D2) do not. Now that we have our formulation in Excel, we are ready to work with Solver.

To access Solver, go to the Data Menu tab in Excel and click on it. If Solver is already installed as an add-in, it will appear to the far right of the Data Menu. If Solver is not installed, refer to instructions below on how to add it.

LOAD THE SOLVER ADD-IN

The Solver add-in is a Microsoft Office Excel add-in (add-in: a supplemental program that adds custom commands or custom features to Microsoft Office) program that is available when you install Microsoft Office or Excel. To use it in Excel, however, you need to load it first.

1. Click the **Microsoft Office** button in Excel 2007 or the Home menu in Excel 2010 and then click **Excel Options**.

2. Click **Add-Ins**, and then in the **Manage** box, select **Excel Add-ins**.

3. Click **Go**.

4. In the **Add-Ins available** box, select the **Solver Add-in** check box, and then click **OK**.

   Tip: If **Solver Add-in** is not listed in the **Add-Ins available** box, click **Browse** to locate the add-in.

   If you get prompted that the Solver add-in is not currently installed on your computer, click **Yes** to install it.

5. After you load the Solver add-in, the **Solver** command is available in the **Analysis** group on the **Data** tab.

Once you have Solver loaded, you will need to click on Solver, and a Solver Parameters dialogue box like the one in Figure 8.7 will appear. Note that in Figure 8.7, we have already indicated three critical fields for our problem. In the Set Target Cell box, we have indicated cell $E$2, which is the cell containing the formula for our objective function. We have clicked on the Max radio button since we want to maximize our objective function. We have also indicated the decision variable range ($B$2:$D$2) for the By Changing Cells box. This means that so far, we have told Solver our objective function, we have indicated it is a maximization problem we are solving, and we have indicated the decision variables whose values can be modified to solve the problem.

The next step is to add the constraints of Equations 8.6 through 8.8. In order to do that, we must first click on the Add button in the Solver Parameters dialogue box. This will open a new dialogue box, the Add Constraint dialogue box, as in Figure 8.8.

FIGURE 8.7   Solver Parameters Dialogue Box

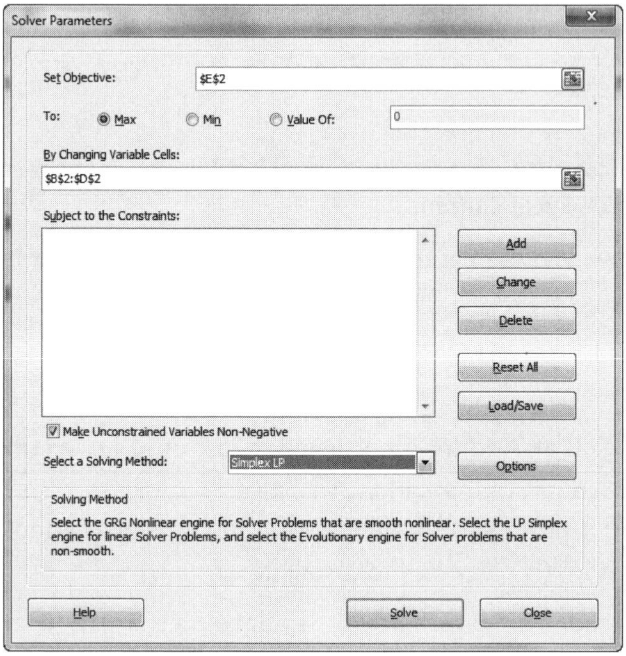

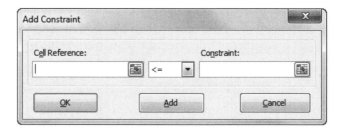

FIGURE 8.8   Add Constraint Dialogue Box

Using the Add Constraint dialogue box, we add the three constraints by referring to the proper cells. For example, for the operating room constraint, we indicate cell $E$5 in the Cell Reference box and cell $F$5 in the Constraint box. The default mathematical symbol between the left-hand side and right-hand side of the constraint is the "≤" sign, so we do not have to alter that. We add all three

FIGURE 8.9 Solver Parameters for Health Care Example

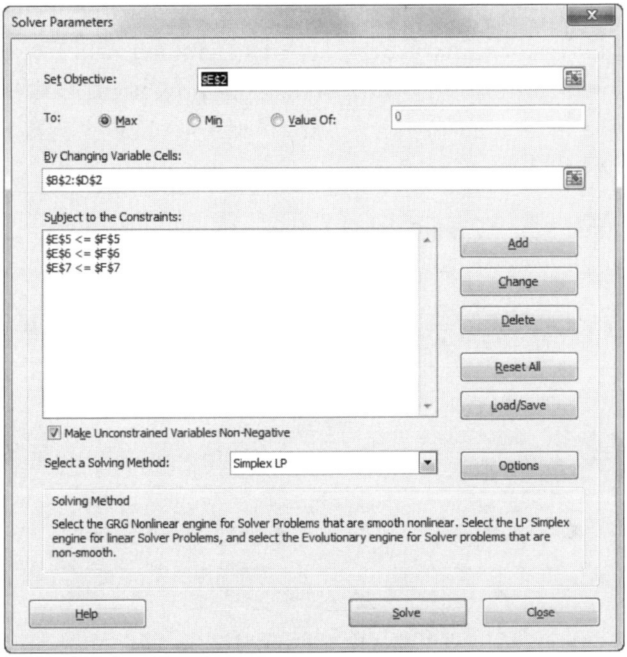

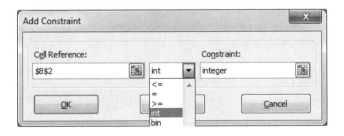

FIGURE 8.10 How to Set Integer Constraints for Health Care Example

constraints and then click OK in the Add Constraint dialogue box. Now our Solver Parameters dialogue box should look like Figure 8.9.

We now have half of our constraints loaded. Remember that we indicated (using Equation 8.10) that we cannot perform partial surgeries, meaning that our decision variables must be integers. In order to add those three constraints, we click on Add in the Solver Parameters dialogue box, and when the Add Constraint dialogue box appears, we provide the appropriate cell reference for each decision variable and indicate "int" using the drop-down menu in the middle of the box.

Figure 8.10 provides an illustration of adding the constraint that decision variable s_1 (whose value is stored in cell $B$2) is integer-valued. Once we click on "int" in the drop-down menu, our Add Constraint dialogue box should look like Figure 8.11.

Now we have loaded all of our constraints. Our Solver Parameters dialogue box should look like Figure 8.12.

FIGURE 8.11   Final Step When Setting Integer Constraints

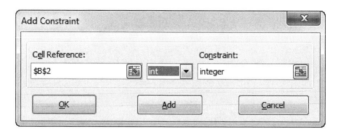

FIGURE 8.12   Final Solver Parameters Dialogue Box for Health Care Example

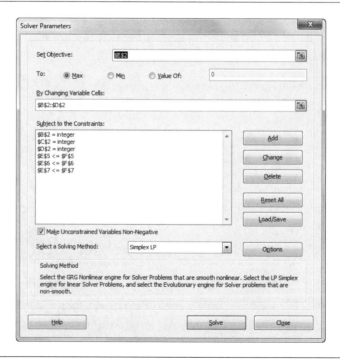

We have one more field whose value we must set in Solver before we can solve the problem. In order to access that field, we need to click on the Options button in the Solver Parameters dialogue box. Once we do that, the Solver Options dialogue box will appear. As indicated in Figure 8.13, we need to uncheck the check box for Ignore Integer Constraints. This will ensure that our model matches the model of Equations 8.5 through 8.10.

Now we are ready to solve. We do this by clicking on the Solve button in the Solver Parameters dialogue box. Once we click Solve, we will notice that Solver has determined optimal integer values for our three decision variables. Those values are $s_1 = 4$, $s_2 = 30$, and $s_3 = 4$. Solver also provides us with the optimal objective function value, which is \$38,000. Thus, in order to optimize use of this operating room subject to the constraints provided, we would want to perform four major surgeries, 30 minor surgeries, and four elective surgeries per week, for a profit of \$38,000.

FIGURE 8.13   Solver Options Dialogue Box

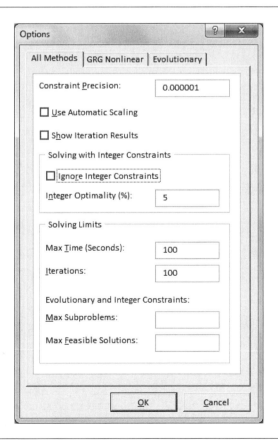

FIGURE 8.14 Final Results for Solver for Health Care Example

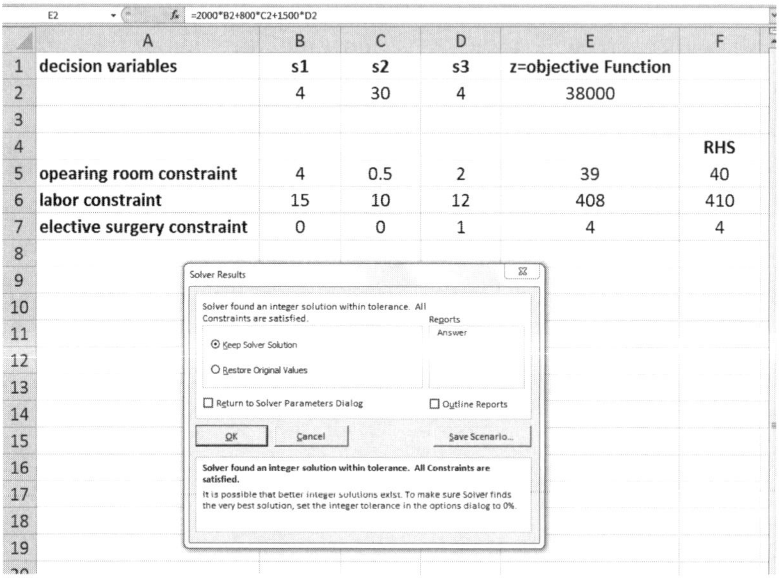

Note that in Figure 8.14 we have a Solver Results dialogue box. In most cases, we would want to click on the Keep Solver Solution radio button in order to preserve the solution we just obtained. Solver also is capable of generating reports, as indicated by the list in the right-hand side of the Solver Results dialogue box. Details on these reports are not provided here, as they are beyond the scope of this book.

OPTIMIZING FACILITY LAYOUT AND DESIGN

For this section, we focus on optimization of process-oriented layouts, since those have the most relevance in health care facilities. As a general rule, it is a good idea to try to minimize the cost of material (patient) handling when optimizing a process layout. This can be done by locating departments with large flows of parts or people between them next to each other.

Let us formulate an optimization problem for layout design with the objective of minimizing a function that is a combination of the number of people moved and the cost of moving them. Keep in mind that the cost we are talking about is the distance-related cost of moving the patient. The further the move, the higher the cost, whether the cost is measured in dollars or time or some other unit.

If we let:

n = total number of departments or work areas

i, j = individual departments

X_{ij} = number of patients moved from department i to department j

C_{ij} = cost to move a patient between department i and department j

our objective function can be given by Equation 8.11:

$$\text{Minimize cost} = \sum_{i=1}^{n} \sum_{j=1}^{n} C_{ij} X_{ij} \qquad (8.11)$$

Given values for the variables listed, we could attempt to use linear programming software to determine an optimal layout; however, we would be successful only if the number of departments, n, was small. When $n = 20$, there are over 600 trillion different possible layouts (Heizer and Render 2004), so it is not possible for a computer program to evaluate and compare all possible layouts.

However, for layout problems involving up to 40 departments, there is software available that can provide good solutions. For example, the Computerized Relative Allocation of Facilities Technique (CRAFT) applies search heuristics to determine good solutions that are feasible. CRAFT systematically evaluates different layout alternatives to find one with low cost. CRAFT cannot guarantee optimality, but it has been shown to perform well (Heizer and Render 2004).

Although determining the optimal layout for an example from health care would require software not covered in this text, there are some lessons that can be learned from applying the cost function of Equation 8.11 to a small health care example.

An Example from Health Care

Consider an outpatient surgery center that is located in a rectangular building that is 90 feet by 50 feet. There are six departments, each of which is 30 feet by 25 feet in size. Using the from-to matrix in Table 8.7, the center was able to

TABLE 8.7 Patient Traffic per Week

	Registration	Exam	Operating	Recovery	Labs/Tests	X-Ray
Registration		100	20	0	40	10
Exam			50	0	20	20
Operating				70	0	0
Recovery					5	5
Labs/tests						20
X-ray						

FIGURE 8.15 Possible Department Layout

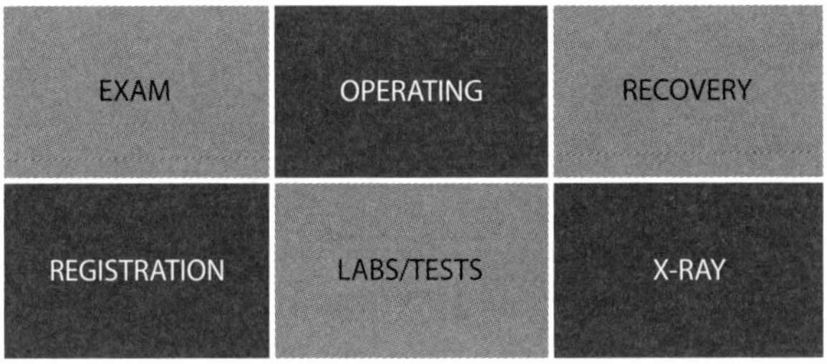

determine the traffic (patients per week) that typically flows among the six departments. An initial layout, which may or may not be optimal, is provided in Figure 8.15. The initial layout was created using the data from Table 8.7 and locating departments with heavy patient flows between them next to each other.

For the proposed layout of Figure 8.15, we can determine its cost using the variables and objective function provided before. We restate them here for clarity:

n = total number of departments or work areas ($n = 6$ for our example)

i, j = individual departments (i = 1 to 6, j = 1 to 6)

X_{ij} = number of patients moved from department i to department j (Table 8.7)

C_{ij} = cost to move a patient between department i and department j (see below)

$$\text{Minimize cost} = \sum_{i=1}^{n} \sum_{j=1}^{n} C_{ij}X_{ij}$$

TABLE 8.8 Patient Movement Costs

From	To	Cost
Registration	Exam	$5 × 100 = $500
Registration	Operating	$5 × 20 = $100
Registration	Recovery	$10 × 0 = $0
Registration	Labs/tests	$5 × 40 = $200
Registration	X-ray	$10 × 10 = $100
Exam	Operating	$5 × 50 = $250
Exam	Recovery	$10 × 0 = $0
Exam	Labs/tests	$5 × 20 = $100
Exam	X-ray	$10 × 20 = $200
Operating	Recovery	$5 × 70 = $350
Operating	Labs/tests	$5 × 0 = $0
Operating	X-ray	$5 × 0 = $0
Recovery	Labs/tests	$5 × 5 = $25
Recovery	X-ray	$5 × 5 = $25
Labs/tests	X-ray	$5 × 20 = $100

For simplicity's sake, let us assume that moving a patient between adjacent departments costs $5 and moving a patient between nonadjacent departments costs $10. Rooms located diagonally to one another are considered adjacent (Heizer and Render 2004). Table 8.8 provides the cost of patient movements for the data values of Table 8.7 and the proposed layout of Figure 8.15.

Our cost is just the sum of the costs in the last column of Table 8.8:

$$\text{Cost} = \$500 + \$100 + \$200 + \$100 + \$250 + \$100 + \$200 + \$350 + \$25$$
$$+ \$25 + \$100$$
$$= \$1,950$$

In order to determine the optimal configuration in terms of minimizing cost, we would need to specify all 36 decision variables (X_{ij}) and all 36 cost coefficients (C_{ij}) and utilize a software package such as Solver.

Health Insurance Portability and Accessibility Act and Optimal Facility Design

Although the *Health Insurance Portability and Accessibility Act (HIPAA)* of 1996 does not impose regulations on facility design, it does have implications that may affect both the layout and the location of employee workstations (www.wbdg.org /design/health_care.php). Privacy must be ensured for all areas where employees deal with medical records and various patient information. HIPAA also impacts patient accommodations, as its regulations place an emphasis on acoustic and visual privacy (Konz 1985).

While it may be straightforward for hospital personnel to ensure visual privacy, acoustic privacy is a bit more complex. As explained in (www.acoustics bydesign.com/venues/hipaa-speech.htm), there are privacy consultants at work in the United States who analyze acoustics of soon-to-be-built medical facilities using acoustical modeling software. Their goal is to ensure that a building's design will not have a negative impact on HIPAA speech privacy compliance. For medical buildings already in existence, these same consultants employ acoustic measurement technology and modeling techniques to analyze the current situation and assess possible solutions if there are concerns about HIPAA compliance.

Additionally, as indicated in Ruano (2003), HIPAA also requires security of those physical components of a facility's infrastructure that support information management. This include facilities. Ruano emphasizes that facilities must protect information by preventing natural elements from damaging the equipment where data are stored. A properly designed facility will provide barriers to unauthorized access. The overall design of medical facilities should be secure and offer protection to employees, equipment, utilities, and other required services.

SUMMARY

This chapter has provided breadth and depth on topics related to facility layout, particularly health care facility layout. Details on various types of layouts were provided, with emphasis on process-oriented layouts that are prevalent in health care facilities. We introduced Muther diagrams as a tool to aid in layout decision making, discussed the evaluation of layouts, and detailed a health care example utilizing the flow criterion of aisles. The chapter introduced the topic of optimization, and presented a detailed description of how to perform optimization using the Excel add-in Solver. This was followed by a section on optimization of facility layout and design, which utilized an example from health care (design of a surgery center).

KEY TERMS

facility layout

Health Insurance Portability and
    Accessibility Act (HIPAA)

Muther diagram

optimization

process-oriented layout

product-oriented layout

DISCUSSION QUESTIONS

1. List six to eight things you need to consider when designing a health care facility.

2. Provide an example of a health care facility you have been in recently whose design could be improved, and explain how it could be improved.

3. In the process of creating a Muther diagram, what are some key questions to consider? Who should be asked these questions?

4. For a health care setting in which you have worked (or any one with which you are familiar), create a Muther diagram for the facility.

5. Consider the discussion of office layout in the chapter. Sketch an optimal design of your working space (office) at home. Clearly indicate placement of different tools, equipment, and so on that you use.

6. When determining which layout is better (Figure 8.2 or Figure 8.3), what would you factor into your decision? What other aspects of the hospital's delivery of care should you factor in?

7. Create a measurable and meaningful criterion to use in evaluating the design of a health care facility. Clearly indicate the information that would be needed to be able to compare two different designs.

8. Use Solver to find the optimal solution to the given integer programming problem.

    Consider the same operating room discussed in the Solver example in the chapter. Suppose that instead of maximizing profit from surgeries, our objective is to minimize the cost incurred due to surgeries. As before, we denote the number of major surgeries scheduled in a week using decision variable s_1, the number of minor surgeries scheduled in a week using decision variable s_2, and the number of elective surgeries scheduled in a week using decision variable s_3.

The relevant data for each type of surgery is:

Surgery Type	Cost	Operating Room Time	Labor Hours
Major (s_1)	$5,500	4 hours	15
Minor (s_2)	$3,000	0.5 hour	10
Elective (s_3)	$4,000	2 hours	12

In addition, for this problem we will assume the facility has only one operating room, which is available 60 hours per week, and the facility has a total of 500 labor hours a week that can be devoted to surgeries.

Prior to using Solver, you may want to formulate your problem (i.e., clearly identify decision variables, objective function, and constraints).

REFERENCES

www.acousticsbydesign.com/venues/hipaa-speech.htm.

www.ateneonline.it/chase2e/studenti/tn/6184–7_tn05.pdf.

www.cbpa.ewu.edu/~pnemetzmills/OMch5/OMFAC.html.

Dowling, R. A., and C. G. Cotner. 1988. "Monitor of Tray Error Rates for Quality Control." *Journal of American Dietetic Association* 88 (4): 450–453.

Gantz, S. P., and R. B. Petit. 1953. "Plant Layout Efficiency." *Modern Materials Handling* 9 (1):65–67.

Heizer, J., and B. Render. 2004. *Principles of Operations Management.* Upper Saddle River, NJ: Pearson Prentice Hall.

Konz, S. A. 1985. *Facility Design.* New York: John Wiley & Sons.

Lin, L. C., and G. P. Sharp. 1999. "Quantitative and Qualitative Indices for the Plant Layout Evaluation Problem." *European Journal of Operational Research* 116:100–117.

Murty, K. 1983. *Linear Programming.* New York: John Wiley & Sons.

Muther, R. 1973. *Systematic Layout Planning.* Boston: Cahners Books.

Nocedal, J., and S. Wright. 1999. *Numerical Optimization.* New York: Springer.

OR/MS Today. 2011. "Linear Programming Survey." (June). Downloaded from www.orms-today.org/surveys/LP/LP-survey.html.

Ruano, Michael. 2003. "Physical Security and HIPAA: What You Need to Know." *In Confidence* 11 (12): 3.

Tompkins, J., J. White, Y. Bozer, and J. Tanchoco. 2003. *Facilities Planning.* 3rd ed. Hoboken, NJ: John Wiley & Sons.

Ulrich, R. 2006. "Evidence-Based Health-Care Architecture." *Lancet* 368:538–539.

www.wbdg.org/design/health_care.php.

PART III

MANAGING

HEALTH CARE

OPERATIONS

QUALITY

CHAPTER 9

MANAGING QUALITY IN A HEALTH CARE SETTING

LEARNING OBJECTIVES

➠ Understand what service quality is and how it is manifested in the health care industry.

➠ Know the concept of quality planning, control, and improvement.

➠ Understand the link between quality and financial performance.

➠ Understand the seven quality tools and how they are applied to health care.

(Continued)

⟼ Understand the concepts of six sigma and how they are applied to health care.

⟼ Understand how lean and six sigma are combined and how they impact health care.

WHAT IS SERVICE QUALITY?

In many cases, the definition of service quality encompasses the identification and satisfaction of customer needs and requirements. Some define service quality as the difference between expected service (patient expectations) and perceived service (patient perceptions). Expectations can be viewed as the patients' wants that they feel a provider should offer. Perceptions are viewed as the patients' evaluation of the service provider or the service provided.

Service quality has also been divided into two categories: functional quality and technical quality. Functional quality is the manner in which the service is delivered to the patient. Patients tend to rely on functional aspects of health care (hospital personnel attitude, quality of food, facility cleanliness, etc.) when evaluating service quality.

Technical Quality

Technical quality is based on technical accuracy and correct procedure. Appropriate medical diagnoses, compliance with professional specifications, and proper testing are all examples of technical quality. Competence of the medical staff, including the surgeons' operating skills and the nurses' familiarity with drug administration, is also considered technical quality.

Functional Quality

However, few patients rely on technical quality when evaluating service quality. Most patients rely on functional quality. Although technical quality is by nature a high priority with patients, many patients are unable to truly evaluate technical quality due to lack of expertise. It is more prevalent for patients to base their evaluation of quality on interpersonal and environmental factors. It is said that patients lean on the caring side of health care instead of the curing side of health care when evaluating service quality.

QUALITY PLANNING, CONTROL, AND IMPROVEMENT

Not only is quality in health care increasingly identified as the main factor in distinguishing between providers and building competitive advantage, but it is also identified through billing transactions and how a health care organization is paid for offering their services (i.e., federal government, Medicare, etc.). However, the health care industry carries with it very high risks, which sets health care service quality planning, control, and improvement apart from other industries.

These risks make planning, controlling, and improving quality in health care more important and more complex. Quality, functional as well as technical, has proven to be a vital element in a patient's choice of hospitals. In turn, health care organizations must embark on continuous efforts to improve the quality service delivery system. However, quality will not improve unless it is properly planned, measured, and controlled. A few strategies to plan, measure, and control quality are:

- Use service quality principles; focus on the patient, not clinicians or institutions.

- Identify and eliminate all steps that do not add value for the patient. (*Note:* Removing wasteful steps not only can increase patient satisfaction and staff satisfaction but also can reduce costs.)

- Support for health care employees and staff from upper management begets improved service quality. The organization's leaders must allocate resources and create systems of reward and compensation for employees and staff that are aligned with the quality mission.

- Create an effective service recovery program that provides action on the spot to resolve problems.

- Partners within the health care supply chain must also be included in the organization's quality mission. In a sense, the health care organization's quality is only as good as its weakest link, and that weakest link should not be a supply chain partner.

- By understanding and simplifying the processes of care, controlling quality, and eliminating waste, cost will be lowered. It has been documented in many other industries (e.g., hospitality management and retailing) that proper planning, control, and continuous improvement in service quality have delivered higher value at lower costs while increasing profit margins.

QUALITY AND FINANCIAL PERFORMANCE

It has been proposed that improving the level of quality reduces operating costs. The quality movement in U.S. manufacturing began in the 1980s and had significant impacts on bottom-line costs.

It can be said that in many health care entities the subject of quality impacting financial performance was not widely discussed unless patient satisfaction numbers decreased. For most clinicians, pleasing patients, improved outcomes, improved clinician satisfaction, and better patient care are the goals and objectives that motivate. However, for administrators and executives, it is all of those areas as well as efficiency with lower costs.

As of late, many entities (business, government, insurance companies) are approaching hospitals to improve quality. In addition, many hospital financial managers rely on the improvements of quality programs as a key to survival and literally a means to get paid.

It has been noted that poor service often involves repetition and misuse of skilled employees, or in other words defects in the service process. These defects raise costs in terms of wasted efforts and resources.

Waste and redundancy are very costly to organizations. American industry finds waste unacceptable as it faces new, aggressive global competition. Almost all manufacturing firms practice continuous improvement, apply the seven principles of quality to everyday operations, and implement in some fashion the tenets of six sigma. Competitive pressures are on the rise in health care not only from other health care organizations, but also from government and business. There is strong evidence that these methods will not only increase patient satisfaction but will also contribute to lower costs. The seven principles of quality along with the principles of six sigma and how they relate to the health care industry are presented in the next main section.

Healthcare Ops and SCM in Action: Service Quality in Surgical Handovers

How are a hospital and a Formula One racing pit crew related? Great Ormond Street Hospital for Children (GOSH) in London, England, and the Ferrari Formula One race car team from Italy teamed up to help each other benchmark their handoff procedures: cardiac care surgery from GOSH and pit stop techniques from the Ferrari team.

Why Benchmark and Why Handovers?

GOSH did not set out to benchmark against anyone, let alone a Formula One pit crew. The link came when two doctors sat down to relax after a long day in surgery. Formula One racing was on TV as they began to wind down, and it dawned on them that a pit stop where a crew changed tires, added fuel, and made other quick modifications looked a lot like what they did when they hand over in surgery (e.g., surgeons, anesthetist, and intensive care unit [ICU] staff transferring the patient, equipment, and information safely and quickly from the operating room to the ICU). The two doctors recognized the importance of teamwork in a highly risky pit stop operation and made the link to their handover process.

Watching the pit crew, the GOSH doctors noticed the value of process mapping, process description, and trying to work out what people's tasks should be. They learned the keys to a successful pit stop:

- The routine in the pit stop is taken seriously.

- What happens in the pit stop is predictable, so problems can be anticipated and procedures can be standardized.

- Crews practice those procedures until they can perform them perfectly.

- Everyone knows his or her job, but one person is always in charge.

In contrast, the GOSH process was more reactive. The medical team's strategy was to wait until something went wrong and then to work out the problem. The GOSH team videotaped their surgery handover and sent it to be reviewed by the Formula One team. The GOSH research team and observers from the Formula One team analyzed the film and noted a great difference in the process map (flowchart). The hospital's process was much longer due to the level of complexity of the medical process. From the analysis came a new 12-page handover protocol. A laminated copy of the protocol was attached at the bedside. If a staff member had not received training in the new process or if someone needed a quick refresher, the posted protocol could be quickly read through.

What Was Learned

Approximately 30 percent of the patient errors occurred in both equipment and information before the new handover protocol was introduced. After the new handover protocol was in place, only 10 percent of the patient errors occurred in those areas. It was also found that the hospital's reaction to the success of the benchmarking effort was very interesting. What made the entire process rewarding was that hospital employees not only were excited that they had improved but they also pushed for continuing improvement.

—This "in action" section was developed from a research paper by Catchpole et al. (2007)

SEVEN TOOLS FOR QUALITY CONTROL

The seven tools for quality control, referred to as the *7 QC tools*, were the work of Kauro Ishikawa. Ishikawa believed that the vast majority of quality issues could be addressed, analyzed, and solved using these seven tools.

The 7 QC tools are: check sheets, flowcharts, cause-and-effect or fishbone diagrams, histograms, Pareto diagrams, scatter diagrams, and control charts.

Check Sheets

Check sheets are a structured form for collecting and analyzing data. A check sheet is a generic tool that can be adapted for a wide variety of purposes. A check sheet minimizes the chance of different users collecting data in different ways. It also forces the quality team to consciously ponder what data to collect, why they are collecting data at all, and what the team plans to do with the data once collected (see Figure 9.1).

Elements of a check sheet include:

- Description of the data being collected.
- Blanks or spaces to enter the data.

FIGURE 9.1 Check Sheet for Admission Delays

Project: Admission Delays				Name:			Shift:	
Location: Emergency Room				Date of Checklist:				
	Date of Delay							
Reason	6/1	6/2	6/3	6/4	6/5	6/6	6/7	Total
Lab Delays	9	4	6	6	3	12	12	52
No Beds Available	2	7	2	4	5	8	3	31
Incomplete Information	2	1	4	7	2	4	5	25
~~	~~~~	~~~~	~~~~	~~~~	~~~~	~~~~	~~~~	~~~~~
Improper Coding	7	3	1	2	2	4	5	24
Total	33	28	36	30	25	47	38	237

- Room for comments.
- Room for descriptive statistical analysis.

Key points to remember when constructing check sheets include:

- Keep the form simple and easy to understand.
- Include only information that you intend to use.
- Pilot test the check sheet before using it on a full scale.

Flowcharts

Flowcharts illustrate the flow of a process. At times they can be referred to as process maps and literally show a picture of a process. Figure 9.2 displays an example of a flowchart for a patient check-in and to room process for a health care facility.

Systems are made up of smaller activities that culminate in an outcome. For a health care facility this could be the check-in process or prescription process. Processes take up time, space, and resources. As health care professionals it is important to begin to characterize processes into their three categories: value-added, non-value-added, and non-value-added but necessary.

From a patient's perspective, these three categories can be described as:

1. *Value-added*—adds form, function, and value (tangible or intangible) to the end product or service and to the patient (e.g., a prescription for antibiotics).

FIGURE 9.2 Example Flowchart for Patient Check-In and to Room Process

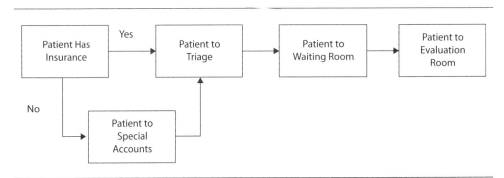

2. *Non-value-added*—does not add form, function, or value to the finished product or service.

3. *Non-value-added but necessary*—does not add value, but may add form or function that is necessary to attain the final value-added product or service.

Process Cycle Efficiency

Process cycle efficiency is defined as the ratio of value-added time to total cycle time. This metric assists in identifying how much of a process actually adds value. It requires the following six steps to compute:

1. Map the process using a flowchart.

2. Identify the value-added steps, non-value-added steps, and the non-value-added but necessary steps.

3. Group the map according to two categories, one for value-added process items and one for non-value-added items.

4. Estimate the time to complete all the activities on the process map.

5. Sum the value-added times and calculate the process cycle time (i.e., the time for the entire process to be completed).

6. Then divide value-added time by cycle time to obtain process cycle efficiency.

For example, we will say for the patient check-in and to room process, the value-added time is 182 seconds and the total cycle time is 860 seconds. Therefore the process cycle efficiency is as shown in Equation 9.1:

$$\text{Process Cycle Efficiency} = \frac{182}{860} = 21\% \qquad (9.1)$$

For the patient check-in example, it can be said that only 21 percent of the process is considered value-added.

Although a very simple exercise, the act of mapping the process and identifying the value-added and non-value-added activities is extremely valuable. This really is the first step into analyzing any process and in turn reducing waste in the process as well as providing a better value and experience for the patient.

Cause-and-Effect or Fishbone Diagram

The *cause-and-effect* or *fishbone diagram* is often referred to by the name of its creator, Kauro Ishikawa. An Ishikawa diagram identifies many possible causes for an effect or a problem and sorts by categories.

The main three components of an Ishikawa diagram, as shown in Figure 9.3, are:

1. At the far right of the diagram (head of the fish) is the defect or deleterious effect, stated in the form of a question. A horizontal line extends from the far right of the diagram to the left of the diagram (the backbone of the fish).

2. Slanted lines extend into the backbone of the diagram. These are considered major bones and are the capstone categories or main groupings of causes.

3. Smaller horizontal lines (typically referred to as minor bones) extend into the major bones from left to right or right to left under each capstone heading.

Common capstone categories do exist. Some common capstone (major bone) categories are:

- People
- Information

FIGURE 9.3 Cause-and-Effect or Fishbone Diagram

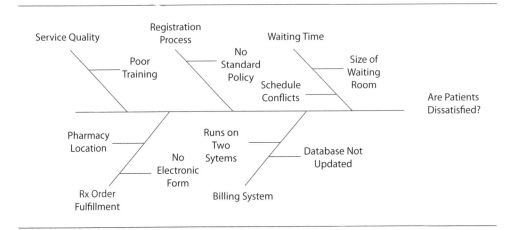

- Equipment

- Methods/procedures

- Environment

- Material

After completing the diagram, it is critically important that you test the logic as a group. Work the bones from top to bottom or bottom to top. For example, logic could follow as: this happens because of J; J happens because of M; and M happens because of Q. If the logic does not work, you have either left a cause out, categorized the cause incorrectly, or misidentified the cause.

Histogram

As was detailed in Chapter 4, *histograms* relate the total number of occurrences for each event in an event space to each other. Each event is represented on the *x*-axis of the histogram while the number of times each event occurs is represented on the *y*-axis. Histograms are very common in everyday life. Many people don't use the term histogram for diagrams depicting the occurrence of events and instead refer to them as graphs.

As a student of health care operations and supply chain management (SCM), you have more than likely seen many histograms throughout your studies.

FIGURE 9.4   Histogram for Delay Times

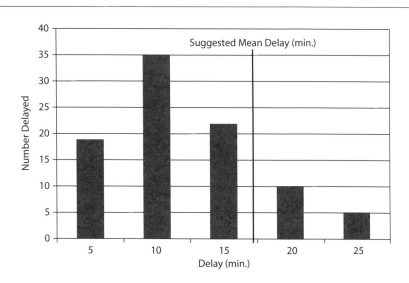

An example could be the distribution of waiting time and the number delayed for any period. A histogram for a daily set of delay times might look something like Figure 9.4.

Histograms are a straightforward, easy-to-construct method of graphical data description that almost everyone understands. All commercial spreadsheet packages have the capability to construct histograms.

Pareto Diagrams

Pareto charts were introduced back in Chapter 4. A *Pareto diagram* or chart is a sorted histogram and is generally shown as a vertical bar graph. The bars represent frequency, and are arranged with the longest bar on the left and the shortest on the right.

The principle is named after Italian economist Vilfredo Pareto, who observed that 80 percent of income in Italy went to 20 percent of the population. Later, Pareto conducted surveys on a number of other countries and found that a similar distribution applied to income in those countries.

Pareto analysis could be characterized as an analytical technique in decision making that is used for the selection of a limited number of tasks that produce significant overall effect. The Pareto Principle, also know as the 80/20 rule,

FIGURE 9.5   Pareto Diagram for Medical Documentation Errors

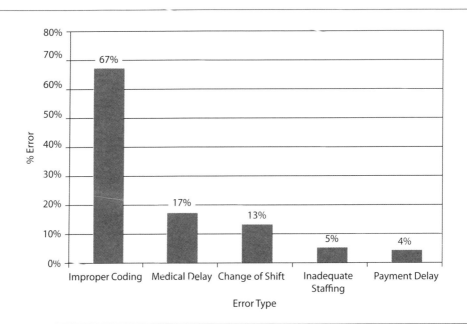

encompasses the notion that by doing 20 percent of the work you can generate 80 percent of the benefit of doing the whole job. Likewise, in terms of quality improvement, a large portion of problems (80 percent) are produced by a few key causes (20 percent). At times these two groups are also referred to as the vital few and the trivial many. Figure 9.5 displays a Pareto diagram for error types in medical documentation.

Scatter Diagrams

Creating a *scatter diagram* is the first step in looking for a relationship between *x* and *y* variables. The scatter diagram graphs data on the *x*-axis and *y*-axis. When the *x* and *y* data are correlated, the points will fall along a line or curve. The more the diagram resembles a straight line, the stronger the correlation and the relationship.

When the diagram shows no relationship, consider whether the independent (*x*-axis) variable varies widely. At times a linear relationship is not apparent because the *y* data points don't cover a large enough range. Think creatively about how to use scatter diagrams to discover a root cause.

FIGURE 9.6   Scatter Diagram of Patients per Day versus Day of the Week

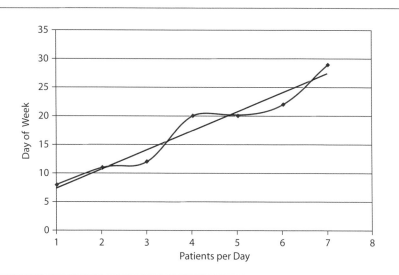

However, it must be noted that even if the scatter diagram shows a relationship, do not assume that one variable caused the other. Both may be influenced by some other variable or variables.

Figure 9.6 displays an example of a scatter plot for patients per day on the *x*-axis versus day of the week on the *y*-axis.

Control Charts

The *control chart* is a graph used to study how a process changes over time. Data are plotted in time order. A control chart always has a central line for the average, an upper line for the upper control limit (UCL), and a lower line for the lower control limit (LCL). These lines are determined from historical data. By comparing current data to these lines, you can draw conclusions about whether the process variation is consistent (in control) or is unpredictable (out of control, affected by special causes of variation). Control charts are a main tool used in statistical process control (SPC).

Control charts for variable data are used in pairs: an x-bar chart and an *R* chart. The x-bar chart monitors the average, or the centering of the distribution of data from the process. The *R* chart monitors the range, or the width of the distribution. Using the analogy of target practice, the average is where your shots are clustering and the range is how tightly they are clustered.

FIGURE 9.7 X-Bar Control Chart Example

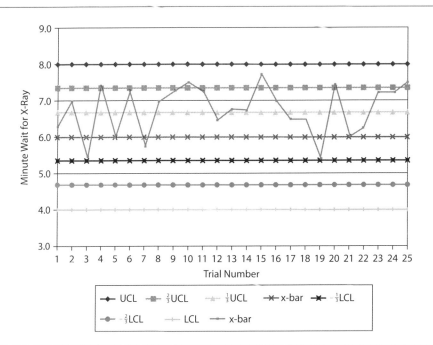

Figure 9.7 displays an x-bar control chart regarding the average wait for a piece of equipment. An abbreviated example of how to create x-bar and R charts is given in the accompanying box. Readers are asked to refer to Chapter 10, as it delves more deeply into quality control and control charting. The concept of six sigma is presented in the next section.

BRIEF EXAMPLE OF X-BAR CONTROL CHART CONSTRUCTION

The following is a step-by-step set of instructions on how to construct an x-bar control chart. R charts are completed in the same manner.

1. Determine what your sample size (n) will be and how many trials you will be conducting. Sample the process using that sample size for the number of trials chosen.

2. Calculate the average of each trial and denote it as $\bar{x}$; also calculate the average of all those averages. Denote this as $\bar{\bar{x}}$. Calculate the range, R (highest

observation value minus lowest observation value), for each sample, and denote this as R. In addition, find the average of all the R's and denote this average as $\bar{R}$. Table 9.1 displays an example of the calculations.

TABLE 9.1 Control Chart Data Set

Trial Number = k	Sample = n					
	1	2	3	$\bar{x}$		R
1	2	3	4	3.00		2.00
2	7	4	6	5.67		3.00
3	2	5	2	3.00		3.00
				$\bar{\bar{x}}$	3.889	$\bar{R}$	2.67

Note: This is a short example; a user would collect more samples and have more trials.

3. Using $\bar{\bar{x}}$ and $\bar{R}$, calculate the process control limits—upper and lower—for the $\bar{x}$ and R charts. These limits are calculated as follows. Use Table 9.2 to locate values for A_2, D_3, and D_4. Remember that n = number of observations. If LCL equals zero, there is no need for construction of the zones below the central line, $\bar{\bar{x}}$. A standard $\bar{x}$ control chart is constructed using the formulas shown in Figure 9.8.

TABLE 9.2 Factors for Determining Control Limits

Sample Size, n	A_2 Factor	D_3 Factor	D_4 Factor
2	1.88	0	3.27
3	1.02	0	2.57
4	0.73	0	2.28
5	0.58	0	2.11
6	0.48	0	2.00
7	0.42	0.08	1.92
8	0.37	0.14	1.86
9	0.34	0.18	1.82
10	0.31	0.22	1.78

4. After construction of the control chart, all sample $\bar{x}$'s should be plotted, with the x-axis being time (or trial number) and the y-axis being in the units of the sample (refer to Table 9.1 or Figure 9.7).

5. Interpret the control chart using the following rules: A process is out of control if any of the following are seen (refer to Figure 9.7):

FIGURE 9.8   Control Chart with Control Limits and Zones

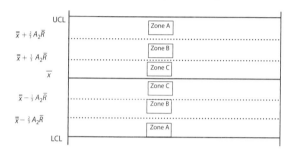

$$\bar{R} = \frac{\Sigma R}{n} \quad \text{and} \quad \bar{x} = \frac{\Sigma x}{n} \text{ and } \bar{\bar{x}} = \frac{\Sigma \bar{x}}{k}$$

For the $\bar{x}$ chart, UCL $= \bar{\bar{x}} + A_2 \bar{R}$ and LCL $= \bar{\bar{x}} - A_2 \bar{R}$

For the R chart, UCL $= D_4 \bar{R}$ and LCL $= D_3 \bar{R}$

- One point beyond the UCL or the LCL.

- Eight points in a row anywhere on one side of the central line.

- Six points in a row steadily increasing or decreasing.

- Fourteen points in a row alternating up and down.

- Two out of three points in a row in Zone A or beyond.

- Four out of five points in a row in Zone B or beyond.

6. An *R* chart should then be constructed using the formulas provided earlier for *R* UCL and *R* LCL. $\bar{R}$ is used as a central line. The *R* chart is then analyzed for trends or points beyond the UCL or LCL. If trends or points beyond the UCL or LCL exist, the process may be out of control or some type of nonrandom cause may have been introduced to the process.

The example presented here is an abbreviated example. Chapter 10 delves more deeply into quality control and control charts.

Quality Principles in a Health Care Organization

Manufacturing firms regularly use quality principles to improve operations, but what about health care organizations? There are many opportunities in health care organizations, but there are also many challenges. Resistance of staff as well as physicians, inefficient communication systems, or even insurance reimbursement processes are all factors that could impact the introduction of quality principles into a health care setting.

One of the nation's top pediatric hospitals, Children's National Medical Center (CNMC) in Washington, D.C., exercises quality principles. For example, Deming's plan-do-check-act cycle, rapid cycle improvement, and failure modes and effects analysis (FMEA) are all employed. Along with many other tools, CNMC promotes quality in all aspects of pediatric care. CNMC's quality model is based on the Institute of Medicine's six aims: safety, effectiveness, efficiency, timeliness, family-centered focus, and equity.

Lessons Learned

It must be noted that success does not come easy. CNMC has identified several important points that have made its quality model successful. The following list of seven lessons learned is provided for others to learn from.

1. Leaders must set the priorities and listen to front-line providers for input.

2. Collaboration at all levels is imperative.

3. Front-line staff must be engaged to make the change.

4. Incentives must be aligned with outcomes.

5. Data must drive the process.

6. Transparency is necessary.

7. Quality must be meaningful and tangible to the provider.

CNMC has seen decreased costs for both the patient and the organization through the implementation of its quality model. In turn, the quality model has become part of its culture and, in a sense, a way of doing business.

—Adapted from Burge (2008)

SIX SIGMA CONCEPTS

Six sigma is designed to significantly reduce organizational inefficiencies and in turn increase profits. The quality improvement methodology was developed and made famous by Motorola in the 1980s. Over the decades since, six sigma has produced significant cost savings and reductions in waste for countless organizations that have embraced it. Motorola developed the methods and implemented them for manufacturing. However, six sigma has expanded into such service industries as the financial sector (Vanguard Group), hospitality (Starwood Hotels & Resorts Worldwide), food processing (PepsiCo), and health care (United Healthcare). Six sigma is even being popularized in the public sector (U.S. military branches) because of its proven track record in private industry.

The concept behind six sigma is to eliminate defects that take time and effort to repair and to eliminate non-value-added aspects of a service that make customers unhappy and waste resources. The overarching management philosophy is to eliminate defects by emphasizing understanding, measuring, and improving processes.

What Does Six Sigma Mean?

The term *six sigma* comes from the statistical concept of six standard deviations away from the mean. At that point processes are working nearly perfectly, delivering only 3.4 defects per million opportunities (DPMO). Standard deviation is a measure of variation (i.e., how much your data set varies from the mean or average; large standard deviations relate to data sets that are spread out around the mean, whereas small standard deviations relate to data sets that are closely grouped around the mean).

For example, if a hospital arrival process were operating at a one sigma level, then that process will produce approximately 690,000 defects per million arrivals or a success rate of only 31 percent. This would be viewed by any health care professional as unacceptable.

Now let's assume the arrival process is operating at a three sigma level. In this case, the process would produce approximately 66,800 defects per million arrivals, delivering a success rate of 93.3 percent. While this level of success is much better, there is still too much waste in the system as well as too many disappointed customers.

Anecdotally it can be said that organizations, manufacturing as well as service, in the United States are operating at three to four sigma quality levels. The losses attributed to this level of success could be up to 25 percent of their total revenues. These losses are somewhat intangible for service industries like health care but would include poor care, return visits, and lost return business.

Six sigma management states that if defects in a process can be measured, there are systematic ways to eliminate them and approach a quality level of zero defects. With that statement in mind, six sigma is the goal, and it is less important than the objective of pursuing continuing process improvement. Six sigma is really an idea or a mind-set. Managers must know the real focus of six sigma is on identifying defects and eliminating their root causes.

Five Phases of Six Sigma Methodology

The *five phases of six sigma* are based on the plan-do-check-act continuous improvement cycle developed by Shewhart and Deming. However, the phases of six sigma are more specific. Figure 9.9 illustrates the two methods juxtaposed with each other.

The five phases are: *define, measure, analyze, improve, and control (DMAIC).* A short definition of each is given next with details following.

1. Define the project goals and customer (internal/external) deliverables.

2. Measure the process to determine current performance. The problem must be quantified.

3. Analyze and determine the root causes of any defects.

FIGURE 9.9 DMAIC Process

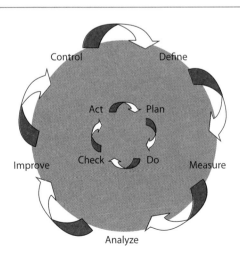

4. Improve the process by eliminating defect root causes.

5. Control future process performance.

Define

For the define phase, the six sigma team selects a project that meets strategic objectives of the organization and meets the needs or requirements of the customer. The project must have a problem to be solved or a process to be improved that has a measurable result. Six sigma projects generally have the following characteristics:

- The project will save or make money for the organization.

- The problem or process being investigated is important to the organization and has a clear link to the organization's strategy.

- Outcomes are measurable.

This phase also contains the definition of project boundaries (project scope—refer to Chapter 13) and process mapping (refer to Chapter 7). In addition, critical to quality (CTQ) characteristics are determined. CTQs are the measurable characteristics of the process that have minimum performance standards per the customer or can be determined by customer desire; for example, all patients want quick service in the emergency room (ER), but a 30-minute or less wait may be the desired standard.

Measure

The measure phase is about documenting the current process, validating the measure of the process, and assessing performance to use as a baseline. Many of the 7 QC tools, such as flowcharts, Pareto diagrams, fishbone diagrams, and scatter plots, are used in the measure phase.

This phase usually gives the user early clues about problems within the process (e.g., 84 percent of patients wait at least 60 minutes in the ER). Metrics for key process output variables (KPOVs) are developed in the measure phase. Key process input variables (KPIVs) are also determined, usually by using a combination of the 7 QC tools (e.g., fishbone or cause-and-effect diagrams and

FIGURE 9.10 Six Sigma DMAIC Process Metrics

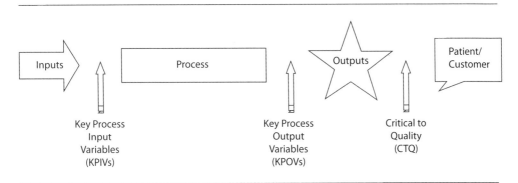

Pareto diagrams). Metrics for the KPIVs are also created and a data collection plan is developed and implemented. Figure 9.10 displays the interrelation of inputs, KPIVs, KPOVs, CTQs, and outputs.

Analyze

The A in DMAIC is about finding the top two or three causes of the problem we are attacking. A well-performed analysis phase begins with input from the team regarding potential causes, and uses statistical methods to isolate the top two or three causes. The most valuable team members to have as part of the team are those who work with the process on a daily basis. Fishbone diagrams as well as Pareto diagrams are a great way to categorize sources of variation.

Isolate the Top Two or Three Causes   One of the most challenging aspects of the analyze phase is if you "can't see the forest for the trees." In other words, it is extremely important to identify the top two or three causes of process variation. Although gathering input from the team is important, the overall goal is to identify the "vital few" causes and eliminate the "trivial many." There are a number of tools to help accomplish this task.

Among the most useful tools we've seen in this area are the Shainin methods (see Shainin and Shainin 1988), hypothesis testing (see Chapter 4), regression analysis (see Chapter 12), and basic design of experiments (DOE). Once the top causes have been identified, they must be confirmed via testing or statistical techniques such as design of experiments.

Improve

Redesigning the process to achieve improved operations is the tenet of the improve phase. The process must be observed with the updated configuration and settings must be implemented before the improve phase is completed. A new baseline with the updated configuration and settings must be made. Common tools in the improve phase include hypothesis testing (refer to Chapter 4), regression analysis (refer to Chapter 12), analysis of variance (ANOVA) (refer to Chapter 4), and simulation (refer to Chapter 6).

Control

Control is the final phase of the DMAIC process. Controlling the critical variables, typically the top two or three that were identified in the analyze and improve phases, is a main goal of the control phase.

The best and longest-lasting product or process design changes generally require no human intervention after the initial change. These types of changes are considered permanent and are the first to consider. For example, if a software change to the patient check-in process adds an error-proofing feature for the desk attendant, the change will be inherent in the software and most likely will not need to be monitored in the future.

However, not all improvements to a process are permanent. Error-proofing or what is sometimes called idiot-proofing a process is the best path to follow. *Poka-yoke* is a Japanese term that captures this notion of mistake-proofing. It must be noted that in error-proofing a process, that fix must be monitored as part of the quality system for the long run. For example, if a testing process takes place in a lab and a new measuring calibration was identified in the improve phase, calibration alarms could be installed on the testing equipment to alert the operator about calibration settings outside acceptable limits.

Poka-yoke can be applied to products, services, as well as processes. A poka-yoke can be as simple as childproof caps for medicine bottles or something as technologically advanced as bar-coding technology in the pharmacy that matches prescriptions with the actual drugs being administered.

Six Sigma Practitioners: Green Belts, Black Belts

Two levels of six sigma practitioners exist: *six sigma black belts* and *six sigma green belts*. Their main charge is to implement process improvement projects within the organization. Green belts and black belts are skilled in the use of the six sigma methodology and tools. In general, black belts complete four weeks of DMAIC in-class training. They are required to demonstrate mastery of the subject matter over a period of four to five months through the completion of projects and an exam.

Green belts have less knowledge of six sigma than black belts have. Green belts complete two weeks of DMAIC in-class training. In addition, over a period of three months green belts are expected to complete a project and an exam. Black belts usually spend 100 percent of their time on six sigma projects, whereas green belts normally devote 25 to 50 percent of their time to six sigma projects.

Misconceptions Regarding Six Sigma

It is a common misconception that only large corporations or organizations with hefty budgets can embark on six sigma. Though large organizations may have the money to pull from a large workforce to train thousands of black belts and green belts, medium and small companies can benefit immensely by securing top management support and training even one employee. It is important to remember that six sigma is not an absolute; it is a vision for continually improving processes and organizations.

SIX SIGMA AND LEAN

At the heart of six sigma is the reduction in costs and the reduction or even elimination of defects. However, six sigma is not as effective in reducing process lead times and variation in the amount of time it takes to complete a process. The reason lies in the heart of six sigma in that it does not focus heavily on reducing process time. Savings from reduction in process time are usually a by-product of reducing defects or waste in the system.

The hallmark of lean is to improve process speed. In order to accelerate improvement, organizations must use both lean and six sigma simultaneously. Six sigma will bring processes under statistical control, and lean will improve process speed. Lean six sigma can help to reduce costs so that the financial issues of the health care system are more transparent.

Processes within health care organizations can always be improved upon. For example, take the case of running lab reports and tests for health care providers.

In most cases, lab reports and tests are performed by individuals at a computer. The lab reports and tests are expensive to run, and human error is always a factor. Six sigma assists in analyzing the lab and testing system and may lead to automation of some of these critical processes. Automation will lead to less human error, which in turn leads to reduced costs. In the case of lean, resources are often limited in health care organizations. Items such as lab equipment are extremely expensive, and with tight budgets there may not be enough resources to purchase additional equipment. The lack of equipment slows down productivity and causes patients to have to wait. The principles behind lean will lead an organization to find ways to make the most of the resources at hand and get the most productivity. Solutions may include repairing broken equipment rather than buying new items, or redesigning an entire patient floor to make things flow more smoothly.

Lean Six Sigma and the Health Care Industry

The tenets of lean six sigma are a fundamental break from Western management ideology. This should not be looked upon as a disadvantage. Western management ideology has consisted of three basic and simplified assumptions:

1. Organizations need to be hierarchical in structure and to maintain a separation between thinking and doing in order to effectively and efficiently perform certain procedures.

2. Defects are inevitable and almost impossible to avoid.

3. Inventory is necessary and important for buffering fluctuations in production. It also provides the health care industry with several basic and standardized solutions for many of its organizational and procedural issues.

Health care organizations are guilty of at least two of these assumptions. The structure of health care organizations is hierarchical, and inventory has been needed in that without it health care professionals could not get their jobs done (i.e., stock up so as to not run out). As far as defects go, obviously the health care system does not assume that when it comes to patients' lives defects are inevitable and okay. However, when it comes to defects or breakdowns in the service process (e.g., extremely long wait times for the ER, improper billing, or inadequate information systems) the health care industry does not have a very good record of ferreting out those defects and taking corrective action.

Lean six sigma provides health care organizations with basic and standardized solutions for addressing process problems. The 7 QC tools coupled with the DMAIC phases and used in conjunction with lean allow a health care organization to define, measure, analyze, improve, and control almost any medical process, whether the process is scheduling of nursing staff or the registration process in the ER. Not only will the complexity and time of the process be reduced, but also the provider can still maintain focus on the patients and serve them with higher overall quality. Chapter 10 contains more on the concept of lean.

SUMMARY

This chapter has presented general topics in quality management within a health care setting. Service quality, quality planning, control, and improvement, along with quality's link to financial performance, were discussed. In addition, the 7 QC tools were detailed and applied to health care. The concepts of six sigma were introduced and followed with a discussion of how they are applied to health care as well as how lean and six sigma can improve health care operations and supply chain management.

Service quality encompasses the identification and satisfaction of customer needs and requirements. Some define service quality as the difference between expected service (patient expectations) and perceived service (patient perceptions). Health care organizations must embark on continuous efforts to improve the quality of the service delivery system. Quality will not improve unless it is properly planned, measured, and controlled.

As of late, many entities (business, government, insurance companies) are approaching hospitals to improve quality. Waste and redundancy are very costly to organizations. Almost all manufacturing firms practice continuous improvement, apply the seven principles of quality to everyday operations, and implement in some fashion the tenets of six sigma. There is strong evidence that these methods will not only increase patient satisfaction but also contribute to lower costs.

The seven tools for quality control, referred to as the 7 QC tools, were the work of Kauro Ishikawa. The 7 QC tools are: check sheets, flowcharts, cause-and-effect or fishbone diagrams, histograms, Pareto diagrams, scatter diagrams, and control charts. At the heart of six sigma is the reduction in costs and the reduction or even elimination of defects. The hallmark of lean is to improve process speed. In order to accelerate improvement, organizations must use both lean and six sigma simultaneously. Six sigma will bring processes under statistical control, and lean will improve process speed.

Readers are encouraged to peruse the reference section at the end of the chapter for further readings on quality control, six sigma, and lean. Deming 1986, Ficalora et al. 2004, Shainin and Shainin 1988, and Shewhart 1939 are all considered to be within the traditional quality control genre, whereas the publications by Barry et al. 2002, Bisgaard 2009, and Kelly 1999 are all works that apply traditional quality control to the health care industry.

KEY TERMS

cause-and-effect or fishbone diagrams

check sheets

control charts

define, measure, analyze, improve, and control
    (DMAIC)

five phases of six sigma

flowcharts

histograms

Pareto diagrams

scatter diagrams

7 QC tools

six sigma

six sigma black belt

six sigma green belt

DISCUSSION QUESTIONS

1. Thirty patients have been tracked as they move through the Medical Direct off-site emergency department. The overall process times are listed in the following table:

Patient #	Process Time (min.)	Patient #	Process Time (min.)
1	28	16	15
2	25	17	56
3	57	18	64
4	82	19	46

Patient #	Process Time (min.)	Patient #	Process Time (min.)
5	90	20	54
6	13	21	16
7	31	22	55
8	73	23	36
9	16	24	42
10	81	25	67
11	76	26	39
12	51	27	16
13	8	28	63
14	64	29	69
15	17	30	54

a. Create a histogram for the data using 5 as the bin width.

b. Create a histogram for the data using 10 as the bin width.

2. The final bills for 40 patients have been collected for a clinic. The overall process times are listed in the following table:

Patient #	Average Clinic Bill	Patient #	Average Clinic Bill
1	$34.76	21	$35.22
2	$45.11	22	$64.52
3	$32.50	23	$27.56
4	$47.21	24	$67.04
5	$102.79	25	$95.31
6	$41.91	26	$31.39
7	$84.64	27	$86.27
8	$37.79	28	$23.76
9	$73.20	29	$78.89
10	$21.68	30	$61.50
11	$85.02	31	$54.23
12	$33.04	32	$61.84
13	$53.36	33	$63.48
14	$38.68	34	$56.67
15	$48.02	35	$82.43
16	$30.79	36	$42.72
17	$17.42	37	$99.33
18	$72.48	38	$45.11
19	$16.63	39	$97.51
20	$30.48	40	$65.35

a. Create a histogram for the data using 10 as the bin width.

b. Create a histogram for the data using 5 as the bin width.

3. The XYZ Clinic is experiencing delays in its accounts receivable. In other words, customers don't pay on time. The clinic has heard that some customers can't pay or they move and don't get the bill sent to their new address. However, there could be many other causes for these delays. Help XYZ develop a fishbone diagram of the accounts receivable dilemma.

4. Create a Pareto diagram from the data in question 2.

5. Memorial Community Hospital runs a day clinic to help patients with minor medical issues. In general, a patient walks into the clinic and registers with a booking clerk. Next, either the patient goes through triage or, if the patient called ahead, he or she goes straight to the main waiting area. Patients who go to triage must wait in another area until seen by a triage nurse; then they are allowed to enter the main waiting room. After some time in the waiting room, the patient is called to see a provider and walks down the hall to an exam room, where a provider sees each patient and gives care. After care is given, the patient exits the exam room, moves to the billing area, and then is called to pay the bill. Upon bill payment (by either cash, credit, or insurance), the patient leaves. Help Memorial Community Hospital flowchart its day clinic process.

6. Jan has noticed that the Blueville Clinic's stockroom is a mess. She sees items that are out of place, items not marked with ID tags, items not unloaded from boxes yet, and items that do not belong to the clinic, as well as many other discrepancies. Jan thinks she could draw a cause-and-effect or fishbone diagram to help her understand why the stockroom is so messed up. Help Jan draw a cause-and-effect diagram for the stockroom's problems.

7. Create a Pareto diagram from the data in question 1.

8. A pharmacy has mapped out its prescription filling process. The pharmacists identified that the total cycle time is on average 27 minutes. The process is broken down into eight steps: (1) patient checks in with pharmacy clerk, (2) pharmacy clerk pulls up order from system or checks customer's paperwork (i.e., handwritten prescription), (3) pharmacy clerk checks with pharmacist regarding dosage and drug preference, (4) pharmacist fills order, (5)

patient waits, (6) pharmacy clerk releases order, (7) pharmacy clerk contacts customer that order is filled, and (8) customer pays for order. The time to complete each step and whether it adds value is listed in the following table:

Step	Completion Time (min.)	Value Added?
Patient checks in with pharmacy clerk.	1	Yes
Pharmacy clerk pulls up order from system or checks customer's paperwork (i.e., handwritten prescription).	3	Yes
Pharmacy clerk checks with pharmacist regarding dosage and drug preference.	3	Yes
Pharmacist fills order.	5	Yes
Patient waits.	5	No
Pharmacy clerk releases order.	1	No
Pharmacy clerk contacts customer that order is filled.	1	No
Customer pays for order.	1	Yes

What is the process cycle efficiency for the pharmacy prescription process?

9. GKS Biologicals tracked its testing process over about 125 days. The subsequent statistical process control (SPC) chart is presented here. Comment on whether GKS's testing process is in control or out of control (i.e., comment on out-of-control points and/or runs in the data).

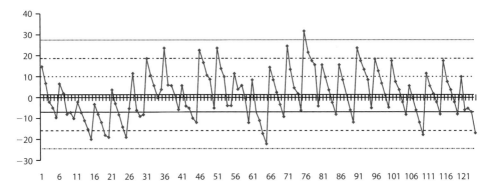

10. Eastern Orthodontics wishes to process its patients on average in around 20 minutes. The orthodontists tracked patient time in the system over about 60 days. The subsequent SPC chart is presented here. Comment on whether Eastern Orthodontics's process is in control or out of control (i.e., comment on out-of-control points and/or runs in the data).

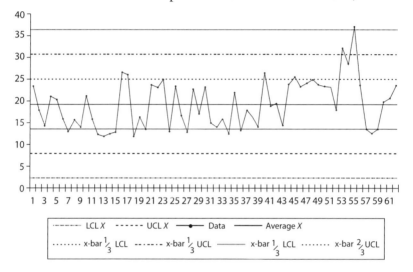

11. The following table displays the average pharmacy bill from 1982 to 2011 for XYZ Pharmacy. The pharmacy assistant thinks there is a trend of increasing bills over the years. Create a linear trend equation and chart for the data.

Year	Average Pharmacy Bill	Year	Average Pharmacy Bill
1982	$7.36	1997	$45.43
1983	$22.85	1998	$41.83
1984	$15.13	1999	$51.08
1985	$26.84	2000	$52.24
1986	$27.80	2001	$60.29
1987	$23.92	2002	$65.16
1988	$27.80	2003	$74.02
1989	$27.58	2004	$51.87
1990	$31.64	2005	$66.46
1991	$30.50	2006	$75.99
1992	$34.55	2007	$93.22
1993	$35.30	2008	$92.00
1994	$45.53	2009	$74.23
1995	$45.58	2010	$94.04
1996	$41.85	2011	$99.31

12. Down East Physical Therapy has mapped out its rehabilitation process. The staff identified that the total cycle time is on average 1 hour and 30 minutes. The process is broken down into nine steps: (1) patient checks in with clerk, (2) pre-appointment screen with triage physical therapist (PT), (3) nurse checks medicine history, (4) patient waits for primary PT recommendation, (5) patient is transferred to respective rehabilitation center, (6) patient waits in respective rehabilitation center for primary PT, (7) primary PT conducts therapy and gives recommendations, (8) nurse checks customer out, and (9) and customer pays for service. The time to complete each step and whether it adds value is listed in the following table:

Step	Completion Time (min.)	Value Added?
Patient checks in with clerk.	2	Yes
Pre-appointment screen with triage PT.	15	Yes
Nurse checks medicine history.	3	Yes
Patient waits for primary PT recommendation.	10	No
Patient is transferred to respective rehabilitation center.	3	No
Patient waits in respective rehabilitation center for primary PT.	2	No
Primary PT conducts therapy and gives recommendations.	45	Yes
Nurse checks customer out.	5	No
Customer pays for service.	5	Yes

What is the process cycle efficiency for the rehabilitation process?

13. The following table displays the average test readings from the last 30 tests (numbered 1011 to 1040). The testing technician believes there is an increasing trend of the test readings and is worried the testing machine maybe miscalibrated. Create a linear trend equation and chart for the data.

Test Number	Average Reading	Test Number	Average Reading
1011	1,031	1026	1,103
1012	1,022	1027	1,090

(Continued)

Test Number	Average Reading	Test Number	Average Reading
1013	1,062	1028	1,057
1014	1,040	1029	1,084
1015	1,027	1030	1,036
1016	1,086	1031	1,059
1017	1,088	1032	1,102
1018	1,076	1033	1,082
1019	1,066	1034	1,102
1020	1,066	1035	1,079
1021	1,022	1036	1,106
1022	1,082	1037	1,107
1023	1,068	1038	1,054
1024	1,038	1039	1,120
1025	1,066	1040	1,059

MINICASE: DELAYED ROOM CLEANING DILEMMA

University Health Systems' Environmental Services department is tasked with cleaning patient rooms. The hospital facility is three floors and is horizontally laid out (i.e., long hallways to traverse between departments and rooms). The Environmental Services department has been experiencing some issues with the room cleaning process. Specifically, the issue is delays in cleaning rooms. While delays cannot be completely eliminated, delays need to be monitored. Leigh, Environmental Services director, has compiled some data over the past three weeks on cleaning delays. She has collected the number of cleaning delays per day and the cause of the delay as written by the room attendant.

Leigh's co-workers believe day of the week plays a role in how many cleaning delays occur. Leigh does not agree and wants to show her co-workers that their team should actually be concerned with the reason(s) for the delays. Leigh also believes there has been a trend upward in the number of delays over the past three weeks. Leigh needs assistance in substantiating her claims.

There are five categories for causes of delays: patient check-out orders delayed, cleaning staff shortage, room occupied, order for patient check-out canceled, or other. Using a scatter plot and a Pareto diagram, help Leigh develop a way to explain her idea to her co-workers. Include dialogue Leigh could use to help clarify her point. Table 9.3 contains the pertinent cleaning delay information.

TABLE 9.3 MiniCase Cleaning Delay Information

Day of the Week	Total Number of Cleaning Delays	Reason Given for Delay				
		Patient Check-Out Orders Delayed	Cleaning Staff Shortage	Room Occupied	Order for Patient Check-Out Canceled	Other
M-Week 1	1	1	0	0	0	0
Tu-Week 1	8	3	2	2	1	0
W-Week 1	9	6	0	0	2	1
Th-Week 1	9	5	1	1	1	1
F-Week 1	21	16	5	0	0	0
M-Week 2	8	0	0	5	2	1
Tu-Week 2	19	5	5	5	2	2
W-Week 2	25	10	0	5	5	5
Th-Week 2	25	7	2	2	12	2
F-Week 2	24	5	5	2	7	5
M-Week 3	29	10	10	5	2	2
Tu-Week 3	19	7	5	0	5	2
W-Week 3	21	12	0	5	2	2
Th-Week 3	19	6	3	1	6	3
F-Week 3	24	4	1	7	7	5

REFERENCES

Barry, Robert, A. Murcko, and C. E. Brubaker. 2002. *The Six Sigma Book for Healthcare.* Chicago, IL: Health Administration Press.

Bisgaard, Soren. 2009. *Solutions to the Healthcare Quality Crisis: Cases and Examples of Lean Six Sigma in Healthcare.* Milwaukee, WI: ASQ Quality Press.

Burge, Ryan. 2008. "Lollipops for Excellence: A Pediatric Hospital's Quality Program." *Industrial Engineer* (August).

Catchpole, K., M. De Leval, A. McEwan, N. J. Pigott, M. J. Elliott, A. McQuillan, C. MacDonald, and A. J. Goldman. 2007. "Patient Handover from Surgery to Intensive Care: Using Formula 1 Pit-Stop and Aviation Models to Improve Safety and Quality." *Pediatric Anesthesia* 17 (5): 470–478.

Deming, Edwards. 1986. *Out of the Crisis*. Cambridge, MA: MIT Press.

Ficalora, Joe, J. Costello, and J. Renaud. 2004. *Combining Lean and Six Sigma Methodologies*. Special publication of the ASQ Statistics Division, Milwaukee, Wisconsin (Spring).

Kelly, D. L. 1999. *How to Use Control Charts for Healthcare*. Milwaukee, WI: ASQ Quality Press.

Shainin, Dorian, and P. Shainin. 1988. "Statistical Process Control" In *Quality Control Handbook*, ed. J. M. Juran and F. M. Gryna. Oak Brook, IL: McGraw-Hill.

Shewhart, Walter. 1939. *Statistical Method from the Viewpoint of Quality Control*. Washington, DC: Department of Agriculture.

CHAPTER 10

QUALITY CONTROL

AND IMPROVEMENT

LEARNING OBJECTIVES

➤ Understand what the design of quality control systems entails.

➤ Become familiar with process quality control.

➤ Understand the basics of variables control charting and be able to create a variables control chart.

➤ Understand what process capability is, how it relates to health care, and how to create and interpret capability ratios and indexes.

➤ Understand the basics of total quality management and continuous improvement.

(Continued)

⇒ Understand what the International Organization for Standardization is and what its certification can do for an organization.

⇒ Understand what the Malcolm Baldrige Award is and what it can do for an organization.

DESIGN OF QUALITY CONTROL SYSTEMS

The health care profession has always been interested in quality. Traditionally the term *quality* referred only to the patient health care outcome (i.e., was the patient's medical problem addressed and/or corrected accurately?). However, the definition of quality and the control systems being employed in health care organizations have been greatly expanded. This expansion of quality within health care arises not just from the need for improved patient outcomes but also from the need for total system improvement (e.g., improved waiting times, improved payment cycles, improved reduction in waste, etc.).

To attain system improvements, *quality control systems* must be designed and implemented throughout health care organizations. Table 10.1 displays areas of interest within an organization where quality control systems could and should exist. When developing control systems, these areas must be investigated.

PROCESS QUALITY CONTROL

As a product or service is being provided, the quality of that service should be monitored. *Process quality control* has two basic objectives: to provide timely information on the service or product regarding whether the product or service meets design specifications and to detect shifts in the process that may signal imperfections within the product or service.

One technique widely used to ensure that processes meet the two aforementioned objectives is statistical process control (SPC). SPC was mentioned in Chapter 9 in the section on the 7 QC tools. This chapter explores the area of SPC

TABLE 10.1   Areas of Interest and Associated Quality Control Systems

Organization Area of Interest	Helpful Tools and Methods
Health care as a process	Diagrams that illustrate flow, interrelationship, and cause/effect; use of 7 QC tools to analyze (refer to Chapter 9).
Variation and measurement	Data recorded over time, analyzed, organized, and explained to those stakeholders responsible for the process where the data originated (e.g., see Chapters 4 and 5—mean, median, mode, standard deviation, and histograms with the eventual use of run charts and control charts).
Collaboration	Managing conflict, building teams, and group learning; implementing quality management systems (e.g., total quality management—see section on TQM later in this chapter).
Teamwork and organization-wide accountability	Becoming ISO certified; working toward the Malcolm Baldrige quality award; documenting unwanted and unnecessary variation; organization-wide sharing of information (see sections on ISO and Baldrige later in this chapter).
Developing new, locally useful knowledge	Adopting six sigma and/or lean (see Chapters 9 and 11 for information on six sigma and lean).

in much more detail. All processes are subject to certain amounts of variability. Walter Shewhart of Bell Laboratories wrote about process variation and identified two separate sources: natural and assignable. He developed a fairly simple yet incredibly powerful tool to separate the two sources of variation.

Natural versus Assignable Variation

A process (product-based or service-based) is said to be in statistical control when the only source of variation is from natural causes. Some level of natural variation occurs in all processes. For example, think about how we all differ when it comes to our patience for waiting in line; most of us will wait for service a reasonable length of time without becoming impatient, but there are some who become impatient very quickly and then there are those who never seem to become impatient.

Assignable variation is the variation that can be traced to a specific reason or cause. Specific reasons or causes may include fatigued workers, untrained workers, or miscalibrated equipment. The goal of an operations and supply chain manager is to identify the causes of assignable variation and reduce if not eliminate it.

Sampling

To monitor variation, SPC uses averages of small samples (e.g., three to eight items). Although individual data points are extremely important, it would be prohibitively expensive (money and time) to sample all products or points in time of a process. SPC charts are built using these samples. The samples are plotted and then examined to distinguish between natural and assignable variation. A product or process could be said to be in statistical control and be capable of producing within the control limits (i.e., the product or process only has natural causes of variation present). A product or process can also be in statistical control but not be capable of producing within the control limits (i.e., only natural variation exists but the product or process cannot meet the specifics for operation set down by the organization). Finally, a product or process can be said to be out of control where assignable causes of variation make the system behave erratically and create errors.

Health Care Operations and Supply Chain Management in Action: Quality Improvement in Nursing Homes

Quality improvement (QI) implementation in nursing homes has increased over the past few decades. A recent study (Berlowitz et al., 2003) has shown that quality improvement implementation is most successful in those nursing homes with an underlying culture that promotes innovation. It was also observed that QI implementation may result in better job satisfaction and care.

Results showed that as more QI practices were adopted, more staff members were satisfied with their jobs. In turn, those employees tended to be more active in the daily care they gave. There has been increased pressure to understand which nursing homes are doing well and how those homes are achieving better outcomes. Although there are differences in the implementation of QI practices, it appears QI initiatives are associated with employee satisfaction and providing better care. Homes that were successful had high levels of organizational culture and capacity for implementing QI initiatives.

VARIABLES CONTROL

Variables are characteristics of a product or process that are continuous in dimension (i.e., they have infinite possibilities). Examples for health care processes include waiting time in an emergency room (ER) and blood pressure measurements. *Variables control* charts for the mean (x-bar or $\bar{x}$) and the range (R) are created to monitor processes.

The x-bar chart monitors the changes that occur regarding the central tendency (e.g., if the specification on average is a 20-minute wait in the ER, how does our process vary around that central number?). The R chart monitors the dispersion resulting from variation within the process (i.e., in any one sample, how far apart are the high and low values being measured?). The two charts must be used in conjunction with each other, as one describes the variation in central tendency, x-bar, whereas the other, R, describes variation in dispersion (refer to Chapter 5 regarding central tendency and dispersion).

Setting Control Chart Limits

Control limits for control charts are calculated using average ranges instead of standard deviations. This is due to the fact that process standard deviations are either not available or very difficult to calculate. The formulas for the upper and lower control limits for an x-bar chart (Equation 10.1) and R chart (Equation 10.2) are as follows:

$$\text{x-bar chart control limits} \quad \begin{aligned} UCL_{\bar{x}} &= \bar{\bar{x}} + A_2\bar{R} \\ LCL_{\bar{x}} &= \bar{\bar{x}} - A_2\bar{R} \end{aligned} \quad (10.1)$$

$$\text{R Chart control limits} \quad \begin{aligned} UCL_R &= D_4\bar{R} \\ LCL_R &= D_3\bar{R} \end{aligned} \quad (10.2)$$

where,

$\bar{R}$ = average range of sample
A_2 = conversion value based on sample size (see Table 10.2)
D_4 and D_3 = conversion value based on sample size (see Table 10.2)
$\bar{\bar{x}}$ = mean of the sample means

TABLE 10.2   Factors or Computing Control Chart Limits (Three Sigma)

Sample Size, n	Mean Factor, A_2	Upper Range, D_4	Lower Range, D_3
2	1.880	3.268	0
3	1.023	2.574	0
4	0.729	2.282	0
5	0.577	2.115	0
6	0.483	2.004	0
7	0.419	1.924	0.076
8	0.373	1.864	0.136
9	0.337	1.816	0.184

Let's take a look at an example. Figure 10.1 displays data taken from an ER waiting room. In brief, patients come to the ER looking for care. They must sign in and then wait to be called in order to see a provider. Sometimes the ER is not very busy and the wait is short, whereas at other times when the ER is busy the wait is longer. The ER staff has monitored wait times, taking four samples randomly for eight trials or periods, and has entered the data into a spreadsheet. This data, along with the calculations necessary for creating the x-bar and R control charts, is included in Figure 10.1. Table 10.3 displays the formulas in Excel that are used to calculate x-bar, x-2bar, R-bar, and so on.

FIGURE 10.1   Spreadsheet for Control Chart Calculations

	A	B	C	D	E	F	G
1	Wait Time in ER (min)		Sample, n				
2	Trial, k	1	2	3	4	x-bar	R (High - Low)
3	1	13	12	15	25	16.25	13.00
4	2	11	13	22	11	14.25	11.00
5	3	24	15	31	14	21.00	17.00
6	4	13	24	21	18	19.00	11.00
7	5	22	41	32	29	31.00	19.00
8	6	11	18	17	10	14.00	8.00
9	7	14	12	19	31	19.00	19.00
10	8	16	22	21	21	20.00	6.00
11					x-2bar	19.31	
12						R-bar	13.00
13			Conversion Table				
14	Sample Size, n	Mean Factor, A₂	Upper Range, D₄	Lower Range, D₃		x-bar	Control Limits
15	2	1.880	3.268	0.000		UCLₓ	28.79
16	3	1.023	2.574	0.000		LCLₓ	9.84
17	4	0.729	2.282	0.000			
18	5	0.577	2.115	0.000		R	Control Limits
19	6	0.483	2.004	0.000		UCL_R	29.67
20	7	0.419	1.924	0.076		LCL_R	0.00
21	8	0.373	1.864	0.136			
22	9	0.337	1.816	0.184			
23							
24							

TABLE 10.3   Formulas for Control Chart Spreadsheet Calculations

Control Chart Calculation	Cell	Formula
x-bar	F3	= AVERAGE(B3:E3) copy down to cell F10
R (high – low)	G3	= MAX(B3:E3)-MIN(B3:E3) copy down to cell G10
x-2bar	F11	= AVERAGE(F3:F10)
R-bar	G12	= AVERAGE(G3:G10)
x-bar UCL	G15	= F11+B17*G12
x-bar LCL	G16	= F11-B17*G12
R UCL	G19	= C17*G12
R LCL	G20	= D17*G12

Figure 10.2 displays the x-bar chart associated with the calculations in Figure 10.1 and Table 10.3, while Figure 10.3 displays the R chart.

Interpreting the x-Bar Chart

It can be seen from Figure 10.2 that trial point 5 lies outside of the upper control limit (refer to circle on Figure 10.2). Since this point is past the upper control limit,

FIGURE 10.2   x-Bar Chart

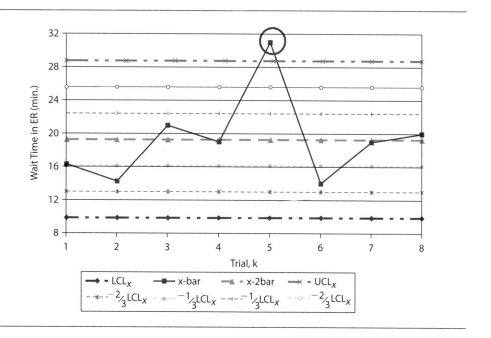

FIGURE 10.3 *R* **Chart**

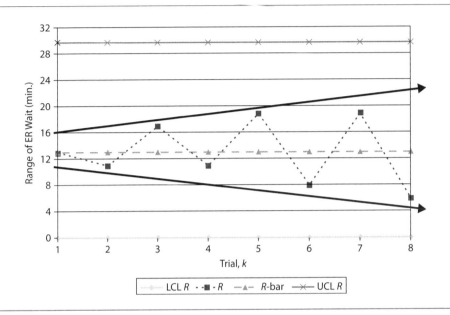

it can be determined that the process is out of control and corrective action needs to be taken. One first step would be to investigate the samples taken for trial number 5 and start asking questions about why those waiting times are longer than normal. All the other trials appear to be within control limits, so it could be possible that the samples that make up trial 5 had some special cause (e.g., the ER was flooded with patients due to a serious auto accident) behind them making the wait time increase. See Table 10.4 for a list of control chart patterns.

Interpreting the *R* Chart

It can be seen from Figure 10.3 that no points appear to be on or outside of the upper or lower control limits. The same patterns used to detect out-of-control points for x-bar charts (see Table 10.4) can be used for *R* charts. However, *R* charts are even more basic to interpret than x-bar charts. The main three patterns one should look for first are:

1. Any points on, above, or below the outer control limits, indicating the process is out of control and corrective action must be taken.

2. A widening of the distance between successive trials, sometimes referred to as the funneling-out effect (see arrows in Figure 10.3). This indicates that the average range of the sample points is increasing with each trial and that the process is beginning to become out of control, so corrective action must be taken.

3. Five points in a row trending upward or downward indicate that the process is out of control due to causes such as employee fatigue or equipment miscalibration.

In Figure 10.3 it can be seen that funneling out is occurring (see arrows). This indicates that the range of the samples is increasing as the process continues to function. In other words, on average the range between the longest waiting time and the shortest waiting time at the ER is increasing. Some special cause is driving this, and the ER team should investigate what is causing the upswing in the range of waiting times.

For example, the upswing in the range of wait times may be due to two disparate groups entering the ER at the same time. A group of seniors from a nursing home needing flu shots and only flu shots may have a very short waiting time (due to only one procedure and appointments set ahead of time), but a group of workers from a local factory who sustained injuries due to an industrial spill may take longer (unspecified injuries, triage needed, protective clothing worn, etc.).

It must be noted that when inspecting only the x-bar chart (Figure 10.2), one would find that the last two trials track very closely to the average signal. If we had not created and examined the R chart, we would have been unaware of the funneling out; the x-bar chart would not have given us any signal of this increasing range between waiting times. This is a good example of why we need to use x-bar and R charts in conjunction with each other. The x-bar chart tracks central tendency while the R chart tracks dispersion.

USING CONTROL CHARTS

When *using control charts*, the assumption of normality is made regarding the data used in the chart. The normal distribution is characterized by two parameters, the mean and standard deviation. The x-bar and R charts are akin to these two parameters. The x-bar chart is sensitive to changes in the process mean, whereas the R chart is sensitive to changes in the process dispersion (i.e., standard deviation). If users track both charts looking for changes, they are tracking any changes that may appear in the process distribution and the process itself.

Steps for Setting Up Control Charts

There are five generally accepted steps in creating x-bar and R charts. They are:

1. Collect samples, n, over a number of trials, k, of a stable process and compute the mean and range of each trial.

2. Compute the overall means, x-2bar and R-bar, and calculate the appropriate control limits using your sample size to find A_2, D_3, and D_4. These limits are said to be the 99.73 percent limits in that we wish to monitor control at the +/–3 sigma level. If the process cannot be deemed stable, use the desired mean instead of x-2bar in your calculations.

3. Graph the sample means and ranges on an x-y scatter plot. Add in the upper and lower control limits as well as the given central lines (i.e., x-2bar and R-bar).

4. Investigate the points you have plotted, looking for patterns or points that are outside the control limits. If out-of-control points or patterns are found, try to assign causes for the variations and resume the process (see the next section, "Control Chart Patterns").

5. Keep collecting samples after corrective action has been taken to revalidate control limits.

Control Chart Patterns

When a process begins to go out of control, certain patterns in the control charts start to appear. Table 10.4 lists some patterns to look for over time.

When patterns such as those described in Table 10.4 arise, corrective action needs to be taken. This corrective action could be as simple as giving an employee a break or recalibrating a blood pressure machine. However, sometimes the entire process must be overhauled if control cannot be maintained. The x-bar and R charts are well suited for continuous type variables, but when a

TABLE 10.4 Control Chart Patterns

Pattern	What to Look For	Conclusion
Outside control limits	One point either above or below the upper or lower control limit	Process is out of control; evaluate immediately, and investigate sample points for special cause.
Trends—upward or downward	Five points in a row trending upward or downward	Employees are experiencing fatigue or equipment needs to be recalibrated or maintenance performed.
Points near control limits	Two points in a row very close to the upper or lower control limits	Investigate for assignable cause (e.g., shift change).
Run above or below central line	Five points in a row on one side of the central line	Investigate for assignable cause (e.g., shift change, poor materials).
Erratic behavior	Large swings by points from upper control limit to lower control limit	Investigate for assignable cause (e.g., machine miscalibration, employee fatigue).

process has an attribute or a discrete outcome, other types of control charts must be employed.

Control Charts for Attributes

Attributes such as being defective or nondefective require a different type of control chart. Measuring attributes involves counting defects (e.g., the number of proper intravenous [IV] insertions). Two types of attribute control charts are commonly used: the p-chart or percent defective chart and the c-chart or number of defects chart.

For brevity, p-charts and c-charts are summarized here and the reader is referred to the end-of-chapter reference section, specifically Shewhart 1939 and Shewhart 1980, to find more information on both of these chart types.

p-Charts

Attributes that can be classified by yes/no or as defective/nondefective are monitored using p-charts. The procedure resembles the procedure used for x-bar charts—we assume that the data distribution can be approximated by the normal distribution. Errors in patient billing or claims processing are two good examples of places where p-charts could be used to monitor a process.

c-Charts

When monitoring a process that is defined by an attribute, the attribute (defect or nondefect) can be aggregated and the number per unit output can be monitored. Control charts for defects are very useful in monitoring processes that could potentially contain numerous errors, but in fact may contain few or none. Defects could be complaints received regarding a health care facility or areas not cleaned properly in a patient room. C-charts differ from x-bar charts and p-charts in that the underlying data distribution is not normal; it is a Poisson distribution.

PROCESS CAPABILITY

Statistical process control (SPC) and control charts provide the means to monitor a process and keep the process in control. However, a process that is in statistical control may not yield output that meets design specifications. The ability to meet design specifications is referred to as *process capability*. A process must be capable of delivering output that meets customer or engineered specifications.

For example, the waiting time in the ER is expected to be 30 minutes with a design specification of +/–10 minutes. In turn, the upper specification limit (USL) would be 40 minutes and the lower specification limit (LSL) would be 20 minutes. The waiting room procedure must be able to operate within these design specifications. If the waiting room process is not capable of meeting these specifications, then customers or staff (or both customers and staff) will not have their requirements met. In other words, the process's performance is not capable.

Capability Ratios and Capability Indexes

Capability ratios and indexes are widely used to determine if a process is able to meet performance specifications. C_p (Equation 10.3), referred to as the capability ratio, and C_{pm} (Equation 10.4), referred to as the Taguchi capability index (Boyles 1991), are typical process capability measures. While C_p works well as a measure of progress for quality improvement and variability reduction, this measure can fail to address the issue of process centering or to distinguish between off-target and on-target processes. In addition, Boyles (1991) shows that C_p is essentially a measure of process yield only. In contrast, C_{pm} discerns between the process target value and the process mean.

$$C_p = \frac{USL - LSL}{6\sigma} \qquad (10.3)$$

$$C_{pm} = \frac{USL - LSL}{6\sqrt{\sigma^2 + (\mu - \mathrm{T})^2}} \qquad (10.4)$$

For our waiting room example, if the target waiting time is 30 minutes and the average waiting time tends to be around the target, then the basic capability ratio can be used. However, if the average wait time is not near the target, then it might be more appropriate to employ the Taguchi capability index. C_{pm} measures process variation from a target and is sensitive to process centering as well as process yield. C_{pm} is calculated using the upper specification limit (USL), lower specification limit (LSL), target (T), and mean and variance of the data.

A process capability index or ratio of at least 1.0 means a process is capable at a +/–3 sigma level. With a process capability index or ratio of 1.0, 2.7 parts per 1,000 can be expected to be out of specification. For our waiting room example, about three patients out of every thousand patients would experience waiting times outside the 20 to 40 minutes specifications. Larger capability values are more favorable, as they are an indication that a process is operating on target and with low variation. Capability values less than 1.0 indicate that a process is highly variable and not operating at or near target. Some health care organizations strive to have process capability of 1.33 as a target. Process capability of 1.33 translates into about 64 parts per million that would be out of specification.

Waiting Room Capability Example

Figure 10.4 displays the spreadsheet that contains the data set and capability calculations for our waiting room example. Table 10.5 presents the formulas used in the spreadsheet.

From Figure 10.4 the capability ratio (refer to cell D8) is 0.1984 and the Taguchi capability index is 0.1968. Both of these values are far below the

FIGURE 10.4   Process Capability Spreadsheet Calculations

	A	B	C	D
1	Observation	Wait Time in ER (min)		
2	1	19	Average Wait (min)	32.14
3	2	1	Wait Standard Deviation (min)	16.80
4	3	35	USL (min)	40
5	4	47	LSL (min)	20
6	5	18	Target - T (min)	30
7	6	45		
8	7	53	C_p-Capability Ratio	0.1984
9	8	11	C_{pm}-Taguchi Capability Index	0.1968
10	9	55		
11	10	24		
12	11	50		
13	12	15		
14	13	42		
15	14	24		
16	15	12		
17	16	49		
18	17	18		
19	18	22		
20	19	10		
21	20	46		
22	21	46		
23	22	39		
24	23	51		
25	24	14		
26	25	24		
27	26	56		
28	27	40		
29	28	41		
30	29	50		
31	30	9		
32				

TABLE 10.5   Formulas for Process Capability Spreadsheet Calculations

Process Capability Calculation	Cell	Formula
Average wait (min.)	D2	= AVERAGE(B2:B31)
Wait standard deviation (min.)	D3	
USL (min.)	D4	= 40
LSL (min.)	D5	= 20
Target—T (min.)	D6	= 30
Capability ratio—C_p	D8	= (D4-D5)/(6*D3)
Taguchi capability index—C_{pm}-	D9	= (D4-D5)/(6*(D3^2+(D2-D6)^2)^0.5)

1.0 value needed to show that the process is capable. Therefore, it can be concluded that the ER waiting room process is not capable of serving patients on average in 30 minutes with 99.73 percent waiting between 20 and 40 minutes.

Take note that the Taguchi capability index is very close to the capability ratio. This is due to the fact that the average waiting time is very close to the expected 30 minutes (e.g., average wait, cell D2, is 32.14). The process appears to be centered but the real problem occurs in the wait standard deviation (refer to cell D3). Waiting times are way too variable or inconsistent to meet the 20 to 40 minutes specification limits. A suggestion to the ER may be to start by mapping its process and then to identify bottlenecks or causes of this variation.

TOTAL QUALITY MANAGEMENT AND CONTINUOUS IMPROVEMENT

The concept of promoting quality on an entire organization level is what is at the heart of *total quality management* (TQM). TQM strives for management buy-in regarding quality and seeks to drive the organization to be excellent in all aspects of its products and services. In general, successful TQM programs incorporate the concepts from the following five areas:

1. *Continuous improvement.* Management promotes a never-ending goal of improving products, processes, and services. *Continuous improvement* techniques include the plan-do-check-act model (refer to Chapter 9) developed by Shewhart (Shewhart 1939) and reinforced by Deming (Deming 1986) and the principle of six sigma (refer to Chapter 9).

2. *Knowledge of TQM tools.* TQM borrows from the 7 QC tools presented in Chapter 9 and stresses that all employees in the organization be trained in these tools.

3. *Benchmarking.* Benchmarking involves selecting products, processes, and/or services that resemble your own organization and comparing (benchmarking) your organization to the other organization.

4. *Just in time (JIT).* Just in time is a philosophy to produce goods or services just as they are needed. JIT also involves continuous improvement coupled

with problem solving to attain shorter setup times, minimal stocks of inventory, streamlined processes, and reduced costs.

5. *Employee empowerment.* This refers to the idea of involving employees in every step of the process. Techniques for fostering employee empowerment include building communication networks that include all employees, developing open and supportive management styles, pushing responsibility down the organizational chart from manager to staff and process workers, encouraging high morale, and creating formal quality entities such as quality circles and quality teams.

TQM, when properly developed and implemented, has been shown to eliminate waste, decrease process variation, and reduce cycle time.

INTERNATIONAL ORGANIZATION FOR STANDARDIZATION CERTIFICATION

The International Organization for Standardization (referred to as ISO) developed and published a series of quality assurance standards called ISO 9000 in 1987. These standards were the first quality standards adopted by all members of ISO. The standards were revised in 1994, updated, and republished in 2000. Currently, the ISO 9000 standards include three main quality standards: ISO 9000, ISO 9001, and ISO 9004. ISO 9000 concentrates on requirements, while ISO 9001 and ISO 9004 present guidelines.

These three quality standards are process oriented, not product oriented. The standards strive to assist organizations to "say what they do" and then "do what they say they do." In other words, the standards indicate how processes should be measured and documented from a quality viewpoint.

Typically an organization goes through a 9- to 18-month *ISO certification* process that involves documenting quality procedures, an on-site assessment, and ongoing audits. In sum, to engage in business globally being listed as ISO certified is critical. However, even if your organization may not conduct business globally, many times your suppliers or customers do, and in turn they may ask you to become ISO certified.

Another ISO standard is the ISO 14000 series. The ISO 14000 series is an environmental management standard that contains six elements: environmental management systems, environmental auditing, environmental performance evaluation, environmental labeling, life-cycle assessment, and environmental aspects in product standards. The standard was established in 1996, revised in 2004, and is now accepted worldwide, with many organizations aligning their ISO 9000 certification with the ISO 14000 standards.

Health Care Operations and Supply Chain Management behind the Scenes

Internationally, many hospitals are ISO certified. However, health care organizations in the United States have been slow to seek certification. There are only a handful of hospitals in the United States that are ISO certified.

Health care organizations can utilize ISO 9001 certification as a vehicle for improvement. These are just a few of the ways ISO certification enhances a health care organization:

- Provides ways to detect and correct errors and problems.

- Helps to maximize customer satisfaction.

- Defines key interfaces between processes, departments, and staff.

- Streamlines work flow and maximizes resource utilization.

- Ensures conformance to and effectiveness of documented processes.

- Focuses on patient and provider needs and expectations.

- Identifies systemic breakdowns and closes gaps or loopholes.

- Prevents problems from occurring proactively.

Hospitals that have implemented ISO 9001 train individuals in the organization to be internal auditors. ISO certification establishes process monitors and evaluates each process at least yearly. In addition, it is key to have the senior management team critique the effectiveness, suitability, and adequacy of all processes.

Significant accomplishments can be made through ISO certification. These are a few examples of what hospitals have achieved by pursuing the ISO 9001 certification:

- Centralization of the product recall process, including medication, equipment, devices, and food.

- Establishment of a yearly review of all physician orders sets and protocols, leading to improved quality and patient satisfaction.

- Creation of an online risk occurrence entry system.

- Cleanup of policies and procedures.

- Cleanup of unnecessary forms and redundant documents.

- Identification and definition of best practices for all hospital-wide patient care processes (outpatient, inpatient, and emergency department) and support processes (e.g., maintenance, calibration, purchasing, receiving, contract management).

Although ISO certification may be viewed as being intended more for manufacturing organizations, hospitals that have embarked on certification have garnered substantial benefits. See Bamford and Deibler 2003 and Naveh and Marcus 2004 for overviews of ISO applied to service industries. In addition, Berlowitz et al. 2003 provides excellent material on quality improvement implementation in a health care setting.

MALCOLM BALDRIGE AWARD

In 1987 the U.S. Department of Commerce established the Malcolm Baldrige National Quality Award. The *Malcolm Baldrige award* was meant to assist organizations to review and structure their quality programs in partial response to slipping quality in U.S. manufacturing; however, the award is not limited to manufacturing firms. The award is named for then Secretary of Commerce Malcolm Baldrige, and winners in the health care field have included SSM HealthCare (St. Louis, Missouri); Baptist Hospital, Inc. (Pensacola, Florida); and Saint Luke's Hospital of Kansas City (Kansas City, Missouri).

The Malcolm Baldrige award's name was changed to the Baldrige Performance Excellence Program in 2010 to reflect the evolution of the field of quality from a focus on product, service, and customer quality to a broader, strategic focus on overall organizational quality.

The award is given to any organization that demonstrates outstanding quality in its products and processes. Up to 18 awards total may be given each year across six sectors: health care, education, not-for-profit, small business, service, and manufacturing. Each submission consists of an application (up to 75 pages) detailing the organization's approach, deployment, and results of its quality activities in six categories: product and service outcomes, customer-focused outcomes, financial and market outcomes, workforce-related outcomes, process effectiveness outcomes, and leadership outcomes.

The applications are scored by total points out of 1,000, with 450 of those points being allocated to results. Organizations scoring above approximately 650 receive site visits. Winners are then honored at an annual awards ceremony in Washington, D.C. One large benefit of applying is in helping organizations determine the most critical areas to measure, create value for stakeholders, and improve performance. The Japanese have a similar award, the Deming Prize, named for Dr. W. Edwards Deming (Deming 1986). Link and Scott 2001 provide an excellent evaluation of the Baldrige program while the NIST website, www.NIST.gov/baldrige/about/baldrige_faqs.cfm, provides an FAQ regarding the Baldrige process.

Additional Quality Tools Used in Health Care

Although this book focuses on six sigma, there are other tools that can be employed to improve processes and quality. Two frequently used tools are quality function deployment and benchmarking. Both tools are briefly described next.

Quality Function Deployment

Quality function deployment (QFD) is a process that identifies customers' needs and wants and translates them into a product or process that meets those needs. QFD was developed to bring a personal interface to manufacturing but has been applied to service-based industries as well. The QFD process employs what is called the house of quality (see Figure 10.5). The house of quality is a structure to organize data in a visible and usable manner. In sum, QFD:

- Aids in understanding customer requirements.

- Links up systems thinking and analysis with feature importance, competitor assessment, and quality specifications.

FIGURE 10.5 House of Quality Example

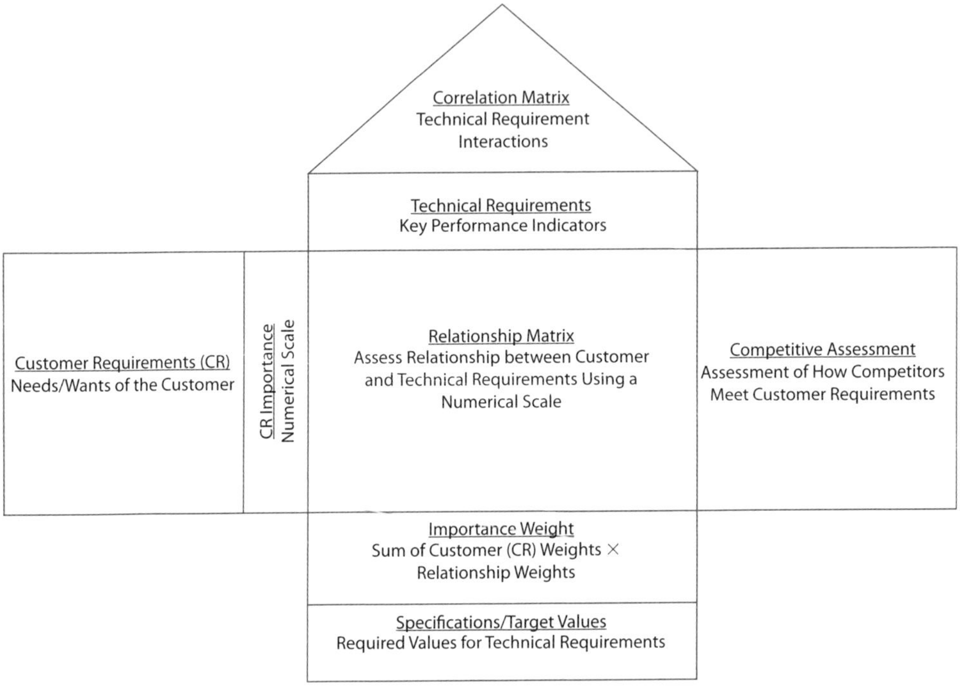

- Maximizes those features and specifications that add value to the customer.

- Provides a comprehensive quality system for customer satisfaction.

- Links the voice of the customer to design for six sigma.

For examples of QFD application in health care, the reader is asked to peruse the following references: Chaplin and Terninko (2000); Jesso-White and Mazur (2010); Mazur, Gibson, and Harries (1995); and Omachonu and Barach (2005).

Benchmarking and the Health Care Organization

The act of comparing performance characteristics between your own organization and separate but often competing organizations with the intent of improving your own organization is the essence of benchmarking. Therefore it can be said that benchmarking:

- Helps organizations to understand their strengths and weaknesses.

- Allows organizations to understand what levels of service are really possible by comparing operations to other similar organizations.

- Promotes change coupled with continuous improvement and provides a road map to deliver improvements in quality, productivity, and service.

- Enables organizations to be cognizant of new developments within their discipline.

In general, benchmarking has been transferred to the health care industry through other industries such as manufacturing. Beginning in the 1990s, benchmarking was being employed to improve quality in the health care field.

Internal and External Benchmarking Benchmarking can be separated into two broad areas: internal and external benchmarking. Internal benchmarking involves communication between departments within the same health care organization. It is advised that internal benchmarking take place before external benchmarking is undertaken.

External benchmarking requires a comparison of internal performance indicators to other organizations. The objective is to gain insight into new ideas, methods, products, and/or services and to continuously improve the internal processes within one's own organization. External benchmarking can be conducted in three ways: on a competitive level, on a functional level, and on a generic level. Competitive benchmarking refers to comparisons made with direct competitors only. Functional benchmarking refers to comparisons made not only with competitors but also with those organizations that are considered best in class no matter what their discipline is (e.g., compare health care service at a hospital to service in the resort tourism discipline). Finally, generic benchmarking refers to comparisons made on business functions that are the same regardless of the industry (e.g., accounting and billing in health care versus accounting and billing in manufacturing). For more information on benchmarking in the health care industry, refer to Kay 2007 in the reference section.

SUMMARY

The term *quality* may be defined differently by different organizations. In the health care field, the definition of quality and the control systems being employed have been greatly expanded. This expansion of quality within health care arises not just from the need for improved patient outcomes but also from the need for total system improvement (improved waiting times, improved payment cycles, improved reduction in waste, etc.).

KEY TERMS

continuous improvement	quality control systems
ISO certification	quality function deployment
Malcolm Baldrige award	total quality management
process capability	using control charts
process quality control	variables control

DISCUSSION QUESTIONS

1. What value of A_2 would be used in an SPC chart with a sample size of 4?

2. Compare and contrast the Malcolm Baldrige award to ISO certification.

3. What values of D_1 and D_2 would be used for an R chart with a sample size of 2?

4. The following table contains 62 trials where during each trial two samples were taken of the processing time (in minutes) of the laboratory technicians. Create an x-bar chart for the data and comment on whether the process is in control.

Trial	Sample 1 (min.)	Sample 2 (min.)	Trial	Sample 1 (min.)	Sample 2 (min.)
1	18	13	32	14	16
2	29	14	33	20	14
3	14	11	34	29	25

4	22	13	35	18	15
5	16	13	36	15	14
6	13	28	37	15	34
7	30	26	38	14	14
8	12	18	39	14	38
9	24	34	40	14	13
10	17	13	41	18	37
11	14	11	42	13	10
12	18	13	43	12	36
13	11	20	44	14	12
14	15	16	45	30	26
15	17	12	46	16	24
16	14	16	47	10	34
17	16	32	48	20	14
18	12	11	49	16	25
19	27	35	50	21	22
20	16	14	51	35	14
21	17	35	52	12	13
22	15	16	53	14	12
23	12	10	54	22	14
24	13	15	55	27	14
25	11	32	56	37	15
26	18	12	57	17	25
27	15	14	58	40	29
28	11	14	59	39	12
29	14	27	60	35	35
30	14	26	61	10	12
31	32	22	62	37	14

5. For the previous table create an R chart for the processing time (in minutes) of the laboratory technicians. Comment on whether the process is in control regarding the R chart, and discuss why x-bar and R charts must be used in conjunction with each other.

6. The processing times for patients at the walk-in clinic are given in the following table. The target processing time is 20 minutes with upper and lower limits of 30 and 10 minutes. Calculate a capability ratio for the data set. Also, calculate a Taguchi capability index, compare it to the capability ratio, and comment on the similarities or differences.

Patient #	Process Time (min.)
1	23.6
2	35.8
3	20.5
4	24.5
5	25.3
6	20.5
7	34.8
8	13.0
9	26.2
10	21.5
11	18.9
12	27.6
13	13.7
14	25.0
15	21.3
16	14.7
17	16.8
18	15.7
19	32.0
20	16.3
21	24.8
22	17.1
23	17.7
24	13.3
25	19.1
26	18.5
27	18.3
28	14.4
29	21.4
30	19.1

7. The same walk-in clinic took data measurements of its processing times on weekends only. Maximum times, with an upper limit of 30 minutes, stayed the same. However, the overall target time, 16 minutes, and the lower limit, 5 minutes, were less than for a full week (which were 20 minutes and 10 minutes, respectively) due to increased staff. Calculate a capability ratio and a Taguchi capability index for the data and compare them, explaining why they are different or similar.

Patient #	Process Time (min.)
1	14.0
2	9.6
3	22.3
4	18.6
5	19.7
6	22.6
7	11.8
8	14.2
9	26.1
10	13.1
11	21.0
12	17.3
13	17.4
14	15.6
15	21.7
16	20.3
17	21.7
18	15.1
19	16.7
20	17.7
21	19.6
22	20.6
23	12.0
24	18.8
25	16.3
26	22.7
27	21.2
28	20.5
29	17.2
30	22.1

8. The following table contains data for room turnaround time by the cleaning staff at the BlackJack/Simpson clinic. Sixty-two trials were conducted with three samples apiece. The clinic manager has heard of a technique called statistical process control and would like to use it to see if the clinic's room turnaround process is in control. Develop an x-bar and R chart for the data, and comment on whether the process is in control or out of control.

Trial	Sample 1 (min.)	Sample 2 (min.)	Sample 3 (min.)	Trial	Sample 1 (min.)	Sample 2 (min.)	Sample 3 (min.)
1	39.0	14.8	39.0	32	39.8	26.5	39.9
2	48.9	48.5	51.5	33	56.2	34.3	58.7
3	51.5	40.3	52.0	34	34.8	40.9	36.4
4	48.0	37.3	49.0	35	19.3	22.3	20.8
5	65.7	41.5	67.9	36	32.3	45.7	33.4
6	34.3	41.9	37.2	37	24.6	47.4	27.2
7	39.0	36.0	40.5	38	49.3	48.7	50.6
8	53.1	66.6	55.8	39	52.0	72.3	54.5
9	43.8	66.5	46.7	40	28.1	31.1	29.6
10	38.5	33.9	38.9	41	35.7	64.7	35.7
11	16.1	16.4	19.0	42	59.1	11.2	59.1
12	31.0	60.4	33.4	43	38.4	48.0	40.3
13	53.3	36.0	55.8	44	28.0	57.7	30.8
14	50.1	42.6	50.7	45	45.2	51.2	45.5
15	40.2	31.9	40.7	46	37.8	64.0	40.1
16	14.5	30.4	16.5	47	41.2	80.4	43.0
17	34.3	44.8	35.0	48	55.2	21.4	55.2
18	18.2	47.2	19.4	49	26.8	52.5	28.9
19	65.7	78.6	66.7	50	46.6	61.2	49.1
20	57.8	52.0	60.5	51	74.6	32.9	74.8
21	43.0	77.7	44.6	52	19.9	57.5	22.6
22	29.2	42.5	32.1	53	21.7	22.7	21.7
23	27.2	57.6	28.3	54	49.5	25.6	51.6
24	39.5	19.7	42.2	55	66.8	28.1	68.1
25	32.0	66.6	33.3	56	75.5	52.1	76.6
26	25.4	18.7	25.6	57	55.0	53.5	57.6
27	46.9	25.3	47.7	58	78.7	70.5	80.8
28	23.3	28.5	24.1	59	79.1	59.9	79.4
29	28.3	36.5	29.1	60	45.1	76.6	45.9
30	23.8	32.9	24.6	61	56.5	20.4	58.1
31	32.3	29.9	32.3	62	66.5	47.2	69.0

REFERENCES

Bamford, Robert, and W. Deibler. 2003. *ISO 9001: 2000 for Software and Systems Providers: An Engineering Approach.* Boca Raton, FL: CRC Press.

Berlowitz, Dan R., Gary J. Young, Elaine C. Hickey, Debra Saliba, Brian S. Mittman, Elaine Czarnowski, Barbara Simon, Jennifer J. Anderson, Arlene S. Ash, Lisa V. Rubenstein, and Mark A. Moskowitz. 2003. "Quality Improvement Implementation in the Nursing Home." *Health Services Research* 38, no. 1, Part 1 (February): 65–83.

Boyles, R. A. 1991. "The Taguchi Capability Index." *Journal of Quality Technology* 23 (1): 17–26.

Chaplin, E., and J. Terninko. 2000. *Customer Driven Healthcare: QFD for Process Improvement and Cost Reduction.* Milwaukee, WI: ASQ Quality Press.

Deming, W. E. 1986. *Out of the Crisis.* Cambridge, MA: MIT Center for Advanced Engineering Study.

Jesso-White, J., and G. H. Mazur. 2010. "QFD to Re-design New Physician Orientation and Induction: Connecting New Physicians into a Healthcare Community." 16th International and 22nd N. American Symposium on QFD.

Kay, J. 2007. "Health Care Benchmarking." *Medical Diary* 12 (2).

Link, A. N., and J. T. Scott. 2001. "Economic Evaluation of the Baldrige National Quality Program." *NIST Planning Report* 01–3 (October).

Mazur, G. H., J. Gibson, and B. Harries. 1995. "QFD Applications in Health Care and Quality of Work Life." 1st International Symposium on QFD.

Naveh, E., and A. Marcus. 2004. "When Does ISO 9000 Quality Assurance Standard Lead to Performance Improvement?" *IEEE Transactions on Engineering Management* 51 (3): 352–363.

www.nist.gov/baldrige/about/baldrige_faqs.cfm.

Omachonu, V., and P. Barach. 2005. "QFD in a Managed Care Organization." *Quality Progress* 38 (11): 36–41.

Shewhart, W. A. 1939. *Statistical Method from the Viewpoint of Quality Control.* New York: Dover.

Shewhart, W. A. 1980. "Economic Control of Quality of Manufactured Product." 50th Anniversary Commemorative Issue. American Society for Quality.

PART IV

PLANNING AND CONTROLLING HEALTH CARE OPERATIONS

CHAPTER 11

LEAN CONCEPTS IN
HEALTH CARE

LEARNING OBJECTIVES

⟫ Understand the concept of lean and the value of creating a lean enterprise.

⟫ Appreciate the benefits of controlling waste.

⟫ Understand how to control flow with kanban systems.

⟫ Recognize what kaizen events are and how they impact a lean enterprise.

⟫ Understand the role value stream mapping plays in a lean enterprise.

⟫ Identify and apply various lean measures and tools.

INTRODUCTION

When it comes to having a fit and healthy body, we all understand what the term *lean* means. Just as a lean body is one with little fat, a lean company is one with little waste. This chapter examines the concept of lean in detail and provides clarification on what it means to be a lean organization. It presents methods for controlling different types of waste, such as waste of motion and waste of time, and explains them in the context of health care settings. Kanban systems, often utilized in production systems, are introduced and an illustration of their success in a health care application is highlighted. Additionally, kaizen events, which were first mentioned in the context of value stream mapping (VSM) in Chapter 7, are explained in detail. The chapter provides several examples of kaizen events in health care taken from the literature. The chapter closes with a summary of various lean tools, most of which were previously explained in Chapter 9.

WHAT IS LEAN?

The core concept of a *lean organization* is that it is an organization that is able to provide maximum value to its customers while minimizing waste (of time, resources, etc.). Lean organizations understand customer value, and they focus key processes to increase it (www.lean.org).

A lean enterprise requires lean thinking, where management shifts its focus from creating optimal silos within the organization to optimizing product flow across the organization. It is a type of systems thinking that examines the impact of changes in technology, policies, and procedures on the entire organization, not just on the area in which the changes are implemented.

According to numerous sources, the term *lean* was coined by a research team headed by Dr. Jim Womack to describe Toyota's business during the late 1980s. The term *lean production* became known worldwide following publication of Womack's book *The Machine That Changed the World* in 1990. Womack continues his work in the area of lean and is the founder and chairman of a nonprofit institution called the Lean Enterprise Institute.

As defined in Chapter 7, the value stream of a product industry or service industry consists of those steps in the production process or service process that add value for the consumer. By working to reduce or eliminate waste along the value stream, companies can refine their processes to reduce capital, space, time, effort, and costs required to deliver products and services. At the same time, quality can be improved, meaning fewer defects and/or fewer customers who are dissatisfied with their service.

In a lean enterprise, production and throughput times are reduced but not at the expense of product or service variety, quality, or cost. Lean is not a business tactic or a cost-reduction program. Lean is a way of thinking and acting across an entire organization (www.lean.org).

Many types of manufacturing and service industries, including health care and governments, utilize lean principles to guide their decisions and actions. It is important to note that lean is not a short-term cost-reduction program, but a manner in which a business chooses to operate. Companies in the process of moving from their old way of thinking to the lean way of thinking are said to be making a *lean transformation*. This transformation requires a complete change in how the company does business. Lean cannot be viewed as just a set of tools or techniques. To be a lean enterprise, a company must not only implement methods, but must also make a broad commitment to a culture change and work to embrace better waste-reducing business habits (Costello 2011).

CONTROLLING WASTE

In order to control waste, you must first identify waste. And to identify waste, you must first accurately map your current processes. Recall in Chapter 7 that we defined and gave an example of a process flow. Additional information that may help modify your process flow into a process map includes how, when, and where products or people move in the process; who the customers are; who the suppliers are; how information is recorded and shared; and how technology is applied (Endsley, Magill, and Godfrey 2006).

From the time of Frederick Taylor's *The Principles of Scientific Management* (1911), companies in the United States have focused tremendous time and effort on optimizing each portion of a production system. While this dissecting of the production system led to significant lessons learned, many companies failed to understand the value in determining and fixing the root causes of production problems and instead only worried about finding suboptimal, narrowly focused solutions to systemic problems.

In Japan, manufacturers took a different approach. There, manufacturing managers worked to eliminate the production of defective items, not just reduce the number of defects per million (Askin and Goldberg 2002). Another strategy derived from Japanese manufacturing that has already been included as a key aspect of lean is elimination of waste. K. Suzaki noted seven sources of waste that should be eliminated (Askin and Goldberg 2002):

1. Waste from overproduction

2. Waste of motion

3. Transportation waste

4. Processing waste

5. Wasted time (queuing)

6. Defective products

7. Excess inventory

In a health care setting, all but the first of Suzaki's list are applicable. Time and motion studies can be utilized on many types of health care workers, from surgeons to housekeeping staff. Motions that do not add value should be eliminated, thus reducing the time to accomplish a task and conserving energy that the worker can use toward more productive endeavors. The Methods Time Measurement Association has developed numerous systems used by industry to measure workers' performance against standards. For health care, they have developed MTM-HC, a standard database devoted specifically to health care activity time standards (Heizer and Render 2004). An analysis of workers' performance against these standards may reveal time standards are not being met due to wasted motions included in performing the task.

An example of transportation waste in a health care setting is the time that nurses must spend retrieving medications for their patients. A patient care unit should be designed in a way that eliminates unnecessary walking between medication storage areas and patient rooms. However, reduction of nurses' wasted steps should not come at the expense of added steps for pharmacy transportation personnel. Chapter 8 examines this issue as related to facility design.

To eliminate processing waste, non-value-added operations should be eliminated. Some emergency departments (EDs) have eliminated the formal triage process that typically occurs when a patient arrives at the ED, replacing it with a two-question assessment done by a registered nurse who then places the patient in a specific room based on the patient's answers to those questions.

Closely linked to the elimination of processing waste is the elimination of wasted time or waiting in line. Using the triage example, patients who are triaged in this manner spend less (or no) time in the ED waiting room. Also, it may be possible to make waiting time value-added time. For example, providing patients in a waiting room with FAQ lists or literature related to their conditions may enable them to determine the questions they need to ask the doctor and expedite the interview process that occurs when they are with the doctor.

As we all know, defective products can lead to increased costs, increased resource consumption, and decreased customer satisfaction. In a health care setting, there is the additional risk of negatively impacting a patient's health. Health care facilities must closely monitor the supply chain for items such as needles, prosthetics, and implants to ensure patient safety and satisfaction.

As these and other health care items typically have a shelf life, facilities must avoid excess inventories or risk having to incur the additional costs that come with disposing outdated items. Also, if storage space is at a premium, then excess inventories of some items can consume space needed to stock adequate quantities of other items.

CONTROLLING FLOW WITH A KANBAN SYSTEM

Kanban production control systems are examples of how simple concepts can have widespread impacts. In a *kanban system*, production is driven by work centers reacting to their customers. When a successor work center has a need, it issues a request for parts to a predecessor work center. When the stock level of completed parts is exhausted, the work center reacts to restock them, maintaining the desired target level of completed parts. The word *kanban* is the Japanese word for card. Kanbans drive the production control system that was perfected by Toyota (Monden 1983).

A sample kanban is shown in Figure 11.1. The kanban, or card, in the figure displays information on the part number and description; the lead time, supplier, and planner; and the quantity authorized and location of all materials needed to create the item. Whereas the original use of kanbans required physical cards,

FIGURE 11.1 Sample Kanban

Part Description		Plastic Fastener	
Part Number		7661325	
Lead time	2 weeks	QTY	25
Supplier	Jones Plastics	LOC	Rack 22W
Planner	T. Johnson		

modern kanbans may be electronic. Regardless of whether the kanbans are electronic or physical, each part type fabricated in a work center has its own set of kanbans, and each kanban authorizes a particular quantity of that part type.

In work centers that produce multiple part types, it may be helpful to associate specific colors with part types and their kanbans. By assigning each part type its own color and developing an association between parts and their colors, it is possible to reduce the likelihood of workers producing the wrong part type.

Managing by means of kanbans has very strict rules that all workers should follow. These five rules are taken from Santos, Wysk, and Torres (2006):

1. Do not send defective products to the following process.

2. The following process removes the product from the current machine and leaves the kanban.

3. Produce only the quantity removed (the number of pieces written in the kanban).

4. Production must be level.

5. The kanban is used to stabilize the production process.

Kanban Example from Health Care

Kanbans transform the scheduling problem into a visual control methodology (Monden 1983). The example provided here, taken from Furrey (2011), does not utilize kanban cards as shown in Figure 11.1, but does employ visual cues that effectively improve communication among workers in a surgery facility.

A catheterization lab was struggling to see the patients it had scheduled and was often forced to reschedule patients who had shown up for their appointments, waited, but not undergone the needed procedures. Management at the facility thought additional beds were needed in the recovery unit or additional staff were needed to improve patient flow.

The industrial engineer tasked with solving the problem decided to observe, investigate, and determine his own conclusions without using the management's preconceived idea that more resources were needed. His analysis led to the conclusion that lack of communication was the number one problem at the facility. Staff were spending too much time on the phone calling to find out if a patient was ready for the next step in the process. It was unclear to everyone which patients were in the building, where they were, what steps they had already completed, and what steps they needed to undergo.

A small decision-support system was developed that allowed staff to input a few pieces of data on a patient, and each patient's status was then available in the system. Using large flat-screen television monitors, patient status information from the system was broadcast to staff areas. Using a color-coding scheme to indicate patient status enabled staff to easily determine which patients were in the building, where they were, what steps they had already completed, and what steps they needed to undergo.

Implementation of this kanban system was successful, and the system is still in use today. The visual cues now allow the staff to know what is going on, and very little time is wasted on phone calls trying to track down patients and learn their status.

KAIZEN EVENTS

Kaizen is the Japanese word for improvement and refers to a philosophy of continuous improvement of processes. Kaizen has its origins in W. Edwards Deming's 14 points. Point five emphasizes the aspect of constant improvement of the system (Deming 1982). By changing activities and processes for the better, kaizen seeks to eliminate waste. The kaizen process begins by questioning current methods (Askin and Goldberg 2002).

Many use the "five whys" as a description of the kaizen process, as the approach typically involves asking "why" five times to discover the root cause or motivation for action—for example, "Why do we store so many syringes?" followed by "Why is it necessary to order syringes in large batches?" followed by "Why can't we find a vendor who will not require such large orders?" The questioning continues on with the goal of identifying alternatives that offer improvement, that can be easily accomplished, and that do not cause complications in other areas of the business.

Kaizen is not something that can be accomplished by management alone. In order to be effective, kaizen must utilize everyone's knowledge to help identify processes that need change and to help implement improvements in an efficient manner.

Kaizen is a term used to describe a set of problem-solving techniques whose goal is process improvement. These techniques range from suggestion systems to scheduled events conducted in the workplace. As with all lean approaches, the goal of *kaizen events* is elimination of waste. The collection of kaizen techniques can be categorized as individual versus teamed and as day-to-day versus special event (www.vitalentusa.com/learn/6-sigma_vs_kaizen_1.php#k_var).

Individual versus Teamed

While most kaizen events are planned occurrences in a workplace and involve a team of employees, there are some kaizen events that occur on an individual basis. *Teian kaizen* is the name given to an event where an individual employee uncovers improvement opportunities while conducting his or her daily work activities (www.vitalentusa.com/learn/6-sigma_vs_kaizen_1.php#k_var). Using the implemented suggestion system, the employee makes management aware of those opportunities. The same term is also used to refer to the situation in which an individual worker uses the kaizen approach to improve his or her own job.

Day-to-Day versus Special Event

Quality circles are an example of a day-to-day kaizen approach. A *quality circle* is a work team that uses its observations about its work processes to identify potential improvements. At scheduled time intervals (perhaps weekly), the team meets and selects a process problem to solve, and then they conduct the analysis and idea generation necessary to develop solutions (www.vitalentusa.com/learn/6-sigma_vs_kaizen_1.php#k_var). Finally, they solve the problem.

Most of the time, kaizen events are planned and require the attention of a large segment of a company's workforce. In these times of events, a process improvement is implemented over a period of days. Such events generally occur at the point where service is being delivered, not at the middle and upper levels of administration.

Kaizen Events in Health Care

Kaizen events in health care have become more prevalent over the past few years. Walsh (2010) provides a brief summary of a 2009 kaizen event held for a physiotherapy department at a hospital in Ireland. The event introduced an electronic system for physiotherapy referrals to replace the existing paper system. The kaizen event included the development of a current state value stream map that enabled the team to identify inefficiencies in the existing handwritten referral process. The future state value stream map provided a vision of achievable improvements. Details on value stream mapping are available in Chapter 7.

Prior to implementation of the new electronic system, training was completed with nursing staff and physiotherapy staff. The decision to cross-train the physiotherapy staff gave them the ability to assist nursing staff with the completion of the electronic referrals. The results included drastic reductions in both referral cycle time and patient waiting time.

Weed (2010) reports on efficiency improvements in the supply system at Seattle Children's Hospital. Using a kanban system, the facility was able to reduce its storeroom to half its original size and also reduced the number of items thrown out due to their age exceeding the expiration date. Prior to the kanban system's implementation, the existing supply system was so unreliable that nurses frequently stockpiled items. After implementation, it now takes only seconds for nurses to find the supplies they need, and their confidence in the system has eliminated their need to stockpile.

Additionally, the hospital implemented a continuous process improvement program called C.P.I. that examines every aspect of patients' stays at the hospital with the goal of uncovering things that could work better for patients and their families. Staff from Seattle Children's Hospital have presented C.P.I. implementation workshops to more than 200 health care professionals.

A recent evaluative study by students at Northern Illinois University (Bartel et al. 2011) examines the need for and benefits of cross-organization kaizen events at Kishwaukee Community Hospital (KCH) in DeKalb County, Illinois. The comprehensive assessment centered on the outpatient services of KCH and its implementation of a kaizen event to implement lean practices. Operational changes resulted from employee-generated initiatives. The project team offered the following recommendations for further improvement of operational quality at KCH:

- Implementation of an organization-wide kaizen suggestion system to direct further process improvements and provide data for future cross-organization kaizen events.

- Implementation of various approaches to increase organizational knowledge of quality improvement.

- Future utilization of industrial engineering and information technology consulting.

VALUE STREAM MAPPING

Chapter 7 of this volume, "Process Improvement and Patient Flow," provides details on value stream mapping (VSM). In relation to creating a lean organization, VSM can enable those working in a system to identify its inefficiencies (current state map) and make adjustments that create a vision of attainable improvements (future state map). Just as kaizen events are employed to provide opportunities for employees to focus on developing a lean organization, kaizen bursts are utilized in future state maps to indicate opportunities for the removal of waste from a current process.

MEASURES AND TOOLS

Lean tools include various processes and strategies that can help identify inefficiencies in the production of goods or delivery of services and reduce those inefficiencies to improve operations. Lean tools enable continual evaluation of a company's processes and to ensure nothing is being wasted (Tatum 2003).

Lean Measures

There are a number of measures that can be used to determine how lean your organization is or to determine the impact of lean approaches. These include, but are not limited to, total cost, total cycle time, throughput, inventory turns, delivery perfor-mance, first-time quality, quality, and safety. Although we will not define each of these measures here, most of them are defined and used in other chapters of this book.

Lean Tools

One lean tool is six sigma (Tennant 2001), which attempts to reduce a process's variability using a combination of statistical data and quality control measures. Six sigma is discussed in detail in Chapter 9.

Pareto analysis is a statistical technique to aid in decision making. It is often used when selecting a limited number of tasks to produce a significant overall effect. It gets its name because it utilizes the Pareto principle, or the 80/20 rule, which has a number of interpretations. In terms of quality improvement, the Pareto principle tells us that a large majority of problems (80 percent) are pro-duced by a few key causes (20 percent). Pareto analysis is covered in Chapter 9.

Cause-and-effect diagrams, also known as *fishbone diagrams*, are used to identify possible causes of an effect or problem. They are often used to add structure to a brainstorming session. They are helpful because they allow for easy sorting of ideas into useful categories. More information on these diagrams is provided in Chapter 9.

Histograms are a useful way to present data that can be classified into several categories. The categories are typically nonoverlapping intervals representing some number of occurrences of a variable value. The graph itself displays adjacent rectangles whose height indicates the frequency of occurrence of the variable value. Histograms are covered in more depth in Chapter 9.

A scatter diagram (also known as a scatter plot or scatter graph) is a graphical representation of the values for two variables for a given set of data. Each point's coordinates on the graph are determined based on the values of the two variables under study. The horizontal axis position is determined by one variable's value and the vertical axis position is determined by the other. Chapter 9 offers additional detail on scatter diagrams.

Often, managers and those involved in kaizen events or observation work to help develop value stream maps will need to collect data in real time. Check sheets provide an organized way to collect data at the location where data are generated. Based on observations, different data values are recorded by making tally marks (or checks) on the check sheet. More information about check sheets is given in Chapter 9.

A *control chart* is a lean tool than enables managers to determine whether a process is operating in a state of statistical control. Using predetermined values for an upper control limit (UCL) and a lower control limit (LCL), process behavior is plotted in two dimensions to determine if there are times when the UCL is exceeded or the process is performing below the LCL. Additional examples involving control charts are presented in Chapter 9.

Another lean tool is 5S, which is a workplace organization approach focused on the concepts of structure, systemize, sanitize, standardize, and self-discipline. The goal of the 5S approach is to create a workplace that enables efficiency and effectiveness. Often, employees who share a workspace are engaged in a directed discussion to determine how to implement 5S in their area. This helps provide ownership of the process to each employee so that each is motivated and has the self-discipline to maintain the improvements made to the workspace.

ADVERSE EFFECTS OF BECOMING TOO LEAN

While we have spent this entire chapter promoting lean concepts and waste reduction, it is also important for health care managers to realize there may be such a thing as becoming too lean. For example, in many health care settings, such as hospitals and emergency departments, demand is unpredictable. If becoming lean reduces inventories too much, then a shortage may arise in the case of an unexpected dramatic increase in demand, such as a bus accident with numerous injured passengers or a natural disaster.

Additionally, many lean concepts are taken from industry and may not translate directly to health care. For example, suppose a nurse is tasked with dispensing medication to her 12 patients as quickly as possible. Dispensing medication to 12 human beings is not the same as performing a one-step maintenance procedure on 12 machines. The human beings (patients) have other needs that the nurse cannot ignore. Often, one of those needs is for attention or a listening ear. Since medication alone is not the only influence on a patient's recovery, it is in the nurse's (and the patient's) best interest for the nurse to provide the extra attention when it is desired or needed. If doing so delays the dispensing of medicine beyond the average time, that extra time should not be considered waste. One must never lose focus on the fact that the main goal of a health care facility and its providers is patient care.

SUMMARY

This chapter has provided an overview of lean concepts in health care. The concept of lean was defined. Since a key focus of lean is the elimination of waste, a section of the chapter was devoted to controlling waste, with examples from health care used to help clarify key concepts. The chapter explained kanban systems in the context of production systems, where they originated. A kanban example from health care demonstrated the approach's relevance to service industries.

Kaizen events were defined and explained, with a number of examples of kaizen events from health care included as well. The chapter provided a summary of lean tools, with reference back to the other locations in the book where they were explained in detail. The notion of a health care facility becoming too lean was discussed. The chapter will close with a minicase related to improving inpatient care.

KEY TERMS

control chart

fishbone diagram

5S

kaizen event

kanban system

lean organization

lean transformation

Pareto analysis

quality circle

DISCUSSION QUESTIONS

1. Provide a good definition of what a lean enterprise is, and explain the value of creating a lean enterprise.

2. Choose two of the types of waste from the following list and explain how these types of waste can be seen in your current work environment. How could these wastes be reduced?

   - Waste of motion

   - Transportation waste

- Processing waste

- Wasted time (queuing)

- Defective products

- Excess inventory

3. Provide an example of how a kanban system (that uses either cards or visual triggers) could be implemented in a health care setting to improve efficiency.

4. Find an example from the past two years of a kaizen event at a health care facility. What were the challenges of holding the event? What were the benefits? Does the description of the event you read about provide any advice for others attempting a similar event?

5. Describe three positive impacts a kaizen event can have on a lean enterprise.

6. Discuss the role value stream mapping plays in a lean enterprise.

7. From the list of lean measures and tools provided in this chapter, select one measure or tool to investigate further. Using a source other than this book, provide enough explanation of the measure or tool to be effective in teaching a classmate about it.

8. Describe how the lean measure or tool you selected for question 7 could be implemented at your current workplace to help reduce or eliminate waste.

MINICASE: USING LEAN CONCEPTS TO IMPROVE INPATIENT CARE

(All information for this case is taken from Béténé [2012].)

Hennepin County Medical Center (HCMC) is Minnesota's premier level I trauma center, with 477 beds and an average daily census of 321. The facility averages 101,070 emergency visits, 10,370 acute psychiatric services visits, and 20,990 discharges per year. Since 2007, the facility has utilized fully integrated electronic health records software.

Leadership at HCMC determined that in order to improve patient care delivery, they needed to change. They made the decision to implement a lean improvement initiative in 2007.

The focus of this case is the inpatient area. Figure 11.2 shows pictures of the actual value stream map created by the team of HCMC employees who worked on the project. Stars represent waste points.

The main observation revealed through the development of the current state map was that lack of a daily schedule was leading to a lot of waste. Staff did not know each patient's daily plan, and neither did the patients and their families. This made it difficult to coordinate care. Although some scheduling tools were in place, they were all localized and nonstandard.

Considering the fact that a typical inpatient at HCMC may need to receive services from as many as a dozen different areas (x-ray, MRI, physical therapy, occupational therapy, dialysis, etc.), how might we apply some lean concepts from this chapter in order to improve the current situation? Provide details on applicable lean methods and tools. Also, how might we be able to gauge the success of any changes that are made to the current process? What is the role of information in our solution?

FIGURE 11.2   Value Stream Map for Hennepin County Medical Center

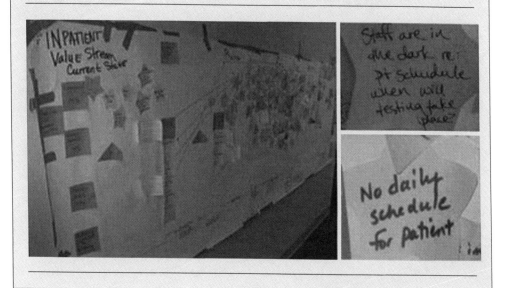

REFERENCES

Askin, R., and J. Goldberg. 2002. *Design and Analysis of Lean Production Systems.* New York: John Wiley & Sons.

Bartel, P., B. Lamb, T. Mighell, I. Polidario, and M. Simko. 2011. "Kaizen in Outpatient Services at Kishwaukee Community Hospital." Report prepared for OMIS 338 Principles of Operations Management, Northern Illinois University.

Bétené, K. 2012. "Keeping Everyone Informed: Scheduling Inpatient Testing and Therapy Appointments." Report from Hennepin County Medical Center, presented at the Society for Health Systems Annual Conference, Las Vegas, NV.

Costello, T. 2011. "Lean: More Than a Shop-Floor Fad." *IT Pro* (May/June): 64.

Deming, W. E. 1982. Quality, Productivity, and Competitive Position. MIT Center for Advanced Engineering Study, Cambridge, MA.

Endsley, S., M. Magill, and M. Godfrey. 2006. "Creating a Lean Practice." *Family Practice Management* 13 (4): 34–38.

Furrey, R. 2011. "Increasing Patient Flow Using Lean Six Sigma and Information Technology." Presentation at the Mayo Clinic Conference on Systems Engineering and Operations Research Applied to Health Care, Rochester, MN.

Heizer, J., and B. Render. 2004. *Principles of Operations Management.* 5th ed. Upper Saddle River, NJ: Pearson Prentice Hall.

www.lean.org.

Monden, Y. 1983. *The Toyota Production System.* Norcross, GA: Industrial Engineering & Management Press.

Santos, J., R. Wysk, and J. Torres. 2006. *Improving Production with Lean Thinking.* Hoboken, NJ: John Wiley & Sons.

Tatum, M. 2003. "What Are Lean Tools?" www.wisegeek.com/what-are-lean-tools.htm.

Taylor, F. 1911. *The Principles of Scientific Management.* New York: Harper & Brothers.

Tennant, G. 2001. *Six Sigma: SPC and TQM in Manufacturing and Services.* London: Gower Publishing, Ltd.

www.vitalentusa.com/learn/6-sigma_vs_kaizen_1.php#k_var.

Walsh, S. 2010. "No More Paper Slips—A Kaizen Event to Introduce an Electronic Referral System for Physiotherapy." www.leadingedgescm.com/news/post/.

Weed, J. 2010. "Factory Efficiency Comes to the Hospital." *New York Times*, July 10, 2010.

Womack, J. 1990. *The Machine That Changed the World.* New York: Rawson Associates.

CHAPTER 12

FORECASTING FOR

HEALTH CARE

MANAGEMENT

LEARNING OBJECTIVES

➠ Understand and know appropriate usage of various time series forecasting models.

➠ Construct moving averages and exponential smoothing models using Excel.

➠ Understand what autocorrelation is and its link to seasonality.

➠ Understand and identify dependent and independent variables and use them in a regression model.

(Continued)

⟫ Develop simple linear and multiple regression models with Excel's Data Analysis package and use it to predict values of the dependent variable.

⟫ Interpret the output from Excel's Data Analysis regression package, including the correlation coefficient R, the coefficient of determination R^2, the F-test, the t-tests, and p-values.

⟫ Understand and speak to multicollinearity, autocorrelation, and heteroscedasticity.

ANALYZING DATA USING TIME SERIES AND REGRESSION MODELS

This chapter reviews techniques for identifying patterns in time series data, introduces models to represent time series data, introduces linear regression models, and shows how to generate forecasts with those models. *Time series* analysis is based on the assumption that successive data points represent consecutive measurements taken at equally spaced time intervals. Linear regression consists of one dependent and one independent variable. The *independent variable* predicts the dependent variable. The *dependent variable*, in turn, is the variable being predicted and is referred to as the criterion variable. Both are common techniques used to forecast within the health care profession.

Goals: Identify and Forecast

This chapter has two main goals: identifying the nature of the situation represented by the time series data and/or regression, and forecasting future values using time series and regression models. Determining the pattern of the observed time series and formally describing that pattern are conditions of these goals. Once the pattern of the data is established, a mathematical model can be used to describe the data and model or predict future data points or events.

Identifying Patterns in Data

Many patterns exist in the health care profession. The age of a patient, type of illness, and even day of the week influence events in the health care industry. Patterns in time series and regression data tend to fall into four distinct components: trend, seasonal, cyclical, and irregular. This chapter discusses the concept of linear trend and multiple linear regression, and also covers seasonal, cyclical, and irregular components.

LINEAR AND NONLINEAR TRENDS

Linear trend is the simple systematic increase or decrease in time series data over a given time range. In addition, simple trend patterns do not repeat themselves. A simple example of a linear trend in health care is the overall cost of health care services. Figure 12.1 displays a trend data pattern.

It is obvious that the line plotted in Figure 12.1 is relatively straight and rises from left to right. The TREND( ) function in Excel can be used to model a data set such as the one in Figure 12.1 as a linear relationship. However, trend can also be nonlinear in nature. In other words, a nonlinear trend must be modeled by using a nonlinear mathematical model.

FIGURE 12.1   Trend Line

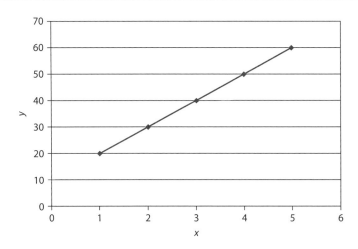

FIGURE 12.2   Nonlinear Trend Data Pattern Example

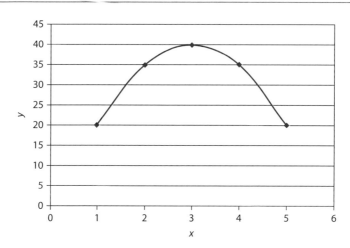

Nonlinear Data

Let's say, for example, the data have a dramatic upward or downward curve or the data seem to oscillate up and then down again. There are many kinds of data that exhibit these characteristics and change over time in a nonlinear fashion. The growth of bacteria from the biology field is a good example of nonlinearity in a data series. Excel's GROWTH( ) function allows for simple nonlinear modeling. Figure 12.2 displays an example of a nonlinear data set.

Although very important to the health care industry, nonlinear trend modeling is not discussed further, as the topic is beyond the scope of this book. Consult the references at the end of this chapter for information on nonlinear modeling.

SEASONALITY IN DATA

The essence of seasonal patterns in time series data is the repetition of the time series in systematic intervals over a given time range. Seasonal patterns may also contain a trend component. In the health care industry, seasonal patterns exist due to the nature of certain illnesses. For example, the colds and flu season is called that due to the seasonal nature of those illnesses. Figure 12.3 displays a seasonal time series pattern.

FIGURE 12.3 Seasonal Data Pattern Example

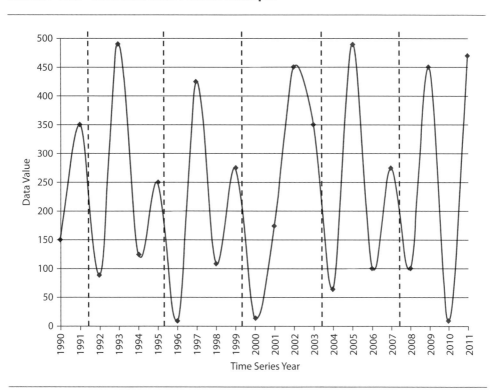

From Figure 12.3 one can see a pattern. The vertical dashed lines split the data at its *seasonality*. In other words, the data repeat every four periods. In actuality, the two categories of patterns in time series do coexist in real-life data.

Figure 12.4 displays a combined trend and seasonal data set. From Figure 12.4 one can see two patterns. The data have a seasonal component and a trend component. The data repeat every four periods and tend to rise from left to right (see dashed lines).

Cyclical Data

Although data may exhibit seasonal and/or trend patterns over the long term, there may exist recurring sequences of points at shorter intervals of time within the data. Any sequence of points that recurs, falling above or below the data's trend, and lasts more than one year can be attributed to the cyclical component of the data.

FIGURE 12.4 Combined Trend and Seasonal Data Pattern Example

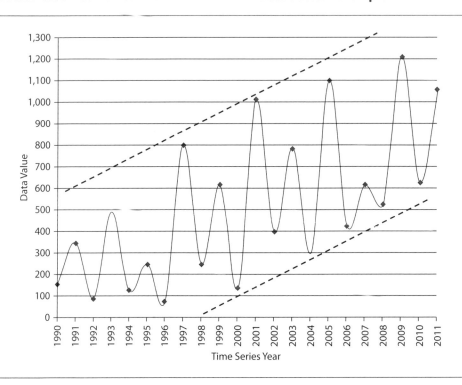

Many data sets contain or exhibit cyclical behavior. Cyclical behavior is most often characterized by regular runs of data points above or below the data's trend line. In most cases, the cyclical component of data is attributed to multiperiod economic movements. For example, in health care, staffing decisions often have a cyclical component to them. Periods of high staffing (i.e., busy times or mandated staff levels by emergency tier level) can be followed by periods of rather low staffing (i.e., slow times or lower emergency tier level). These individual data points alternate above and below the generally increasing trend.

Irregular Data

At times the irregular component is referred to as the random component. It encompasses the residual (the difference between the actual and predicted values) or random variability in the data. Irregular variations do not follow any discernible pattern. They can be caused by short-term, unanticipated, and/or nonrecurring factors that affect the data. Since the nature of this time series component is random, we do not attempt to predict its impact.

General Forms of Models to Explain the Data

In general, two forms of models exist: multiplicative and additive. For now we will assume that the model is attempting to predict the demand for some health care product or service. The multiplicative model is the most widely used, and it assumes that demand is the product of the four time series components. It is expressed as:

$$Demand = Trend \times Seasonal \times Cyclical \times Irregular$$

The additive model simply adds the components together:

$$Demand = Trend + Seasonal + Cyclical + Irregular$$

It should be noted that most real-world forecasters assume the irregular component will average itself out over time, and they concentrate only on the trend, seasonal, and cyclical components.

Analyzing Patterns in Data

There are no automated techniques for analyzing and interpreting models. In fact, many of the techniques that exist to analyze data require substantial computational effort and statistical insight. Forecasters expend effort in building and choosing the proper models and apply insight in interpreting the output from the models.

There exist a set of techniques called time series techniques that assist in modeling data. The next sections detail a number of these models, including the latest period or naive model, trend analysis, smoothing techniques such as moving averages and exponential models, as well as multiple regression models. In general, moving average and exponential smoothing models are referred to as time series models whereas regression techniques are referred to as causal models.

TABLE 12.1 Example Data Set for Hospital (Beds Demanded)

Year	Demand (Yearly Beds)	Year	Demand (Yearly Beds)
1990	52,034	2001	83,180
1991	59,014	2002	87,050
1992	56,046	2003	84,790
1993	54,028	2004	73,490
1994	65,033	2005	76,230
1995	75,023	2006	96,540
1996	62,015	2007	95,080
1997	74,047	2008	87,050
1998	81,031	2009	96,020
1999	98,030	2010	98,900
2000	87,040	2011	83,230

Table 12.1 contains a set of yearly demand data (yearly beds demanded) for a hospital over a 22-year period.

NAIVE FORECASTING

This method may be the simplest method available. In this method a forecaster uses the value of the latest period to forecast the next period. This method is sometimes referred to as the naive method because it uses just one piece of data when other relevant data are available.

Figure 12.5 contains the naive forecast for the beds data in Table 12.1. The active cell in Figure 12.5 is cell C3. Take note that the formula in cell C3 is =B2. The forecast for the next period (e.g., 1991) using the naive method is just the value of the last period (e.g., 1990) or, as referred to earlier, the latest period. Following the naive method's logic, the forecast for 2012 would be 83,230 (i.e., the yearly bed demand for 2011).

Trend Analysis

If the time series has a pattern akin to the one shown in Figure 12.1, the analysis is not very difficult. These time series exhibit a trend component that is consistently increasing. Excel's TREND( ) function can be used to easily model these types of time series (see the material later in this chapter on linear regression).

FIGURE 12.5 Naive Forecast for Beds Demanded

	A	B	C
	Year	Demand (Yearly Beds)	Naive Forecast
1	Year	(Yearly Beds)	Forecast
2	1990	52,034	
3	1991	59,014	52,034
4	1992	56,046	59,014
5	1993	54,028	56,046
6	1994	65,033	54,028
7	1995	75,023	65,033
8	1996	62,015	75,023
9	1997	74,047	62,015
10	1998	81,031	74,047
11	1999	98,030	81,031
12	2000	87,040	98,030
13	2001	83,180	87,040
14	2002	87,050	83,180
15	2003	84,790	87,050
16	2004	73,490	84,790
17	2005	76,230	73,490
18	2006	96,540	76,230
19	2007	95,080	96,540
20	2008	87,050	95,080
21	2009	96,020	87,050
22	2010	98,900	96,020
23	2011	83,230	98,900
24			83,230

However, if the trend is not as distinct as the one in Figure 12.1 or contains considerable noise, then the time series may need to be adjusted to help identify the trend. This adjustment process is generally referred to as smoothing.

Smoothing

Smoothing always incorporates some form of averaging of the time series data. The most common smoothing techniques are the moving average and exponential smoothing. The moving average technique is presented first followed by exponential smoothing.

MOVING AVERAGES

Moving averages tend to be the easier technique to use. The technique calculates a forecast at any period of the data set by averaging several observations in the time series. For example, if one wanted to smooth the data for the years of 1990, 1991, and 1992 (referred to as a three-year moving average), a forecast for 1993's bed demand could be developed. This forecast would be calculated by averaging the data points from 1990, 1991, and 1992.

A four-year moving average can be developed by using the bed demand data from 1990, 1991, 1992, and 1993. The longer a moving average is, the smoother the data set becomes. In fact, one can control the effect of smoothing on the time series data by using a longer or shorter averaging period. The formula for calculating a moving average (MA) is shown in Equation 12.1:

$$MA_n = \frac{\sum_{i=1}^{n} D_i}{n} \tag{12.1}$$

where

n = number of periods in a moving average

D_i = data in period i

Moving Average Example Using Excel

To illustrate the concept of smoothing using moving averages, let's analyze the hospital bed data set listed in Table 12.1.

We will demonstrate three-year and five-year moving averages on the data set provided in Table 12.1 using Excel's Moving Average tool. The following steps should be completed to create a moving average in Excel:

1. Be sure to have Excel's Data Analysis package loaded (see Microsoft Help menu).

2. In Excel, go to the Data tab and from the Analysis group choose Data Analysis.

FIGURE 12.6   Data Analysis Dialogue Box

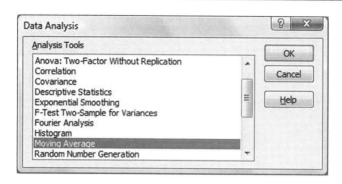

3. From the dialogue box displayed in Figure 12.6, choose Moving Average and click OK.

4. Excel displays a dialogue box that prompts you for an input range, interval, and output range. This dialogue box, accompanied by the time series data, is shown in Figure 12.7.

5. Enter the bed demand data range in the Input Range edit box by highlighting the data or typing in its reference.

6. Click on the Labels in First Row box if the data set contains a label in the first row.

7. Enter the number of periods to be included in the moving average in the Interval edit box.

8. Click on the Output Range edit box and enter the address of the cell or click on the cell where you want the output to start. The author suggests juxtaposing your forecasted values with your actual values. For our data set, cell C3 should be selected for the three-year MA and cell D3 for the five-year MA. This positioning of the output matches up the forecasted values with the actual values of the same time period.

9. Click OK.

Excel will fill in the formulas for the moving average. The moving average will begin with the term #N/A. There will be as many #N/A terms as the number of

FIGURE 12.7 Excel's Moving Average Dialogue Box

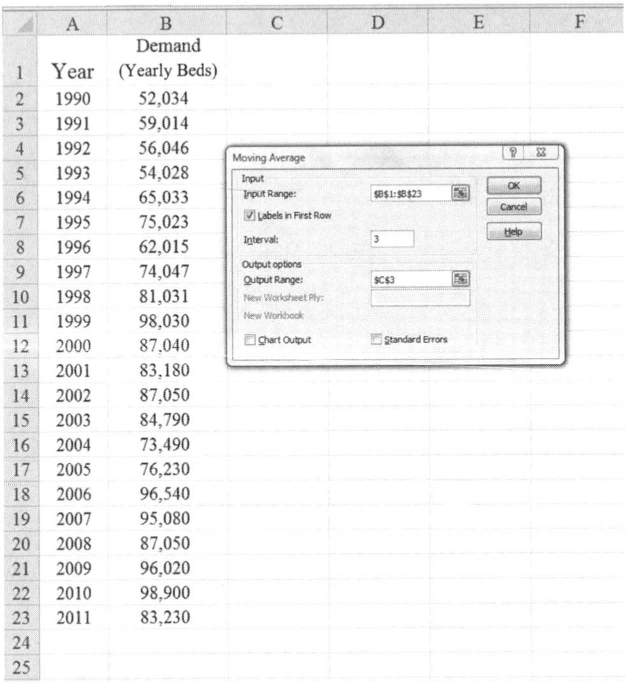

	A	B	C	D	E	F
1	Year	Demand (Yearly Beds)				
2	1990	52,034				
3	1991	59,014				
4	1992	56,046				
5	1993	54,028				
6	1994	65,033				
7	1995	75,023				
8	1996	62,015				
9	1997	74,047				
10	1998	81,031				
11	1999	98,030				
12	2000	87,040				
13	2001	83,180				
14	2002	87,050				
15	2003	84,790				
16	2004	73,490				
17	2005	76,230				
18	2006	96,540				
19	2007	95,080				
20	2008	87,050				
21	2009	96,020				
22	2010	98,900				
23	2011	83,230				
24						
25						

Moving Average

Input
Input Range: $B$1:$B$23
☑ Labels in First Row
Interval: 3

Output options
Output Range: $C$3
New Worksheet Ply:
New Workbook
☐ Chart Output   ☐ Standard Errors

OK
Cancel
Help

intervals you specified, minus 1. Excel does this because there is not enough data to calculate an average for those observations that number less than the interval. Figure 12.8 displays the results of the three- and five-year moving averages on the bed demand time series data (see Table 12.1).

Using Excel's charting feature, it is very simple to create a graph of the bed demand baseline data, the three-year moving average, and the five-year moving average all on one graph. Figure 12.9 displays such a graph.

From Figure 12.9 it is apparent that the longer the moving average interval is, five-year versus three-year, the smoother the forecast is. In addition, it can be seen that the moving averages lag behind movements in the baseline. This is because the moving averages are based on prior data points. In other words, longer moving averages tend to smooth data more and also tend to lag behind movements in the underlying baseline more.

Overall, moving average techniques tend to work best on stable data (i.e., no pronounced ups or downs). However, this is a bit ironic, in that if a time series is

FIGURE 12.8 Three- and Five-Year Moving Averages for Bed Demand Time Series Data

	A	B	C	D
1	Year	Demand (Yearly Beds)	3-Year MA	5-Year MA
2	1990	52,034		
3	1991	59,014	#N/A	#N/A
4	1992	56,046	#N/A	#N/A
5	1993	54,028	55,698	#N/A
6	1994	65,033	56,363	#N/A
7	1995	75,023	58,369	57,231
8	1996	62,015	64,695	61,829
9	1997	74,047	67,357	62,429
10	1998	81,031	70,362	66,029
11	1999	98,030	72,364	71,430
12	2000	87,040	84,369	78,029
13	2001	83,180	88,700	80,433
14	2002	87,050	89,417	84,666
15	2003	84,790	85,757	87,266
16	2004	73,490	85,007	88,018
17	2005	76,230	81,777	83,110
18	2006	96,540	78,170	80,948
19	2007	95,080	82,087	83,620
20	2008	87,050	89,283	85,226
21	2009	96,020	92,890	85,678
22	2010	98,900	92,717	90,184
23	2011	83,230	93,990	94,718
24			92,717	92,056
25				

more stable, smoothing techniques may not have to be used at all. It should be noted that a moving average is a simple average of the data over a time frame. All data points are weighted the same. This may or may not be desirable for a decision maker. Therefore, weighted moving averages are an extension to moving averages. Weighted moving averages allow a decision maker to weight data; they are covered next, followed by exponential smoothing.

WEIGHTED MOVING AVERAGES

As previously mentioned, in using a simple moving average, all weights assigned to the data points are assumed to be equal. Weighted moving averages are a variation on simple moving averages that allow the forecaster to choose the

FIGURE 12.9 Graph of Baseline, Three-Year, and Five-Year Moving Averages

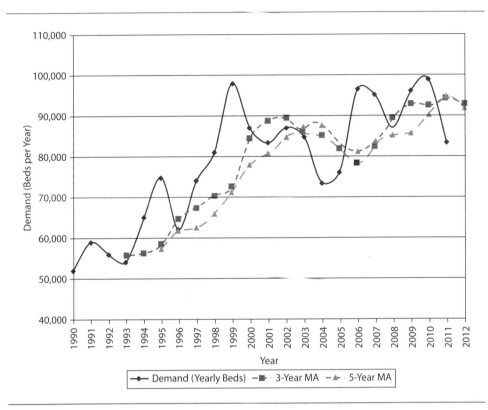

weights assigned to the data points. A weighted moving average (WMA) can be expressed as shown in Equation 12.2:

$$WMA = \frac{\sum (\text{weight for period n})(\text{demand for period n})}{\sum \text{weights}} \qquad (12.2)$$

Weights can be used to place more emphasis on recent data or more emphasis on older data. The weighting scheme chosen makes the technique more responsive. In general, more weight is applied to the recent data. Let's use the bed demand data from Figure 12.8 to calculate a weighted three-year moving average with the most recent data point receiving three times as much weight as the oldest data point, while the middle data point receives twice as much weight as the oldest data point (i.e., the weight for the 2011 bed demand data would be

⅜ or ½, the weight for the 2010 bed demand data would be ⅔ or ⅓, and the weight for the 2009 bed demand data would be ⅙).

The forecast for 2012 would be as follows:

$$\text{WMA 2012 sales} = \frac{3*83,230 + 2*98,900 + 1*96,020}{6} = 90,585$$

Note that for the weighted moving average the sum of the weights is equal to 1.0. This is also true for a three-year simple moving average where each weight was ⅓. Recall that the forecast using a three-year simple moving average was 92,717 beds.

One advantage to weighted moving averages is that the technique allows a decision maker to choose individual weights. However, as the length of the moving average gets bigger, choosing weights becomes burdensome. Therefore a smoothing technique, exponential smoothing, is introduced that allows for multiple weights but does not require the decision maker to choose more than one initial weight.

EXPONENTIAL SMOOTHING

Exponential smoothing (ES) is another smoothing technique, one that calculates a forecast at any period by using past observations. Specifically, exponential smoothing combines a prior forecast with a weighted error measurement. This error measurement comes from the difference between the prior forecast and the actual observation at the time of the prior forecast.

The basic equation is shown in Equation 12.3:

$$F_{t+1} = F_t + \alpha e_t \tag{12.3}$$

Given that t is time, F_t is the forecast at time t, α is a smoothing constant (a value between 0.0 and 1.0, inclusive), and $e_t = A_t - F_t$, where A_t denotes the actual observation at time t, Equation 12.3 can be rewritten as follows:

$$F_{t+1} = F_t + \alpha(A_t - F_t) \tag{12.4}$$

With some mathematical manipulation, Equation 12.4 can be rearranged to yield Equation 12.5:

$$F_{t+1} = (1 - \alpha)F_t + \alpha A_t \qquad (12.5)$$

Equation 12.5 describes the forecast at period $t + 1$ as a proportion of the forecast at period t plus a proportion of the actual observation at period t. If α is 1.0, the forecast at period $t + 1$ is the actual observation from period t. Conversely, if α is 0.0, the forecast at period $t + 1$ is the forecast from period t.

Exponential Smoothing Example Using Excel

To illustrate the concept of exponential smoothing, let's analyze the same hospital bed demand data set previously listed in Table 12.1. We will use $\alpha = 0.1$ and $\alpha = 0.3$. Take note that Excel uses what is called a damping factor. The damping factor is equal to 1 minus the smoothing constant. See step 6 for further discussion. The following steps should be completed to create an exponentially smoothed model in Excel:

1. Be sure to have Excel's Data Analysis package loaded (see Excel Help menu).

2. Choose the Tools menu in Excel and then the Data Analysis option.

3. From the dialogue box displayed in Figure 12.10, choose Exponential Smoothing and click OK.

4. Excel displays a dialogue box that prompts you for an input range, a damping factor, and an output range. This dialogue box accompanied by the time series data is shown in Figure 12.11.

FIGURE 12.10   Data Analysis Dialogue Box

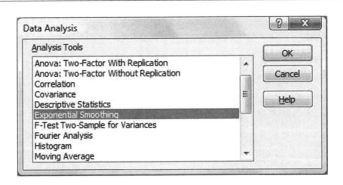

FIGURE 12.11   Excel's Exponential Smoothing Dialogue Box

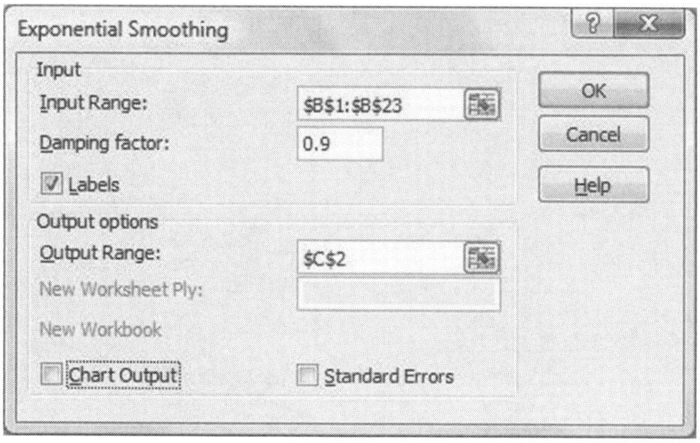

5. Enter the bed demand data range in the Input Range edit box by highlighting the data or typing in its reference.

6. Enter the value of $1 - \alpha$ in the Damping factor edit box. Excel requests a damping factor instead of a smoothing constant. The damping factor is equal to 1 minus the smoothing constant (i.e., 1 − Smoothing constant = Damping factor). We will use a damping factor of 0.9 for the example.

7. Click on Labels box if the data set contains a label in the first row.

8. Click on the Output Range edit box and enter the address of the cell or click on the cell where you want the output to start. Refer to the Help menu in Excel for more details regarding output range selection. For our example cell C2 is chosen.

9. Click OK.

Excel will fill in the formulas for the exponentially smoothed model. The exponentially smoothed forecasts will begin with the term #N/A. There will be one #N/A term. Excel does this because there is not enough data to calculate an exponentially smoothed forecast for the first observation. Figure 12.12 displays the results of the exponentially smoothed models for $\alpha = 0.1$ and $\alpha = 0.3$.

We see from Figure 12.12 that the higher the smoothing constant α is, the smoother the forecast is. In addition, we see that the exponentially smoothed

FIGURE 12.12   Graph of Baseline and Exponentially Smoothed Bed Demand Data

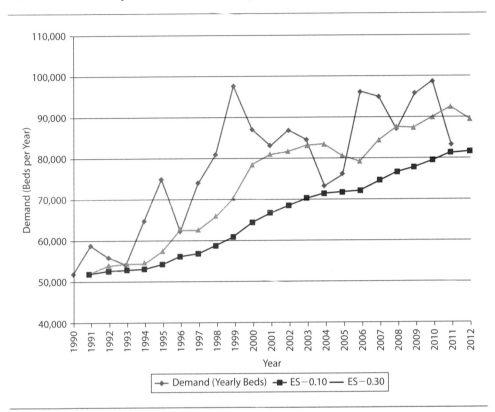

forecasts lag behind movements in the baseline. This is because the exponentially smoothed data is based on a weighted average of prior data points and the present data point.

Choosing a Smoothing Constant

In general, the higher the smoothing constant α, the smoother the forecast will be. Standard forecasting nomenclature recommends that the smoothing constant should be between 0.1 and 0.3. This recommendation is based on the following: If exponential smoothing appears to work significantly better when a larger smoothing constant is chosen, the improved results are likely to be due to a substantial amount of autocorrelation in the time series data.

AUTOCORRELATION

Autocorrelation occurs when there is dependency between time series data points. In other words, a current time series data point could be dependent on a time series data point or points a number of time periods earlier. For our example, the number of beds demanded in one period may be dependent upon the number of beds demanded in a previous period. This is very likely to occur in a hospital setting. This type of dependency describes the essence of a seasonal time series. Autocorrelation is key to forecasting seasonal time series.

Identifying Autocorrelation

Autocorrelation can be calculated by lagging a data set against itself. If the data points in a time series are paired with the data points that immediately precede them, you can calculate the correlation ρ between the two data sets. If the correlation is strong, $\rho > 0.5$, then there is a substantial amount of autocorrelation in the time series. The Excel function CORREL( ) calculates the correlation between sets of time series data. Figure 12.13 displays an example of a lagging time series data set and the corresponding correlation coefficient, ρ. Cell B26 uses the following formula: =CORREL(B2:B24, C2:C24).

It is seen from Figure 12.13 that the correlation is relatively high for the lagged variables since $\rho = 0.77$. This leads us to believe there is dependency between the time series data points. In turn, this may lead one to believe there is a seasonal component to the time series.

Autocorrelation and Seasonality

Measuring autocorrelation can identify seasonality in a set of time series data. Figure 12.14a displays the hospital bed demand data but now it is provided in a quarterly format (we asked IT for more data and they gave it to us!). The data appears to have a pronounced seasonal component. Figure 12.14b provides a graph of the data in Figure 12.14a, and one notices peaks and valleys at regular intervals in the bed demand data.

If one wishes to forecast future bed demand, then seasonal variations in the time series must be identified. For example, many data sets tend to be seasonal in nature. Sales of flu shots tend to peak around February or March during the height of the colds and flu season.

FIGURE 12.13 Lagged Time Series Example and Correlation Estimate

	A	B	C
		Demand	Lagged Demand
1	Year	(Yearly Beds)	(Yearly Beds)
2			52,034
3	1990	52,034	59,014
4	1991	59,014	56,046
5	1992	56,046	54,028
6	1993	54,028	65,033
7	1994	65,033	75,023
8	1995	75,023	62,015
9	1996	62,015	74,047
10	1997	74,047	81,031
11	1998	81,031	98,030
12	1999	98,030	87,040
13	2000	87,040	83,180
14	2001	83,180	87,050
15	2002	87,050	84,790
16	2003	84,790	73,490
17	2004	73,490	76,230
18	2005	76,230	96,540
19	2006	96,540	95,080
20	2007	95,080	87,050
21	2008	87,050	96,020
22	2009	96,020	98,900
23	2010	98,900	83,230
24	2011	83,230	
25			
26	Correlation ρ =	0.77	
27			

Figure 12.14a notes the seasonality of the bed demand data to be at regular intervals of four years. The data points in bold are the highest sales for the respective four-year seasonal period. A trend can also be seen as the data points create peaks and valleys at regular intervals in Figure 12.14b.

Seasonal Adjustments

A number of methods for adjusting seasonal time series exist. The author suggests a simple weighting method for developing seasonal factors (SFs) of a data set. The method consists of dividing the actual demand for a single period by the total demand over the entire seasonal period. The basic equation for this calculation is shown in Equation 12.6:

FIGURE 12.14a   Seasonal Data for Hospital Bed Example

	A	B
		Average Quarterly
1	Year	Demand (Beds)
2	2005	17,116
3	**2005**	**20,335**
4	2005	19,455
5	2005	19,198
6	2006	23,213
7	**2006**	**24,833**
8	2006	24,350
9	2006	24,202
10	2007	22,646
11	**2007**	**25,045**
12	2007	24,946
13	2007	24,913
14	2008	20,937
15	**2008**	**22,073**
16	2008	21,960
17	2008	21,914
18	2009	22,046
19	**2009**	**25,303**
20	2009	24,217
21	2009	24,111
22	2010	24,721
23	**2010**	**25,514**
24	2010	24,869
25	2010	24,810

$$SF_i = \frac{D_i}{\sum_{i=1}^{n} D_i} \qquad (12.6)$$

where

SF_i = seasonal factor for period i

D_i = demand for period i

Basically, Equation 12.6 calculates the portion of total demand assigned to each seasonal period. These seasonal factors are then multiplied by the forecasted

FIGURE 12.14b   Graph of Seasonal Data for Hospital Bed Example

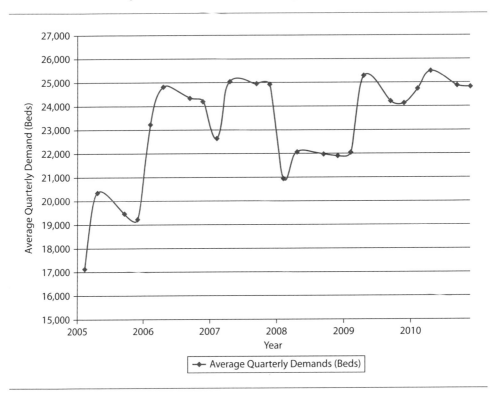

demand to yield seasonally adjusted forecasts. The forecasted demand is obtained by using a linear regression model on the original data. An example using the hospital bed data starting in 1995 from Figure 12.13 is presented next.

Seasonal Adjustment Example

Figure 12.15 depicts the data starting in 2005, sorted by seasonal period. In this case, there are four seasonal periods labeled 1, 2, 3, and 4. The sum of each column and the total sum have been computed. The seasonal factors are computed by dividing each seasonal period (column) demand total by the overall total demand.

The following calculations exhibit the seasonal factors (Equations 12.7 through 12.10):

$$SF_1 = \frac{130,679}{552,727} = 23.6\% \qquad (12.7)$$

$$SF_2 = \frac{143,103}{552,727} = 25.9\% \qquad (12.8)$$

$$SF_3 = \frac{139,797}{552,727} = 25.3\% \qquad (12.9)$$

$$SF_4 = \frac{139,148}{552,727} = 25.2\% \qquad (12.10)$$

These seasonal factors then must be multiplied by the forecast for the upcoming period. Overall, there seems to be an upward trend in the amount of beds demanded each year. This can be seen in the last column of Figure 12.15, as demand for beds steadily rises from around 76,000 to almost 100,000. Therefore, it would be reasonable to use linear trend to predict the upward trend component of the time series and adjust it for seasonality.

Trend and Seasonal Adjustment

A linear trend line is calculated to forecast bed demand for 2011 using yearly demand data from 2005 to 2010. The trend equation for the data, where x_1 is in

FIGURE 12.15   Seasonally Sorted Demand Data

	A	B	C	D	E	F
1						
2			Demand (Beds)			
3			Seasonal Period			
4		1	2	3	4	Totals
5	2005	17,116	20,335	19,455	19,198	76,104
6	2006	23,213	24,833	24,350	24,202	96,598
7	2007	22,646	25,045	24,946	24,913	97,550
8	2008	20,937	22,073	21,960	21,914	86,884
9	2009	22,046	25,303	24,217	24,111	95,677
10	2010	24,721	25,514	24,869	24,810	99,914
11		130,679	143,103	139,797	139,148	552,727
12						

years, is calculated using the TREND( ) formula in Excel. In the Excel spreadsheet displayed in Figure 12.15, type in any blank cell the formula =TREND(F5:F10,A5:A10,2011). The array F5:F10 identifies the bed demand totals as the known y's, and the array A5:A10 identifies the year as the known x's; the 2011 is the value of the new x (year) we wish to forecast for. The actual trend equation is shown in Equation 12.11 with the forecasted bed demand for 2011 listed:

$$\hat{y} = -5,965,997.62 + 3017.74 * x_1 \tag{12.11}$$

Therefore, the forecast for 2001 is as shown in Equation 12.12:

$$\hat{y} = -5,965,997.62 + 3017.74 * 2011 = 102,683.27 \tag{12.12}$$

The bed demand forecast produced from Equation 12.12 predicts that approximately 102,684 beds will be demanded in 2011. The number produced by the equation is rounded up, as it is not feasible to have 0.27 of a bed demanded.

Using this forecast for bed demand for 2011, the seasonally adjusted forecasts SF_i for the four quarters of 2011 are as follows (Equations 12.13 through 12.16):

Note: The final seasonal forecast numbers are rounded up.

$$SF1 = (0.236)(102,683) = 24,277 \tag{12.13}$$

$$SF2 = (0.259)(102,683) = 26,585 \tag{12.14}$$

$$SF3 = (0.253)(102,683) = 25,971 \tag{12.15}$$

$$SF4 = (0.252)(102,683) = 25,850 \tag{12.16}$$

Figure 12.16 displays the combined graph of the original time series and the new forecasts. The new forecast is represented in the graph by the $\times$ data symbol. It is apparent that these forecasts reflect both the seasonal variation and the upward trend in the bed demand time series.

FIGURE 12.16   Combined Graph of Original Time Series and Forecasted Data

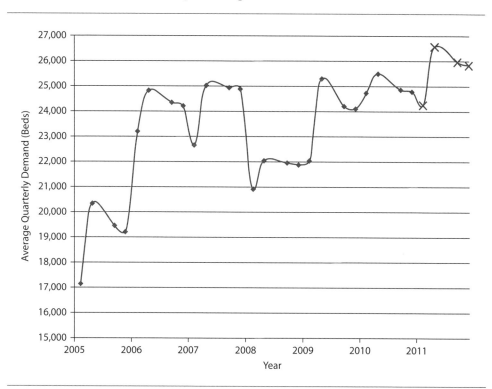

Seasonality and Regression

The previous section illustrated how a simple linear trend coupled with a seasonal index can be used to forecast future demand for beds at a health care facility. Although the TREND( ) function in Excel was employed, the concept of linear regression must be discussed in more detail. The next section explains regression and its accompanying concepts.

REGRESSION AS A FORECASTING TECHNIQUE

Regression is one of many forecasting techniques used in the health care profession to predict future events. The purpose of forecasting is to reduce the level of uncertainty. Some methods are better at predicting short-term events whereas others predict better in the long term. Regression is one of the most popular methods. The regression analysis helps determine the relationship between the dependent variable (y) and one or more independent variables (x).

You might have tried to predict, for example, the average length of stay (LOS) of patients at your facility. In a regression model, length of stay would be the dependent variable and the type of illness/procedure, age of the patient, and overall health could be the independent variables. Many health care professionals use regression models to predict health care–related events. The level of inventory in the pharmacy might be the dependent variable and an indicator such as the time of year (i.e., maybe it is colds and flu season) might be the independent variable.

In reality, it might not be this simple, as there are many factors influencing a possible outcome. However, regression analysis provides the tools for helping model such predictions. There are many reasons why forecasters choose a linear relationship:

- Simple representation

- Ease of use

- Ease of calculations

- Many linear relationships in the real world

The clue is to start simply and eliminate relationships that do not work. This chapter is designed to introduce regression analysis to the reader. It gives basic regression information; presents examples of where regression is being used; and looks at regression modeling steps, scatter plots, and hypothesis testing to make sure all readers have the same statistical background before going on to analyze the data.

Health Care Operations and Supply Chain Management behind the Scenes: History of Regression

Egyptians, Greeks, and Romans and Statistics

Statistics can be traced back to the early years of the Egyptians, Greeks, and Romans. Until 1850 the word *statistics* was used in a different sense than it is used today. It meant information about political states, the kind of material that is nowadays to be found assembled in *The Statesman's Yearbook*.

Pearson, Galton, Gauss? Where Did It All Start?

The technique of regression analysis is not new; it's a standard statistical tool for comparing the relative behavior of two or more variables. Regression analysis originated in Great Britain in the late nineteenth century, and it has been revised and reconstructed since then to take the present form of $y = a + bx$.

The origin of regression first stemmed from the "Theory of Errors," or Gaussian model (named after K. F. Gauss), which was devised for a measurement problem in astronomy and took the form $m = Xb$. This model was later revised by J. Neyman in 1934 and A. C. Aitken in 1935 and became known as the linear model. The most prominent scientists in developing the regression model were Franc Galton, Francis Ysidro Edgeworth, George Udny Yule, and K. F. Gauss.

Pearson, Gauss, and the Theory of Correlation

In 1896, Karl Pearson presented regression and correlation as aspects of the multinormal distribution, hence the entrance of the theory of correlation. Pearson's formulas for the multinormal regression were identical to those developed by Gauss for the "least squares" technique, except that the variables x and y in the Gaussian model were not correlated. To further enhance the technique of regression analysis, G. U. Yule in 1897 extended the linear regression specifications to cases of skew correlation and least squares.

Fisher and the Standard Regression Model

Eventually, in 1922, Ronald Aylmer Fisher synthesized the regression theory of Pearson and Yule with the least squares theory of Gauss to introduce the fixed x regression model. As time passed, mathematicians and scientists have debated over the intricacies of the regression model. It is up to you to decide whether regression analysis will best suit your statistical needs.

Scatter Plots

In a spreadsheet there are two variables, x and y. These variables are plotted in a pair (coordinates). The variable x is plotted horizontally, and the variable y is plotted vertically. These coordinates are the points in the scatter plot. When the slope is large, the line is steep. When the slope is small, the line is almost flat.

The relationship can be positive, negative, or curved—or there can be no relationship at all. However, if the line is perfect, one should be suspicious.

A person interested in predicting future events would want to determine if the variable y would increase, decrease, or stay the same when x changes. It is important to find out whether the relationship forms a straight or curved line and how steep the line is. The scatter plot patterns (x-y data plots) that one can encounter are illustrated in Figures 12.17 to 12.20.

FIGURE 12.17   Scatter Plot of a Perfect Positive Linear Relationship

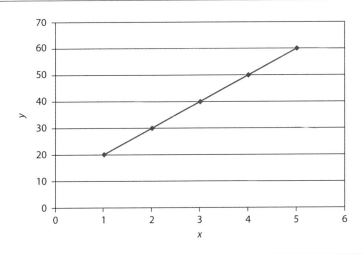

FIGURE 12.18   Scatter Plot of a Perfect Negative Linear Relationship

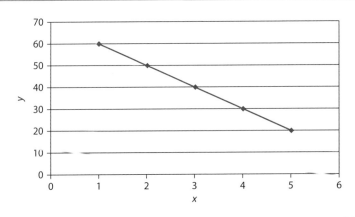

FIGURE 12.19   Scatter Plot Depicting a Curvilinear Relationship

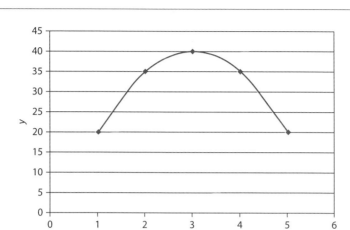

FIGURE 12.20   Scatter Plot Depicting No Linear Relationship

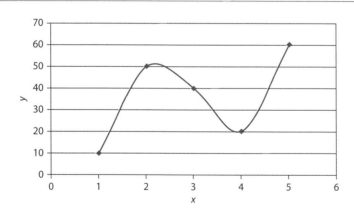

From Figure 12.17, it can be seen that when x increases, so does y in a perfect linear relationship. A straight line can easily be drawn between the data points.

In Figure 12.18, the data points form a perfect negative relationship. When x increases, the variable y decreases in a perfect relationship. A straight line can also be drawn between these data points.

Figure 12.19 shows a curved relationship. It is not possible to draw a straight line though these data points.

Finally, Figure 12.20 shows no linear relationship between the x and y data pairs.

Simple Linear Regression Equation

A linear regression consists of one dependent and one independent variable. The independent variable predicts the dependent variable. The dependent variable, by contrast, is the variable being predicted and is referred to as the criterion variable. The regression equation of a sample, which is the equation of a straight line, is expressed as shown in Equation 12.17:

$$\hat{y} = b_0 + b_1 x_1 + \varepsilon \qquad (12.17)$$

where

$x =$ the dependent variable

$x_1 =$ the independent variable

$b_0 =$ intercept

$b_1 =$ individual independent variable contributions

$e =$ error term

The slope is defined as the change in y for every one-unit change in x. When data are tested with the regression model, the slope is expected to change in response to when the predictor increases by one unit. Equation 12.18 displays the *simple linear regression model* without the error term.

$$\hat{y} = b_0 + b_1 x_1 \qquad (12.18)$$

The intercept is defined as the value of the response, y, expected when the predictor, x, equals zero.

The symbol b is referred to as the population parameter. Looking at the graph presented in Figure 12.21, we see that b_0 represents the point where the line crosses the vertical y-axis. The symbol b_1 represents the slope of the line. Figure 12.21 displays a simple linear relationship and the equation for a line in slope-intercept form.

FIGURE 12.21 Simple Linear Representation

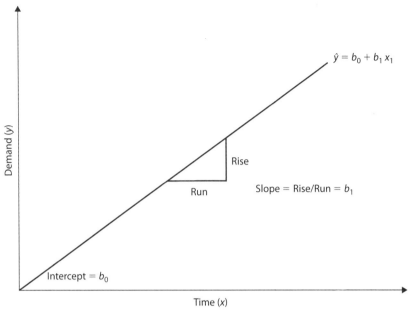

Simple Linear Regression Example

Suppose a manager at a health care facility samples the hospital charges and length of stay for the last six patients. Data in Table 12.2 have been found for length of stay and total hospital charges, where y = total hospital charges, and x = length of stay. The calculations necessary to find b_0 and b_1 are shown next.

The slope of the linear regression curve is given by Equation 12.19:

$$b_1 = \frac{n\sum_{i=1}^{n} x_i y_i - \sum_{i=1}^{n} x_i \sum_{i=1}^{n} y_i}{n\sum_{i=1}^{n} x_i^2 - \left(\sum_{i=1}^{n} x_i\right)^2} \tag{12.19}$$

and for our example (Equation 12.20):

$$= \frac{6(175,000) - (30)(32,000)}{6(168) - (30)^2} = \frac{-90,000}{108} = 833.33 \tag{12.20}$$

The intercept can be calculated as follows, with Equation 12.21 calculating the mean of x and Equation 12.22 calculating the mean of y.

$$\bar{x} = \frac{30}{6} = 5 \qquad (12.21)$$

and

$$\bar{y} = \frac{32,000}{6} = 5333.33 \qquad (12.22)$$

In turn, the intercept is calculated by Equation 12.23:

$$b_0 = \bar{y} - b_1\bar{x} = 5,333.33 - (833.33)(5) = 1,166.67 \qquad (12.23)$$

The least squares regression line for these data is found to be as shown in Equation 12.24:

$$\hat{y} = 1,167.67 + (833.33)x \qquad (12.24)$$

Therefore, if the next patient had a length of stay of seven days (i.e., $x = 7$) then the total hospital charges are calculated using the linear regression equation as shown in Equation 12.25:

$$\hat{y} = \$1,167.67 + (\$833.33)7 = \$7,000.00 \qquad (12.25)$$

TABLE 12.2 Hospital Charge/Length of Stay Data for Linear Regression Computation

Data Point	Total Hospital Charges = y_i	Length of Stay = x_i	$y_i x_i$	x_i^2
1	$5,000	6	$30,000	36
2	$3,000	3	$9,000	9
3	$8,000	8	$64,000	64
4	$6,000	5	$30,000	25
5	$6,000	5	$30,000	25
6	$4,000	3	$12,000	9
Sum	$32,000	30	$175,000	168

From the linear regression, the manager can estimate a seven-day length of stay to be equivalent to $7,000 in total hospital charges.

Health Care Operations and Supply Chain Management in Action: The Scientists of Regression

Many have studied regression analysis over the years. A few of the famous scientists who have studied regression include: Franc Galton, George Udny Yule, Karl Pearson, Ronald Aylmer Fisher, and Francis Ysidro Edgeworth. A brief bio of each is given next.

Franc Galton (1822–1911)

Galton showed early signs of intellectual prowess. His major contributions to statistics were in connection with genetics and psychology. The fact that the regression of y on x differed from that of x on y worried him. In 1877 he discovered a solution. By normalizing x and y in terms of their own variability, he solved the problem. The regression coefficient he then called the correlation coefficient. Since it was a regression, Galton called it simple r, hence the modern one-word name.

George Udny Yule (1871–1951)

Yule was born in Beech Hill near Haddington, Scotland, and at the age of 16 he began engineering studies at University College, London. Yule laid the foundations for the autoregressive series and invented the correlogram. The terms *Yule process* and *Yule distribution* are well known in the statistical literature.

Karl Pearson (1857–1936)

Pearson was educated at University College School and at Kings College, Cambridge. Through his many papers, Pearson studied the likelihood function, $\square^2$ goodness-of-fit test, frequency curves, and the errors of movements. Pearson expressed the goal of the statistician in this way: "The imagination of man has always run riot, but to imagine a thing is not meritorious unless we demonstrate its reasonableness by the laborious process of studying how it fits experience."

Ronald Aylmer Fisher (1890–1962)

In 1912, Fisher published a paper on the maximum likelihood theory. He was able to prove that using the sample mean instead of the population mean was equivalent to reducing the dimensionality of the sample space by one. This concept became known as the degrees of freedom concept.

Francis Ysidro Edgeworth (1845–1926)

Edgeworth's original contributions to mathematical, or analytical, economics include the indifference curve, the contract curve, the law of diminishing returns, and the determination of economic equilibria. His statistical contributions included work on index numbers, the law of error, the theory of estimation, correlation, goodness of fit, and probability theory.

MULTIPLE REGRESSION MODEL

In a *multiple regression*, the linear equation is the same as in simple linear regression, except that more than one independent variable is present (Equation 12.26).

$$y = b_0 + b_i x_i + \ldots + \varepsilon \quad \text{for } i = 1 \text{ to n} \tag{12.26}$$

where

$\hat{y}$ = the dependent variable

x_i = the independent variable(s)

b_0 = intercept

b_i = individual independent variable contributions for $i = 1$ to n

e = error term

This is a more realistic model for health care applications, as real-life situations are not as easy and simple as a simple linear regression (i.e., trying to predict using only one independent variable). Usually more than one independent variable is necessary to explain the dependent variable.

Multiple regression models also have an underlying set of equations for the intercept and corresponding independent variable contributions. Due to the

TABLE 12.3 Patient Satisfaction Data for Linear Regression Computation

Data Points	Patient Satisfaction	Length of Stay (LOS)	Number of Previous Admissions
1	102	7	5
2	100	4	3
3	95	3	3
4	103	3	4
5	115	4	6
6	117	3	5
7	92	2	2
8	69	1	1
9	62	3	2
10	66	2	1
11	91	4	2
12	100	3	3
13	105	4	3
14	125	5	4
15	138	5	5

operational nature of this chapter, we will not present the derivation of those equations here but refer the reader to the references at the end of the chapter.

Instead of the multiple regression equation derivations, we will move directly into a health care example using Excel's regression analysis package. The example is detailed next.

Multiple Linear Regression Example

A health care manager wants to determine whether patient satisfaction scores are affected by length of stay (LOS) and the number of previous admissions. This example (Table 12.3) involves two independent variables. A total of 15 data points have been found. This problem is solved using Excel's regression package.

Excel Output for Multiple Regression Example

The regression output created by Excel is presented in Figure 12.22. A tutorial on the use of regression in the Data Analysis package is presented later in this chapter. For brevity, readers are referred to the tutorial regarding how to enter

FIGURE 12.22 Regression Output from Excel for Patient Satisfaction Example

	A	B	C	D	E	F	G
1	SUMMARY OUTPUT						
2							
3	*Regression Statistics*						
4	Multiple R	0.8291842					
5	R Square	0.687546438					
6	Adjusted R Square	0.635470844					
7	Standard Error	12.8334619					
8	Observations	15					
9							
10	ANOVA						
11		*df*	*SS*	*MS*	*F*	*Significance F*	
12	Regression	2	4.348.960402	2.174.48	13.2029	0.000930493	
13	Residual	12	1.976.372931	164.698			
14	Total	14	6.325.333333				
15							
16		*Coefficients*	*Standard Error*	*t Stat*	*P-value*	*Lower 95%*	*Upper 95%*
17	Intercept	59.41412284	9.258005653	6.41759	3.3E-05	39.24266134	79.5855843
18	Length of Stay (LOS)	1.246781905	3.158217741	0.39477	0.69994	−5.634383428	8.12794724
19	Number of Previous Admissions	10.66752483	3.000861998	3.55482	0.00396	4.129208205	17.2058414
20							

data and how to obtain the regression output. The explanation of the output from the regression analysis is presented next.

The regression output is displayed in Figure 12.22. The regression equation is found by combining the values in the Coefficients column in cells B17 (intercept-b_0), B18 (x_1 coefficient-b_1), and B19 (x_2 coefficient-b_2) from Figure 12.22. Following the multiple linear regression equation form, the regression equation for this example is as shown in Equation 12.27:

$$\hat{y} = 59.41 + 1.25x_1 + 10.67x_2 \tag{12.27}$$

Therefore, if the health care manager were to assume a patient's LOS is four days (i.e., $x_1 = 4$) and the patient's previous admissions are 5 (i.e., $x_2 = 5$), then the predicted patient satisfaction score would be as shown in Equation 12.28:

$$\hat{y} = 59.41 + 1.25(4) + 10.67(5) = 117.74 \tag{12.28}$$

or approximately 118.

Regression analysis is very valuable for predictions such as the example just given. However, we really have no idea whether the underlying regression model is performing well. In order to determine whether the regression model is actually a good model, some performance measures must be analyzed.

Performance Measures

A number of statistical performance measures must be analyzed to decide whether the regression model is an adequate or good model. The following sections investigate the R, F, and t statistics.

R-Squared

R-squared is referred to as the *coefficient of determination*. *R*-squared is also another measure of correlation. This value should be close to 1.0. The scale ranges from 0.0 to 1.0. R^2 indicates the percentage of variation in the dependent variable that results from the independent variable.

It is basically a measure of how well the independent variables explain the dependent variable. It is referred to as the measure of goodness of fit. R^2 can never decrease when a new independent variable is introduced to the model. The reason is that the method of least squares minimizes the explained sum of squares. This basically means we could increase R^2 regardless of whether the independent variable relates to the dependent variable. The formula for R^2 is shown in Equation 12.29:

$$R^2 = \frac{\sum_{i=1}^{n} (\hat{y}_i - \bar{y})^2}{\sum_{i=1}^{n} (y_i - \bar{y})^2} \tag{12.29}$$

If we look back at Figure 12.22 and examine the regression output from the patient satisfaction example, R^2 equals 68.75 percent (cell B5 in Figure 12.22). This means that 68.75 percent of the total variance in the dependent variable around the mean has been accounted for by the two independent variables in the estimated regression function. This also means the independent variables are doing a good job of explaining the dependent variable.

Multiple R

Multiple *R* represents the strength of the linear relationship between actual and estimated values. The scale ranges from 0.0 to 1.0. It is preferable to have a value close to 1.0 because this indicates a good fit. The patient satisfaction regression model presents a value of 82.92, which is good, and now we can continue on to the next test.

Adjusted R-Squared

This value is supposed to give the researcher a clearer estimate of how much the independent variable in a regression analysis explains the dependent variable. It differs from R^2 in that it adjusts R^2 for the size of the sample (i.e., how many data points are being used in the regression). If sample size is very small (i.e., 5 to 10 data points), then the adjusted R-squared will vary greatly from the standard R^2. Again, this estimate is a measure of strength of the regression. From Figure 12.22 (cell B6), the adjusted R-squared is 63.55 percent, which is within the boundaries of differences in R^2 and adjusted R-squared.

t-Statistic

The *t-statistic* looks at individual variables and shows how they affect y singularly. The t-statistic is the value that is compared to the critical region. A critical region is an area in a sampling distribution representing values that are critical to a particular study. They are critical because, when a sample statistic falls in that region, the null hypothesis can be rejected. The null hypothesis, in general for any independent variable that is being tested, is:

$$H_0: b_i = 0$$

In words, we are testing to see if a particular coefficient of contribution (b_i) is actually different from zero. If the t-statistic is deemed significant, we reject this hypothesis. Acceptance or rejection of the underlying hypothesis is next.

The rule of thumb says the t-statistic should be greater than 2. However, to be more accurate, the t table can be used to find the real value. It is possible to conduct a one-tailed test or a two-tailed test. For our example, looking up the t-distribution in a table, we find the number of degrees of freedom is 12. When the critical value of t is at the 5 percent level of significance, it shows a value of 2.179. This is the value for a two-tailed test. Our t-values, from Figure 12.22, are 0.3948 for x_1 (LOS) and 3.55 for x_2 (number of previous admissions). The null hypothesis is therefore rejected for x_2 since the associated value falls within the reject regions, but for x_1 the number does not fall in the reject region; consequently, we are uncertain about the impact LOS has in the model. More investigation must be completed regarding LOS and its relationship to patient satisfaction.

F-Statistic

The *F-statistic* measures the significance of statistical joint relationships among independent variables, and it looks at the model as a whole. For the most part, the F-statistic is associated with the analysis of variance (ANOVA).

The null hypothesis that is being tested is as follows:

$$H_0: b_0 = b_1 = b_2 = \cdots b_n = 0$$

In other words, we are testing to see if any of the coefficients of contribution (*b*'s) actually are different from zero. If F is deemed significant, we reject this hypothesis. Acceptance or rejection of the underlying hypothesis is next.

F is automatically calculated when a regression analysis is run. In earlier years, one had to refer to an F-distribution table to look up the value. The rule of thumb is that the F-statistic should be greater than 4 to be considered significant. The equation for the F-test is as shown in Equation 12.30:

$$F = \frac{\text{mean square of regression}}{\text{mean square of error}} = \frac{\text{variance of regression}}{\text{variance of error}} \qquad (12.30)$$

Figure 12.22 shows an F-value of 13.21, which is greater than 4. This means the F-value meets the criterion. Looking up the exact value of F, find it to be 3.88. The result is that the null hypothesis is accepted.

p-Value

The *p-value* is another way to interpret t-statistics. The rule of thumb is: If the *p*-value is less than the level of significance, the variable is statistically significant.

Standard statistical nomenclature is that the *p*-value should be less than 0.05, which means there would be less than a 0.05 chance that the data have been produced by chance. In addition, the *p*-value goes hand in hand with the t-statistic. This value is often viewed as the minimum level of significance. Referring back to Figure 12.22, the p-value for x_1 is 0.6999 and for x_2 is 0.0039, which verifies what the t-statistics claimed: x_1 is not significant in the model while x_2 is significant.

Other Assumptions within Multiple Linear Regression

There are a few other assumptions within linear regression models that must be mentioned. These areas are multicollinearity, autocorrelation, and hetero-scedasticity. Each of these assumptions is briefly discussed next, but for more detail on each of these areas please refer to the references section at the end of this chapter.

Multicollinearity

When using a multiple regression model, the user assumes that the independent variables are not collinear. However, *multicollinearity* can exist when two or more variables are highly correlated. Multicollinearity increases the uncertainty of the parameter estimates. This makes it difficult, if not impossible, to deter-mine the parameters' separate effects on the dependent variable.

Multicollinearity is something that should be avoided if possible. Excel can help test for collinearity. In trying to solve or test for the problem of multi-collinearity, one can:

- Rethink the impetus of linear regression.

- Drop one of the correlated variables.

- Use stepwise regression to screen variables (SPSS is a software application that can help eliminate factors).

- Look for new variables that can better explain the model.

Autocorrelation

When using a multiple regression model, the user also assumes that the residuals or error terms are not correlated. As previously mentioned, residuals are the difference between the actual and the predicted values. Users must test for autocorrelation. Basically, the larger the autocorrelation or residuals are, the less reliable the results of the regression analysis will be.

A Durbin-Watson statistic must be calculated to measure autocorrelation. It measures the correlation of each residual and the residual for the time period immediately preceding the one of interest. It is desirable that the Durbin-Watson statistic be above 2 and greater than the upper range. As the autocorrelation increases, the Durbin-Watson statistic goes down.

Heteroscedasticity

Finally, when using a multiple regression model the user assumes that the residuals (error terms) have constant variance, homeoscedasticity. *Heteroscedasticity* is the term used when the residuals of a linear regression model do not have constant variance. An easy method to test for heteroscedasticity is plotting the residuals in a graph. From the graph it can be determined whether there is a pattern (trend upward or downward, funneling inward or outward, etc.).

Each of these assumptions—collinearity, correlation, and constant variance of the residuals—must be studied to determine the strength of the underlying linear regression model. Next, the concept of model accuracy is discussed.

MEASURING ACCURACY

The R, F, and t statistics are used to determine whether the underlying regression model is a good fit. However, when different forecasting models, including regression models, are compared to each other, a set of accuracy measures must be looked at.

This is an important process for the researcher because this strategy will lead to valid and useful results for the industry, future students, degree holders in this field, universities, investors, and others. The example that follows illustrates how the computations are completed for the error measurements by using formulas in an MS Excel spreadsheet.

To evaluate and compare multiple regression models, four forecasting error techniques will be used to evaluate the forecasting method. These are mean square error (MSE), mean absolute error or mean absolute deviation (MAD), mean percentage error (MPE), and mean absolute percentage error (MAPE).

These methods measure the accuracy of the models and tell the researchers which method is the best. They are used for model comparison.

MSE is a method that provides a penalty for large forecasting errors because it squares each error or residual. The formula is shown in Equation 12.31:

$$\text{MSE} = \frac{\sum_{i=1}^{n} (y_t - \hat{y}_t)^2}{n} \tag{12.31}$$

MAD measures the forecast accuracy by averaging the magnitudes of the forecast errors. This technique is most useful when you want to measure forecast error in the same units as the original series. The formula is shown in Equation 12.32:

$$\text{MAD} = \frac{\sum_{i=1}^{n} |y_t - \hat{y}_t|}{n} \tag{12.32}$$

MAPE is a method that tries to find the absolute error in each period. MAPE provides an indication of how large the forecast errors are in comparison to the actual values of the series. In addition, MAPE can be used to compare the accuracy of the same or different techniques on two entirely different series. The formula is shown in Equation 12.33:

$$\text{MAPE} = \frac{\sum_{i=1}^{n} \frac{|y_t - \hat{y}_t|}{y_t}}{n} \tag{12.33}$$

MPE is an excellent method to determine whether a bias exists. This tells us if the method is consistently forecasting too low or too high. The formula is shown in Equation 12.34:

$$\text{MPE} = \frac{\sum_{i=1}^{n} \frac{(y_t - \hat{y}_t)}{y_t}}{n} \tag{12.34}$$

Consider the scenario of predicting patient satisfaction. The four error esti-mates to test the model have been used. The result of the residual calculations from Excel will be used. Excel automatically creates the Observation, Predicted Patient Satisfaction, and Residuals/Error columns when the regression is run. The Actual Patient Satisfaction, $Error^2$, |Error|, |Error|/Actual, and Error/Actual col-umns have to be created manually. Refer to Figure 12.22 for the residual information.

The results of the Excel calculations are:

$$MSE = 131.76$$

$$MAD = 8.97$$

$$MAPE = 0.10$$

$$MPE = -0.02$$

The formulas for the manually created columns E, F, G, and H in Figure 12.23 are displayed in Table 12.4.

FIGURE 12.23 Excel Output for Residual/Error Calculations

	A	B	C	D	E	F	G	H
1	RESIDUAL OUTPUT							
2								
3	Observation	Actual Patient Satisfaction	Predicted Patient Satisfaction	Residuals/ Error	Error ^{2}	|Error|	|Error| Actual	Error Actual
4	1	102	121.48	-19.48	379.44	19.48	0.19	-0.19
5	2	100	96.40	3.60	12.93	3.60	0.04	0.04
6	3	95	95.16	-0.16	0.02	0.16	0.00	0.00
7	4	103	105.82	-2.82	7.98	2.82	0.03	-0.03
8	5	115	128.41	-13.41	179.73	13.41	0.12	-0.12
9	6	117	116.49	0.51	0.26	0.51	0.00	0.00
10	7	92	83.24	8.76	76.69	8.76	0.10	0.10
11	8	69	71.33	-2.33	5.42	2.33	0.03	-0.03
12	9	62	84.49	-22.49	505.78	22.49	0.36	-0.36
13	10	66	72.58	-6.58	43.23	6.58	0.10	-0.10
14	11	91	85.74	5.26	27.71	5.26	0.06	0.06
15	12	100	95.16	4.84	23.45	4.84	0.05	0.05
16	13	105	96.40	8.60	73.89	8.60	0.08	0.08
17	14	125	108.32	16.68	278.28	16.68	0.13	0.13
18	15	138	118.99	19.01	361.55	19.01	0.14	0.14
19				Averages	131.76	8.97	0.10	-0.02
20								
21	MSE:	131.76						
22	MAD:	8.97						
23	MAPE:	0.10						
24	MPE:	-0.02						
25								

TABLE 12.4 Excel Formulas for Error Calculations

Cell	Formula
E4	=D4^2 (Copied down to cell E18)
F4	=ABS(D4) (Copied down to cell F18)
G4	=ABS(D4)/B4 (Copied down to cell G18)
H4	=D4/B4 (Copied down to cell H18)
E19	=AVERAGE(E4:E18)
F19	=AVERAGE(F4:F18)
G19	=AVERAGE(G4:G18)
H19	=AVERAGE(H4:H18)
B21	=E19
B22	=F19
B23	=G19
B24	=H19

Looking at the results, we can conclude that there is little or no bias taking place because MPE has a value close to zero.

Next we detail how to install and use Excel's Analysis ToolPak and Regression add-ins.

Excel Tutorial: Using Add-Ins

Microsoft Excel contains add-in statistical functions that help the researcher with the analysis of data. Excel's Analysis ToolPak contains add-ins that are pre-programmed functions that simplify the job of forecasting and creating regression models. Data analysis is still left up to the researcher, since no statistical programs can perform this function.

Installing Excel's Data Analysis ToolPak

This section details the procedure for installation and use of Excel's Data Analysis ToolPak. The procedure is as follows:

1. Click on the File tab in Excel (see Figure 12.24).

2. Click the Excel Options button (refer to the left menu area of Figure 12.24). Choose the Add-Ins menu in the left pane, and a screen resembling Figure 12.25 will be displayed.

FIGURE 12.24   Excel File Tab

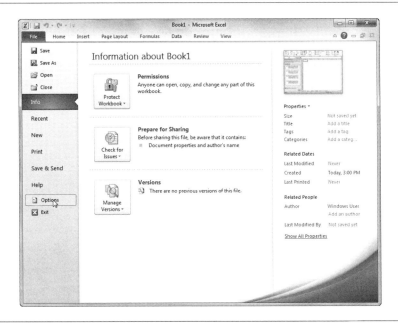

FIGURE 12.25   Excel Options Add-Ins Menu

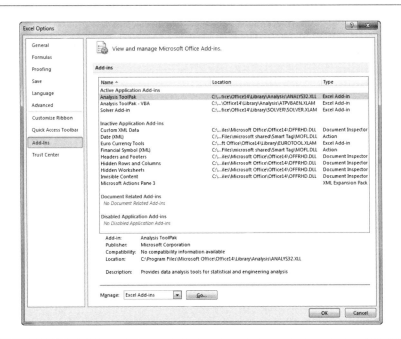

FIGURE 12.26 Add-Ins Dialogue Box

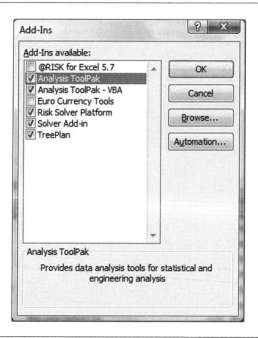

3. Next click on the Go button located in the bottom center of Figure 12.25. A screen resembling Figure 12.26 will appear.

4. Select Analysis ToolPak and Analysis ToolPak—VBA (refer to Figure 12.26).

5. Click OK. The Data Analysis tool is now ready to be used.

Excel Tutorial: Regression Analysis

Now that the Data Analysis ToolPak is installed, let's take a look at another regression example via Excel. In this example, glucose area is the dependent variable, whereas age and body mass index (BMI) are the independent variables influencing the dependent variable. A total of 30 observations have been gathered. Excel will be employed to create the regression result. Enter the data into Excel (Figure 12.27 shows the data for the example).

1. On the ribbon in Excel, click on the Data tab and the Data Analysis option in the Analysis group (see Figure 12.28).

FIGURE 12.27 Glucose Area Data Set

	A	B	C	D
1	Data Point	Glucose Area	Age	BMI
2	1	6,862.90	19	20
3	2	9,915.79	31	30
4	3	10,498.67	41	34
5	4	6,438.38	20	24
6	5	7,257.86	22	23
7	6	10,616.71	45	37
8	7	11,272.11	62	39
9	8	9,715.84	30	28
10	9	7,151.46	24	25
11	10	10,510.69	40	29
12	11	11,032.34	65	35
13	12	7,305.05	25	25
14	13	7,097.70	20	21
15	14	10,055.86	34	26
16	15	11,564.76	70	41
17	16	6,795.27	19	25
18	17	6,932.04	22	24
19	18	10,195.39	37	28
20	19	10,490.55	38	37
21	20	6,648.47	22	25
22	21	7,010.57	24	20
23	22	10,039.41	32	30
24	23	10,561.02	42	31
25	24	6,838.14	24	26
26	25	7,032.28	21	24
27	26	10,519.35	41	35
28	27	11,072.55	67	37
29	28	6,917.30	23	21
30	29	7,405.10	24	21
31	30	1,0627.38	39	34
32				

2. Select Regression from the list and click OK (Figure 12.29).

3. The input and output options available are explained next with reference to Figure 12.30.

Input Options

- Input Y Range: Highlight the *y* range; this is the dependent variable in the example (Glucose Area, cells B1:B31).

FIGURE 12.28 Data Analysis Option in Excel

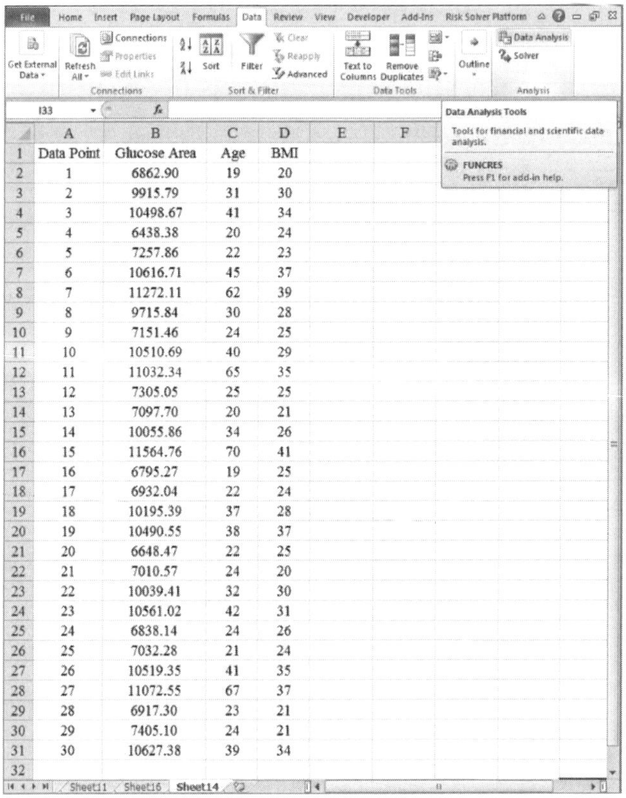

- Input X Range: Highlight the *x* range; these are the independent variables in the example (Age and BMI, cellsC1:D31). Note that the independent variables can span multiple rows and the column headers are included (see next bullet point).

- Labels: This is optional; however, it will make it easier to identify the variables later when analyzing the data. For this example we are including the dependent and independent labels, so click the check box.

- Confidence Level: This is set at 95 percent; however, it can be changed.

- Constant is Zero: This should not be checked, as it would force a regression line through the origin, and for our purposes we wish to estimate an intercept.

FIGURE 12.29 Data Analysis Options Menu

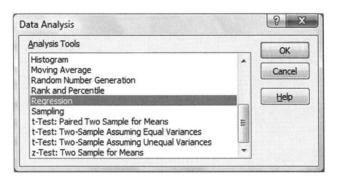

FIGURE 12.30 Data Analysis Regression Menu

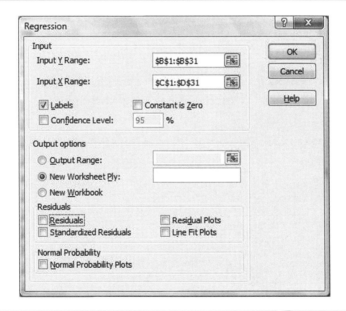

Output Options

- Output Range: Select this box if you would like the regression result to be placed in the same worksheet as the raw data.

- New Worksheet Ply: Selecting this box will move the result into a new worksheet. Remember to name the sheet if you are going to create many of them.

● New Workbook: This will place the regression result in a new workbook.

Residuals

● Residuals: A residual is the difference between the actual y and the predicted y value.

● Residual Plots: These graphs compare the actual y with the predicted y for each of the predictors. These plots can be used to analyze heteroscedasticity.

● Standardized Residuals: Selecting this combines the residuals into a unit normal distribution with the mean of 0 and standard deviation of 1. These plots can be used to analyze heteroscedasticity.

● Line Fit Plots: These graphs show the difference between the actual and predicted values of y. These plots can be used to analyze multicollinearity.

Normal Probability

Selecting Normal Probability Plots will generate a chart of normal probabilities. The assumption of normality can be tested using these plots.

FIGURE 12.31   Regression Output for Glucose Data Set

	A	B	C	D	E	F	G
1	SUMMARY OUTPUT						
2							
3	*Regression Statistics*						
4	Multiple R	0.90319997					
5	R Square	0.81577018					
6	Adjusted R Square	0.80212353					
7	Standard Error	824.326187					
8	Observations	30					
9							
10	ANOVA						
11		*df*	*SS*	*MS*	*F*	*Significance F*	
12	Regression	2	81,239,990.87	40,619,995	59.77804	1.20881E-10	
13	Residual	27	18,346,868.87	679,513.7			
14	Total	29	99,586,859.74				
15							
16		*Coefficients*	*Standard Error*	*t Stat*	*P-value*	*Lower 95%*	*Upper 95%*
17	Intercept	2,538.93333	936.1347336	2.712145	0.011488	618.1435142	4,459.72314
18	Age	45.4627098	21.76994418	2.088325	0.046331	0.79447399	90.1309456
19	BMI	168.075542	53.08231404	3.166319	0.003807	59.15962972	276.991453
20							

When you have selected all the options you want, click OK, and the regression result will be generated (Figure 12.31). An explanation of the Summary Output follows.

Multiple *R*

Multiple *R* represents the strength of the linear relationship between the actual and the estimated values for the dependent variables. The scale ranges from −1.0 to 1.0, where 1.0 indicates a good direct relationship and −1 indicates a good inverse relationship. Multiple *R* is found to be 90.32 percent, which means there is a strong linear relationship.

R-Squared

In simple linear regression models, R^2 is referred to as the coefficient of determination. However, in the case of multiple regression models the term coefficient of determination is modified, due to multiple independent variables being defined within the model. In turn, R^2 is defined as the coefficient of multiple determination and describes the relationship between a dependent variable and the independent variables. It tells how much of the variability in the dependent variable is explained by the independent variables. R^2 is a goodness-of-fit measure, and the scale ranges from 0.0 to 1.0.

This study shows R^2 is equal to 0.8158. This means that 81.58 percent of the total variance in the dependent variable around its mean has been accounted for by the independent variables in the estimated regression function.

Adjusted *R*-Squared

In the adjusted *R*-squared, R^2 is adjusted to give a truer estimate of how much the independent variables in a regression analysis explain the dependent variable. Taking into account the number of independent variables makes the adjustment. The adjusted *R*-squared is found to be 80.21 percent, and is a measure of strength.

Standard Error of Estimates

The standard error of estimates is a regression line. The error is how much the research is off when the regression line is used to predict particular scores.

The standard error is the standard deviation of those errors from the regression line. The standard error of estimate is thus a measure of the variability of the errors. It measures the average error over the entire scatter plot.

The smaller the standard error of estimate, the higher the degree of linear relationship between the two variables in the regression. The larger the standard error, the less confidence can be put in the estimate. For this data set, the standard error of estimates equals 824.33. This indicates that the y value falls 824.33 units away from the regression line. This measure is okay since the magnitude of our variable is in the thousands.

t-Test

The rule of thumb says the absolute value of t should be greater than 2. To be more accurate, the t table has been used. When the critical value of t is at the 5 percent level of significance, it shows a value of 2.052. The critical values can be found in the back of most statistical textbooks. The critical value is the value that determines the critical regions in a sampling distribution. The critical values separate the obtained values that will and will not result in rejecting the null hypothesis.

Referring back to the regression results, we need to determine whether the coefficients of contribution are significantly different from zero at the 5 percent significance level. From the data, we can see that the Age variable's t-statistic equals 2.088 and for BMI the t-statistic equals 3.166. We can conclude that the null hypothesis cannot be rejected for either the Age variable or the BMI variable. This means the variables Age and BMI are doing a good job of explaining the dependent variable Glucose Area.

F-Statistic

The F-distribution shows 2 and 27 degrees of freedom. Looking at the F-distribution table at the 5 percent level of significance, we find the value 3.35. In the results, it can be seen that the critical value equals 59.78 and is greater than the F-statistic of 3.35.

The result is that H_0: $B_1 = B_2 = 0$ is to be rejected. This implies in this study that the explanatory variables in the regression equation are doing a good job of explaining the variation in the dependent variable y.

p-Value

The *p*-value should be less than 0.05, which would mean there would be less than a 0.05 chance that the data have been produced by chance. In this case, both variables meet the criterion, as the Age variable *p*-value is 0.0463 and the BMI variable *p*-value is 0.0038. The *p*-value can be viewed as the minimum level of significance that can be chosen for the test and result in rejection of the null hypothesis. Overall, it could be said from the regression analysis that Age and BMI do a very good job of predicting Glucose Area.

Excel Tutorial: Correlation

To run a correlation analysis, follow these steps:

1. Enter the data into Excel as in Figure 12.27.

2. On the ribbon in Excel, click on the Data tab and the Data Analysis option in the Analysis group (see Figure 12.32).

3. Select Correlation from the Data Analysis list and click OK (Figure 12.33). A Correlation menu will appear (Figure 12.34).

4. Insert the Input Range, which consists of the independent variables (Age and BMI, cells C1 to D31). Note: the data should be grouped by Columns.

FIGURE 12.32   Data Analysis Menu Option in Excel Ribbon

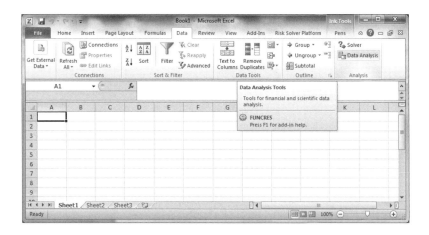

5. Check the Labels in First Row box; this will make it easier when you are interpreting the results.

6. Check the New Worksheet Ply box; this will create a separate sheet for your correlation matrix.

7. Click OK when you are done, and a table resembling Figure 12.35 will appear in a new worksheet containing the correlation matrix for Age and BMI.

It must be noted that Age and BMI are correlated and the user would have to address this correlation in the overall model. For brevity we will allow

FIGURE 12.33   Data Analysis Dialogue Box in Excel

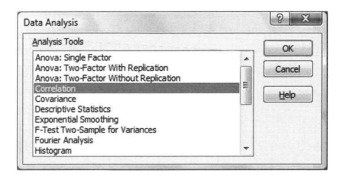

FIGURE 12.34   Correlation Menu in Excel's Data Analysis Package

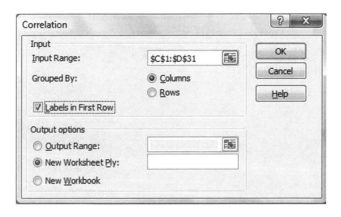

FIGURE 12.35 Correlation Matrix for Age and BMI

	A	B	C
1		*Age*	*BMI*
2	Age	1	
3	BMI	0.884227	1
4			

TABLE 12.5 Error Measurements for Glucose Example

Error Measurement	Error Value
MSE	611,562.30
MAD	652.70
MPE	–0.01
MAPE	0.07

readers to investigate that topic on their own. Next, we analyze the regression model's error.

MEASURING FORECASTING ERRORS

Measuring the forecasting error is a technique used to compare and evaluate forecasting techniques. As mentioned earlier in this chapter, there are four common methods for evaluating these forecasting techniques: mean absolute deviation (MAD), mean squared error (MSE), mean absolute percentage error (MAPE), and mean percentage error (MPE); they are presented here. The errors are calculated from the residuals, and can be seen in Table 12.5.

It is further found that no bias exists in the models since the MPE is close to zero. The MAPE indicates that an appropriate size has been chosen to test the relationship with since the MAPE is less than 10 percent.

The reason for getting such a large error on the MSE is the data chosen. The dependent variable (Glucose Area) is presented in actual numbers and is large in magnitude (in the thousands).

Forecasting and Use of the Regression Model

To forecast one year ahead, the regression equation is utilized to create a forecast, for example, using data for Age and BMI. Equation 12.35 is the equation for the regression (rounded):

$$\hat{y} = 2538.93 + 45.46x_1 + 168.08x_2 \tag{12.35}$$

Therefore, when x_1 (Age) $= 40$ and x_2 (BMI) $= 38$, the Glucose Area that the linear regression model predicts is 10,744.40, as shown in Equation 12.36.

$$\hat{y} = 2538.93 + 45.46(40) + 168.08(38) = 10744.40 \tag{12.36}$$

SUMMARY

From this case, it can be concluded that the independent variables can be used to predict the glucose area based on age and BMI. The independent variables chosen for this example do a good job of explaining the dependent variable. It is very useful to be able to predict future events, as health care professionals can use the information as a guideline for what the future may hold.

Further, when able to understand which variables have an effect on the subject being studied, health care professionals can use the information to determine future work situations and decide courses of action to assist patients. In addition, the chapter has discussed such factors as the number of observations, degrees of freedom, critical value of F and the t-test, R^2, adjusted R^2, and the standard error of estimates.

Time series analysis techniques such as moving averages and exponential smoothing are also effective tools to identify and confirm trends. This chapter provides health care professionals with methods to identify situations that are suitable for analysis with these techniques and how the analysis should be applied.

The advantages of using these techniques must be weighed against the disadvantages. Both moving average and exponential smoothing techniques are trend following, or lagging, indicators that will always be a step behind. This is not necessarily a bad thing. Once in a trend, moving averages and exponential smoothing techniques inform you about that trend, but also give late signals. Moving averages and exponential smoothing are simple but effective tools for basic forecasting, but must be coupled with sound health care acumen to achieve superior forecasting results.

Readers are encouraged to peruse the references listed at the end of the chapter. Specifically, for regression analysis see Dielman 1996, Mendenhall and Sincich 1996, and Montgomery and Peck 1992; for forecasting using spreadsheets see Hanke and Reitsch 2008 and Kros 2011; and for general statistical analysis applied to forecasting see Vogt 1998.

KEY TERMS

autocorrelation

coefficient of determination R²

correlation coefficient R

dependent variable

exponential smoothing

F-statistic

heteroscedasticity

independent variable

moving averages

multicollinearity

multiple regression

p-value

seasonality

simple linear regression model

t-statistic

time series

DISCUSSION QUESTIONS

1. Refer to the following data set for nurse staffing hours in Hospital XYZ.

1992	34,084	1997	41,008	2002	47,000	2007	70,456
1993	37,051	1998	41,817	2003	51,206	2008	87,865
1994	36,845	1999	46,815	2004	78,456	2009	75,084
1995	37,815	2000	45,845	2005	62,559	2010	77,615
1996	39,908	2001	46,036	2006	68,048	2011	81,084

   a. Using the latest period or naive method, compute the forecast for nurse staffing hours in 2012.

   b. Model the time series using Excel's TREND function.

2. Using Excel, compute the three-year and five-year moving averages for the data set from question 1 and determine the expected nurse staffing hours for

2012. Now compute a three-year weighted moving average using ½, ⅓, and ⅙ for the weights of the most recent, second most recent, and third most recent periods.

3. Using Excel, create an exponentially smoothed model from the data set in question 1. Assume $\alpha = 0.1$.

4. Refer to the following data set for hourly wages for housekeeping staff in Hospital XYZ.

2004	$9.20	2008	$11.18
2005	$10.14	2009	$11.43
2006	$10.40	2010	$12.03
2007	$11.12	2011	$12.09

a. Forecast the 2012 hourly wages using a three-year moving average.

b. Forecast the 2012 hourly wages using a five-year moving average.

5. Referring to the data set in question 4:

a. Forecast the 2012 hourly wages using exponential smoothing with $\alpha = 0.1$.

b. Forecast the 2012 hourly wages using exponential smoothing with $\alpha = 0.4$.

6. Refer to the following quarterly data set for nurse staffing hours in Hospital XYZ.

2007–1	19,023	2008–2	16,694	2009–3	16,518	2010–4	24,061
2007–2	13,387	2008–3	21,966	2009–4	24,778	2011–1	21,082
2007–3	16.909	2008–4	26,360	2010–1	19,404	2011–2	16,217
2007–4	21,137	2009–1	22,525	2010–2	20,180	2011–3	17,838
2008–1	22,845	2009–2	11,263	2010–3	13,971	2011–4	25,947

a. Compute the seasonal factors for each quarter.

b. Use a simple linear trend to forecast the demand for nursing hours in 2012.

7. The overall mean number of days in inpatient care per admitted patient is known to be normally distributed with a standard deviation of 2. A sample

of six patients is taken, and they are kept in the hospital for the following number of days: 4, 2, 8, 7, 1, 5. Can we say with 95 percent confidence that the mean is above 2.5?

8. Refer to the following quarterly data set of salaries and years of experience of the emergency room (ER) physicians at Hospital XYZ.

Years of Experience	Salary
7	$294,034
1	$194,453
28	$403,489
18	$320,034
12	$275,495
3	$210,453
6	$280,435

a. Show the equation for the linear regression relating years of experience and salary.

b. Using linear regression, predict the salary of an ER physician at Hospital XYZ with 20 years of experience.

c. Hospital XYZ is planning to hire a new ER physician and plans to use this linear regression to determine what salary to offer. The hospital is considering two physicians for the job. Dr. A is fresh out of residency and will accept any offer above $190,000. Dr. B has been practicing for 15 years and will accept any offer above $300,000. What will Hospital XYZ's offers be to each physician, and what would be each one's response?

9. Hospital XYZ's new director of medicine has decided to begin taking into account the quality of each ER physician's past performance as well as the physician's years of experience. She has a measure of quality from 0 to 100, which she also uses.

Years of Experience	Quality of Performance	Salary
7	70	$294,034
1	57	$194,453
28	99	$403,489

(Continued)

18	70	$320,034
12	52	$275,495
3	42	$210,453
6	86	$280,435

a. Using Excel, compute the multiple regression output.

b. Predict the starting salary of a new physician with 17 years of experience and a quality of performance of 93.

c. List and explain the assumptions used in this regression.

10. Referring to question 9, calculate R^2, multiple R, and adjusted R^2. Describe what these figures mean.

11. Referring to question 9, compute the t-statistic, F-statistic, and p-value for both years of experience and quality of performance. Using a 5 percent critical value, determine if these independent variables have significant impacts on salary.

12. Hospital XYZ has the following data measuring patient satisfaction levels with the patients' length of stay and their number of prior hospital admissions the past five years.

Length of Stay (Days)	Number of Previous Admissions	Patient Satisfaction Rating
5	3	84
2	5	98
14	7	72
8	2	75
3	4	90
4	6	89
4	1	80

a. Using Excel, compute the multiple regression output.

b. Predict the satisfaction of a patient with a length of stay of four days who has been admitted to the hospital twice before.

c. List and explain the assumptions used in this regression.

13. Referring to question 12:

a. Calculate R^2.

b. Calculate multiple R.

c. Calculate the adjusted R^2.

d. Compute the t-statistic for each independent variable.

e. Compute the F-statistic for each independent variable.

f. Compute the p-value for each independent variable.

14. Referring to question 9:

a. Calculate MSE and explain its meaning.

b. Calculate MAD and explain its meaning.

c. Calculate MAPE and explain its meaning.

d. Calculate MPE and explain its meaning.

15. Referring to question 12:

a. Calculate MSE and explain its meaning.

b. Calculate MAD and explain its meaning.

c. Calculate MAPE and explain its meaning.

d. Calculate MPE and explain its meaning.

REFERENCES

Dielman, T. E. 1996. *Applied Regression Analysis for Business and Economics.* 2nd ed. Pacific Grove, CA: Duxbury Press.

Hanke, J. E., and A. G. Reitsch. 2008. *Business Forecasting.* 9th ed. Upper Saddle River, NJ: Prentice Hall.

Kros, J. F. 2011. *Spreadsheet Modeling for Business Decisions.* 3rd ed. Dubuque, IA: Kendall/Hunt.

Mendenhall, W., and T. Sincich. 1996. *A Second Course in Statistics: Regression Analysis.* 5th ed. Upper Saddle River, NJ: Prentice Hall.

Montgomery, D. C., and E. A. Peck. 1992. *Introduction to Linear Regression Analysis.* 2nd ed. New York: Wiley Interscience.

Vogt, P. W. 1998. *Dictionary of Statistics & Methodology.* 2nd ed. Thousand Oaks, CA: Sage.

PROJECT

MANAGEMENT

➠ Comprehend the basic concepts of project management.

➠ Understand the definitions and roles of project planning and control.

➠ Apply the basic concepts of project scheduling.

➠ Understand the critical path method and be able to apply it.

➠ Understand Gantt charts and be able to create a Gantt chart for a simple project.

➠ Understand and apply Program (or Project) Evaluation and Review Technique.

INTRODUCTION

Project management involves the application of various planning, organizing, and managing techniques and tools in order to complete a project on time, at or below cost, and at a level of quality that satisfies the customer. Project management evolved as its own discipline separate from the traditional management discipline during the 1950s (Cleland and Gareis 2006). Today it is viewed as an essential endeavor for most successful companies. The expanded popularity of project management can be seen in the explosion in membership of the Project Management Institute (PMI), "the world's leading not-for-profit membership association for the project management profession, with more than half a million members and credential holders in more than 185 countries" (www.pmi.org/About-Us.aspx).

Projects differ from the day-to-day operations of a business. They consist of a set of temporary activities performed by an ad hoc team and usually involve greater risk and uncertainty than daily tasks (Olson 2004). The team is led by a project manager, who coordinates the team members' efforts. The team will often utilize one or more project management tools, such as Gantt charts, critical path method (CPM), or Program (or Project) Evaluation and Review Technique (PERT), each of which is explained in sections of this chapter.

ROLE OF PROJECT MANAGER

Although most of this chapter is devoted to methods project managers may use to plan, control, manage, and monitor their projects, there are numerous other aspects and responsibilities related to project management that need to be addressed here as well. The role of a project manager is critical because he or she provides the leadership and guidance to keep a project on track. Effective project management is the only way a project will be completed on time, within budget, and to the satisfaction of the customer.

Two dimensions exist within the project management process. One dimension includes the sociocultural side. Leadership, teamwork, organization, and communication skills are all part of the sociocultural dimension.

Sociocultural Dimension: Leadership, Teamwork, Organization, and Communication

Project managers are leaders and must build a cooperative team among divergent entities with different standards, commitments, reward systems, and perspectives.

Project managers must ensure that the project team has the proper composition. This involves more than just identifying the types of knowledge and expertise that are needed. An effective project manager will also identify the personality types on the team and determine appropriate methods of motivation for each.

Organization is another key skill that a project manager must possess. At any time, a project manager may be in charge of multiple projects or one large project. In either case, keeping project teams on schedule, on budget, and working toward the end goal requires organization skills. Meetings must be scheduled, planned, and executed effectively so as not to waste the valuable time of stakeholders. The availability of resources must be synchronized with the project schedule, with flexibility to adapt to unexpected delays due to weather or other events. Financial records must be kept up-to-date and include contingency plans for unanticipated expenses.

Communication skills are essential for any project manager. This includes both oral and written forms of communication. A project manager must be able to communicate project needs to the project team and project accomplishments to supervisors and clients.

Technical Dimension: Planning, Scheduling, and Controlling

The second dimension of project management is the more concrete technical side. This dimension consists of more formal, logical parts such as planning, scheduling, and controlling projects. Creation of a set of deliverables and a work breakdown facilitates planning and in turn monitoring the progress of the project. Project control is linked to the original schedule developed from the project scope statement and the work breakdown.

Project managers have a lot of responsibility. While the remainder of this chapter provides methods they may employ to help them plan, control, manage, and monitor their projects, it is important that the other skills and abilities just mentioned are not overlooked, as they are critical to the success of any project manager.

OBJECTIVES AND TRADE-OFFS

When undertaking any project, there will always be multiple objectives, and often two or more of these objectives are in conflict with each other. For example, if we want to design a car that rates high in safety but is inexpensive, that may be difficult. The features we must incorporate to make a car safe will add to its cost; thus these two design objectives are in conflict with each other.

As an example from health care, we may want to refine our room cleaning process so that patient rooms at a hospital are available more quickly, but we cannot sacrifice patient safety. We cannot remove essential steps of the cleaning process even if some of those steps are quite time consuming. If a patient contracts an infection while in his or her hospital room, it is bad not only for the patient, but also for the hospital since as of October 1, 2008, the federal government (i.e., Medicare) will no longer pay for care related to hospital-acquired infections (www.premierinc .com/safety/topics/guidelines/cms-guidelines-4-infection.jsp#HAC-PO).

Project managers and the project team must work with the client to determine priorities. If project objectives are prioritized, then appropriate trade-offs can be considered in order to meet high-priority objectives. Several approaches exist for establishing the client's priorities. Two of them, direct ranking methods and weighting methods, are discussed next.

Direct Ranking Methods

A direct ranking method requires that the clients be surveyed about their preferences on the project's objectives. Direct ranking may be simplified using the method of paired comparisons, where the clients are asked which objective out of a pair they consider to be more important (Blanchard and Fabrycky 2006). The method assumes transitivity of preferences, meaning if objective one is more important than objective two and objective two is more important than objective three, then objective one is more important than objective three. Table 13.1 provides a summary of an example of preference comparisons. Following the notation of Blanchard and Fabrycky (2006), a "P" in the chart means the objective identified by the row is preferred to the objective identified by the column, and an "=" entry means the two objectives are equally important to the decision maker (client).

TABLE 13.1 Direct Ranking Method Example

Objective	1	2	3	4	5	Times Preferred
1			P	=		1+
2						
3	P	P			=	2+
4	P	P	P			3
5	=		P	=	P	2++

This method may not always lead to a clear-cut prioritization of objectives. As can be seen from Table 13.1, objective 4 receives the highest score and is preferred to all objectives except objective 5. However, while no objective is preferred to objective 5, it does not attain the highest score using this method.

Weighting Methods

Sometimes it is better for the decision maker to weight all of the objectives at one time instead of using only pairwise comparisons. No matter how many objectives are being considered, the weights must add up to 100 percent. The easiest approach is to ask the client to weight the objectives so that the weights sum to 100 percent. However, if the client wishes instead to simply attach a subjective importance rating to each objective, then weights can be determined by adding the ratings and using their sum as the denominator to determine the percentage of weight the objective carries. See Table 13.2 for an example.

Many other methods exist for weighting or ranking objectives. No matter what method is employed, once the objectives have been ranked, it is then critical to identify trade-offs that may need to occur in order to ensure that the most critical objectives are met. These trade-offs may call for the utilization of additional resources even if it means additional cost, or a reduction in the size of the project team even if it means extending the time to project completion.

PLANNING AND CONTROL IN PROJECTS

Planning

Planning can be defined as the work done to predetermine a course of action (Chang 2004). Today's world of rapidly changing technology, globalization of

TABLE 13.2 Deriving Weights from Importance Ratings

Objective	Importance Rating	Derived Weight
1	6	6/30 = 0.200
2	8	8/30 = 0.267
3	10	10/30 = 0.333
4	4	4/30 = 0.133
5	2	2/30 = 0.067

the business environment, and high turnover in many business organizations makes planning a critical step in managing any project.

Two basic types of *project planning* are strategic planning and operational planning. A company's strategic plan defines its goals, purpose, and direction and generally considers a five-year time horizon. Strategic plans often fail. Reasons for such failure include the following (Chang 2004):

- Not thinking in the long term

- Not correctly identifying critical success factors

- Not having long-term commitment from management

- Not leaving enough flexibility in the plans

- Not communicating the plan well

While it is true that project managers may not be heavily involved in developing a company's strategic plan, it is critical that they are aware of the plan and align the goals and results of their projects with the strategic plan.

When the goals of a strategic plan are broken down into short-term objectives, the actions required to accomplish these objectives are known as the operational plan. From a health care perspective, an outpatient surgery center may establish its strategic plan by determining its target market, potential partnerships, profit goals, and service-level goals. As the center carries out its day-to-day operations, one of its objectives related to service-level goals may be that at least 90 percent of its patients undergo surgery on the original day surgery was scheduled. Of course, many tasks related to scheduling, surgery, recovery, and room turnaround must be carried out correctly in order for the surgery center to meet the objective.

There are a number of tools that can be used to assist with planning. They include market research, SWOT analysis, financial modeling, what-if analysis, benchmarking, technology forecasting, and product life-cycle analysis.

Market research allows a company to determine the preferences of its customers. For a health care facility, market research might impact a facility's chosen hours of operation or the method of communication used for appointment reminders. A SWOT analysis enables a company to determine its strengths, weaknesses, opportunities, and threats and modify its course of action appropriately. A rehabilitation clinic may perform a SWOT analysis and realize it has too few speech therapists for its expected increasing demand in the upcoming quarter, thus allowing the facility to adjust staffing to the appropriate level in a timely fashion.

Using spreadsheets, financial modeling and what-if analysis can be conducted to better plan for an uncertain future. Specifically, three kinds of what-if analysis tools come with Microsoft Excel: scenarios, data tables, and Goal Seek. Scenarios and data tables work with given sets of input values to determine achievable results. A scenario can handle many variables, but will accommodate only up to 32 values for those variables. Somewhat in contrast, a data table can work with only one or two variables, but it can handle many different values for those variables. Goal Seek works differently from both scenarios and data tables. Goal Seek starts with a given result and determines the possible input values that will produce that result.

In addition to scenarios, data tables, and Goal Seek, there are add-ins you can install to help perform what-if analysis. One such add-in, Solver, is similar to Goal Seek but can accommodate more variables. An example using Solver is included in Chapter 8. For more advanced models, Excel has an Analysis Pack add-in.

Control

As detailed earlier, planning focuses on setting goals and directions. Control is focused on guiding the efforts of the project toward achievement of these goals through the effective use of resources and the detection and correction of problems (Olson 2004).

Although a majority of activities related to *project control* are administrative in nature, it is critical that one understands the strategic importance of such activities. If efficient implementation is lacking, the best-laid strategic plan becomes useless. Control also is a necessary complement to delegation (Chang 2004).

There are a number of ways to exercise control. These include but are not limited to setting performance standards, benchmarking (both internally and externally), measuring performance, evaluating performance, and correcting performance. Further details on these topics can be found in Chang (2004).

PROJECT SCHEDULING

There are several tasks that must be accomplished before a project schedule can be created. These tasks may include creation of a work breakdown structure (WBS), development of estimates for the effort required to complete each task, and a formation of an exhaustive resource list that includes availability of each resource.

A work breakdown structure is a product- or service-oriented family tree that allows for identification of the various activities, tasks, subtasks, and work packages required for completion of a given project. It displays the system/product to be developed, produced, operated, and supported, as well as all elements of work to be accomplished (Blanchard and Fabrycky 2006). Figure 13.1 provides an example of a generic WBS. In the end-of-chapter questions, you will be asked to create a specific WBS for a project from your work.

Once the WBS is complete, the next goal is to determine the amount of effort (person-hours or machine hours) that will be needed to complete each task. Usually there are some data available or some previous knowledge of the expected time to complete the task that can be used to establish effort estimates. It is also generally the case that the skill level and experience of human resources and the reliability of machinery factor into the effort estimates. For example, a triage nurse with 20 years of experience may be able to assess emergency department patients more quickly than a triage nurse with two years of experience.

One additional step that should be taken prior to the establishment of a project schedule is the creation of a list of resources and their availability. If the human resources and machinery needed for the project are not available at the time and for the duration they are needed, the project schedule will undoubtedly face delays.

The person or group of persons responsible for project scheduling varies depending on the industry and the size of the organization. Often at large

FIGURE 13.1   Generic Work Breakdown Structure

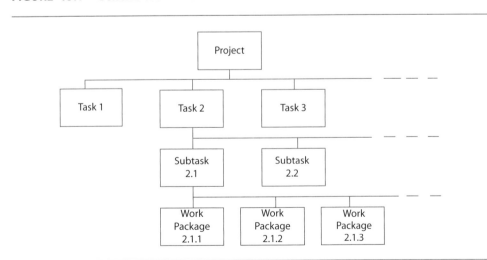

construction or engineering firms, development of project schedules and their maintenance are the job of a full-time scheduler or team of schedulers. At smaller companies or in settings where fewer resources are devoted to projects, such as most health care settings, the project scheduling duties may fall on the shoulders of the project managers or those leading process-improvement efforts.

There are several approaches to and techniques for project scheduling. As classified by Olson (2004), there are quantitative project scheduling methods (critical path method, project crashing, resource leveling, resource smoothing) and probabilistic project scheduling models (Program Evaluation and Review Technique, simulation). The quantitative methods are explained in detail in the critical path method section that follows. Likewise, Project Evaluation and Review Technique (PERT) has a section of this chapter devoted to it. Recall that simulation is the feature topic of Chapter 6.

Microsoft Project is one of many software tools that may be utilized to assist with project scheduling. This popular scheduling tool has numerous features, including those listed here (www.microsoft.com/project/en/us/project-standard -2010-benefits.aspx):

- Ability to work with summary data or more detailed data

- Time line view that provides a clear view of the progress on project tasks, milestones, and phases

- Capability to view resources and work over time

- Ability to resolve schedule conflicts

- Ability to compare budgeted expenses versus actual expenses versus forecasted expenses for the project

- Ability to perform what-if analysis

Other popular project-scheduling software tools include WorkZone, HyperOffice, Quintiq, FastTrack, and Zoho Projects. The best software for your needs will likely depend on the size of your company, the size of the projects you face, and the budget allotted for software purchases. It is important to note that before project managers can use any of the project scheduling software tools, they must understand the concepts behind the WBS, resource allocation, critical paths, Gantt charts, and so on.

CRITICAL PATH METHOD

Given a list of a project's activities, their estimated durations, and information on which activities serve as immediate predecessors for others, one can employ the *critical path method (CPM)* to determine how fast the project can be completed and which project activities are likely to be bottlenecks. An immediate predecessor is defined as an activity that must be completed before the activity in question can begin, and there are no other activities between the predecessor and the activity in question (Olson 2004).

As an example, let us consider a project consisting of five activities. All of the information needed to apply CPM is provided in Table 13.3. In the subsections that follow, we will apply CPM to determine this project's critical path.

Early Start Schedule

To begin, we will develop what is called an early start schedule. For this schedule, we will schedule each activity to start as soon as possible. That means the activity will start when the project starts or at the maximum early finish time of all of its predecessors. Early finish time is the sum of the early start time plus the activity duration (see Table 13.4). We calculate early start and early finish times for all

TABLE 13.3   Data for Example Project

Activity	Duration	Predecessors
A = estimate project completion cost	8 weeks	None
B = secure person/machine power for project	2 weeks	A
C = build system	28 weeks	B
D = train system users	12 weeks	B
E = implement system	4 weeks	C, D

TABLE 13.4   Early Start Schedule

Activity	Early Start	Early Finish
A = estimate project completion cost	0	0 + 8 = 8
B = secure person/machine power for project	8	8 + 2 = 10
C = build system	10	10 + 28 = 38
D = train system users	10	10 + 12 = 22
E = implement system	max{38,22}	38 + 4 = 42

project activities. The project's early completion time is the maximum early finish time for all activities. From the data in Table 13.4, we can see this project's early completion time is 42 weeks.

Often it is helpful to use a network to graphically display the relationships among the project's activities (see Figure 13.2). Although networks are not necessary for creating the early start schedule, they can be useful when sorting out relationships for the late start schedule. Networks may also serve as visual aids for project managers who are attempting to identify relationships among activities.

Late Start Schedule

Now we turn our attention to development of the late start schedule. The late start schedule provides the latest time at which each activity can be scheduled without delaying the project's completion time. Usually, the desired completion time is based on a contractual deadline. If the contractual deadline is earlier than the project early finish time, the project is infeasible, meaning it cannot be completed on time. If the contractual deadline is later than the project early finish time, then activities in the project will have slack, or spare time. If the contractual deadline and the project early finish time are the same, then there exist at least one critical path connecting activities with zero slack (Olson 2004).

The late start schedule is calculated by starting with the last activity of the project and working in reverse order. Assuming we know the contractual deadline or early finish time, we can back off of this time and schedule all activities to start

FIGURE 13.2 Network for Simple Project Example

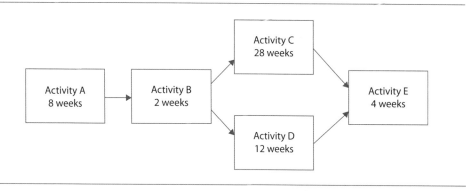

at the latest possible time. The late finish time for each activity is either the project end time or the minimum of the late start times for all activities that follow it (see Table 13.5).

Slack

The difference between the late start time of an activity and the early start time of an activity is referred to as that activity's slack. Critical activities are those with zero slack (see Table 13.6). A critical path is a chain of critical activities from project start to project finish. If any of the critical activities are delayed, then the project's completion time is delayed.

A critical path for a project may not be unique. A project network, similar to the one given in Figure 13.2, can assist with the identification of all critical paths. For the example we have been using, slack exists only for activity D (see Table 13.6).

So, for the tasks depicted in Figure 13.2, the critical path is A − B − C − E. Task D has slack; thus it is not critical. This means that a delay in when task D starts and/or ends will not necessarily result in a delay of the project completion time.

TABLE 13.5 Late Start Schedule

Activity	Late Finish	Late Start
E = implement system	42	42 − 4 = 38
D = train system users	38	38 − 12 = 26
C = build system	38	38 − 28 = 10
B = secure person/machine power for project	min{10,26}	10 − 2 = 8
A = estimate project completion cost	8	8 − 8 = 0

TABLE 13.6 Slack for Project Activities

Activity	Early Start	Early Finish	Late Start	Late Finish	Slack
A	0	8	0	0	0
B	2	10	8	min{10,26}	0
C	10	38	10	38	0
D	10	22	26	38	16
E	max{38,22}	42	38	42	0

Critical path method enables the identification of the earliest a project can be completed and which activities are critical. Obviously, critical activities should be managed more closely than noncritical activities. Any delay experienced on a critical activity will delay the project completion time. In contrast, a delay in a noncritical activity, such as activity D of our example, will not impact project completion time until 16 spare days (slack) are consumed. Note that once all of an activity's slack is exhausted, that activity becomes critical.

Project Crashing

Sometimes it is possible to acquire additional resources in order to complete crucial project activities more quickly. A trade-off must be made regarding the acquisition of more expensive resources in order to save time. Risk also factors in, as many activities are subject to unanticipated delays, so it is less risky to finish tasks ahead of time than to schedule them to be finished at a deadline. The concept of crashing a project identifies the least-cost method of reducing the duration of activities on the critical path (i.e., those with no slack time in their scheduled completion time) one time unit at a time (Olson 2004).

To demonstrate *project crashing*, let us revisit the example project we have been discussing throughout this section. We know that for the tasks given in Figure 13.2, the critical path is A − B − C − E. Let us assume that it is not possible to accomplish tasks B, C, and E any faster than the durations provided in Table 13.3. Let us also assume that there is a $200 per week penalty for taking longer than 40 weeks to complete this project.

Since the only activity that can be accomplished faster than the duration provided in the original schedule is activity A, we will focus our crashing activity on activity A. If we added another person to the team tasked with accomplishing activity A, then it would be possible to finish activity A in fewer than eight weeks. Let us assume that it will cost $150 per week to secure the additional person to help accomplish activity A. Let us also assume that each week this additional person works on activity A, it will reduce the time to complete activity A by one week.

If we utilized an extra person on activity A for one week, the cost would be $150 and the project completion time would drop from 42 weeks to 41 weeks. We would reduce our penalty for being late from $400 to $200, so the $150 investment would save us $200 ($50 net savings).

If we utilized an extra person on activity A for two weeks, the cost would be $300 and the project completion time would drop from its original value of 42 weeks to 40 weeks. This would reduce our lateness penalty from $400 to $0. So, the $300 investment would save us $400 ($100 net savings).

If we utilized an extra person on activity A for three weeks, the cost would be $450 and the project completion time would drop to 39 weeks. We would save $400 since we would not have to pay a lateness penalty; however, it would cost us $450 to save $400, so we do not want to do this. We should utilize the extra person on activity A for only two weeks, with a net savings of $100.

Table 13.7 summarizes what has just been explained. The first column provides the three scenarios investigated, along with the original problem for which we did not add any resources to activity A. The second column shows the resulting project completion time, which drops by one week for each week we add a person to activity A. The penalty cost is given in the third column; there is no penalty if the project is completed in 40 weeks or less. The fourth column indicates the resource cost, calculated at $150 per week for use of the additional person on activity A. The values given in the net benefit column, the final column, are calculated for each row using the formula ($400 − Penalty cost − Resource cost).

Resource Leveling

The concept of *resource leveling* involves spreading out the early start schedule in order to reduce the maximum number of a specific required resource (Olson

TABLE 13.7 Project Crashing Example

Scenario	Project Completion Time	Penalty Cost	Resource Cost	Net Benefit
Original problem	42 weeks	$400	$0	—
Add person to activity A for 1 week	41 weeks	$200	$150	$50
Add person to activity A for 2 weeks	40 weeks	$0	$300	$100
Add person to activity A for 3 weeks	39 weeks	$0	$450	−$50

2004). It looks at the most effective way to extend an existing schedule so that particular resources are not overbooked. For example, if the same person or machinery is needed for both activity C and activity D of Figure 13.2, then those two tasks cannot be accomplished concurrently. Either activity C or activity D must be delayed.

It is not always easy to determine what should be delayed. There are a few good rules of thumb that project managers typically employ. The first is to schedule critical tasks first. Additionally, if there are multiple critical tasks that share a scarce resource, you may want to schedule the longest task to occur first. These and other leveling heuristics are usually built into project management software, but packages will vary in the rules they employ (Olson 2004).

Let us consider a project similar to the simple project example given in Table 13.3, but modify and extend it to fit a health care project. Suppose our project involves developing a forecasting model for a local rehabilitation facility. Table 13.8 lists the activities of this project, their durations, and their predecessors. Figure 13.3 provides a network diagram for the health care project example.

TABLE 13.8 Health Care Project Example

Activity	Duration	Predecessors
A = collect relevant data	2 weeks	None
B = build forecasting model	6 weeks	A
C = model testing/validation	2 weeks	B
D = code development	8 weeks	C
E = interface development	4 weeks	C
F = user training	2 weeks	E
G = implementation	1 week	D, F

FIGURE 13.3 Network for Health Care Project Example

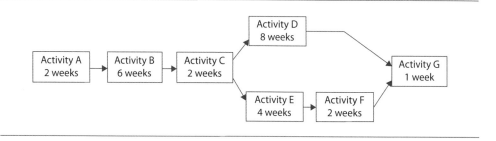

FIGURE 13.4 Gantt Chart for Health Care Project

	A	B	C D E F G H I J K L M N O P Q R S T U
1		wks	
2	Activity	Duration	1 2 3 4 5 6 7 8 9 10 11 12 13 14 15 16 17 18 19
3	A	2	x x
4	B	6	x x x x x x
5	C	2	x x
6	D	8	x x x x x x x x
7	E	4	x x x x s s s s
8	F	2	x x s s
9	G	1	x

FIGURE 13.5 Resource Leveling—Delaying Activity D

	A	B	C D E F G H I J K L M N O P Q R S T U V W X Y
1		wks	
2	Activity	Duration	1 2 3 4 5 6 7 8 9 10 11 12 13 14 15 16 17 18 19 20 21 22 23
3	A	2	x x
4	B	6	x x x x x x
5	C	2	x x
6	D	8	x x x x x x x x
7	E	4	x x x x
8	F	2	x x s s s s s s
9	G	1	x

Although Gantt charts are not discussed until the following section, one is included here (Figure 13.4) to quickly indicate that this project will take 19 weeks to complete. Additional explanation of the Gantt chart is provided in the next section.

If we now add in the assumption that activity D and activity E require the same person, then we are faced with an example of resource leveling. Either D or E must be delayed. Since this is a small example, we can examine our two options to determine which is preferred.

If we delay D, then it cannot start until week 15, when activity C is completed and the resource person needed for both activities has completed activity E. As we can see from Figure 13.5, a delay in D will delay the completion time of the project from 19 weeks to 23 weeks.

If we delay E, then it cannot start until week 19, when activity C is completed and the resource person needed for both activities has completed activity D.

FIGURE 13.6 Resource Leveling—Delaying Activity E

	A	B	C	D	E	F	G	H	I	J	K	L	M	N	O	P	Q	R	S	T	U	V	W	X	Y	Z	AA
1		wks																									
2	Activity	Duration	1	2	3	4	5	6	7	8	9	10	11	12	13	14	15	16	17	18	19	20	21	22	23	24	25
3	A	2	x	x																							
4	B	6			x	x	x	x	x	x																	
5	C	2									x	x															
6	D	8											x	x	x	x	x	x	x	x							
7	E	4																				x	x	x	x			
8	F	2																								x	x	
9	G	1																										x

As we can see from Figure 13.6, a delay in E will delay the completion time of the project from 19 weeks to 25 weeks.

If we are forced to delay either activity D or activity E due to a resource leveling issue, we are better off delaying activity D. That modification to the schedule will result in a four-week extension to the project completion time, which is preferred to the extra six weeks needed if we delay activity E.

Resource Smoothing

The goal of *resource smoothing* is to adjust schedules in order to obtain a level amount of work for a given resource. Schedule adjustments may include extending or compressing activity times to make work volume more even. Smoothing may also include recognizing where there are gaps in the work schedule that management might be able to fill with extra work (Olson 2004).

It is inevitable that all projects will experience both gaps in work as well as periods of critical resource shortage. While reducing idle time or work gaps is important in project management, priority should be given to making sure the critical activities have the resources they require. A schedule that enables a project team to complete their jobs correctly, on time, and within budget is what is needed, and the managerial decision to smooth a schedule should not come at the detriment of these three key aspects of project delivery.

One should be aware that there is a bias in projects (Olson 2004). Though activity delays accumulate, gains from finishing activities ahead of schedule do not (Goldratt 1997). This bias results from the fact that when an activity is late, all activities for which it is a predecessor start later than scheduled. But if an activity is completed ahead of its scheduled finish time, this rarely works to the project

FIGURE 13.7 Project Data

	A	B	C	D	E	F	G	H	I
1	Activity	Activity Description	Predecessor Activities	Time in Weeks	Early Start	Early Finish	Late Start	Late Finish	Slack
2	A	estimate completion cost	none	8	0	8	0	8	0
3	B	secure project resources	A	2	8	10	8	10	0
4	C	build system	B	28	10	38	10	38	0
5	D	train system users	B	12	10	22	26	38	16
6	E	implement system	C, D	4	38	42	38	42	0

team's advantage since it is usually the case that different personnel and materials have to be gathered and coordinated to start subsequent activities ahead of schedule. Since an early finish time is not usually known very far ahead of the activity's completion, it is difficult to gather all of the required resources in order to start any subsequent activities early.

GANTT CHARTS

A *Gantt chart* is a graphical illustration of a project's schedule. It displays the desired schedule versus time. Using Gantt charts, it is possible to show the current schedule status using percent-complete shadings as well as to indicate project status at the current time (i.e., today) using a vertical line.

We will begin by taking a previous example and generating the project data (early start time, early finish time, late start time, late finish time, slack) for each activity using Excel. Then we will examine how to create a Gantt chart of a different format (different from Figure 13.4) in Excel. Recall our simple project example depicted in Figure 13.2.

We can use Excel to calculate values for the early start time, early finish time, late start time, late finish time, and slack for each activity. Figure 13.7 presents all of these data for the simple project example. Figure 13.8 indicates the formulas needed to make each calculation.

Creating a Gantt Chart in Excel

Kros (2011) provides good step-by-step instructions on how to create a Gantt chart in Excel. The main points of his instructions are provided here.

FIGURE 13.8 Project Data Formulas

	A	B	C	D	E	F	G	H	I
1	Activity	Activity Description	Predecessor Activities	Time in Weeks	Early Start	Early Finish	Late Start	Late Finish	Slack
2	A	estimate completion cost	none	8	0	E2+D2	H2-D2	G3	G2-E2
3	B	secure project resources	A	2	E2+D2	E3+D3	H3-D3	MIN(G4,G5)	G3-E3
4	C	build system	B	28	E3+D3	E4+D4	H4-D4	G6	G4-E4
5	D	train system users	B	12	E4+D4	E5+D5	H5-D5	G6	G5-E5
6	E	implement system	C, D	4	E5+D5	E6+D6	H6-D6	F6	G6-E6

FIGURE 13.9 Intermediate Step—Gantt Chart Creation

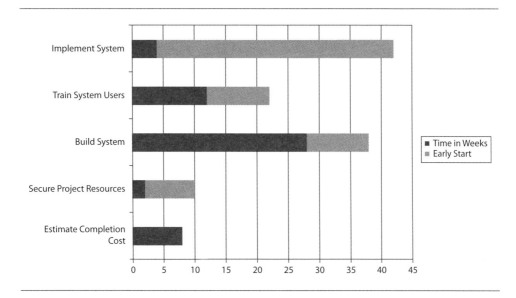

Step 1: From the data loaded to create Figure 13.7, select the columns for activity description, time in weeks, and early start (columns B, D, and E).

Step 2: Select the Insert tab from the top ribbon in Excel and click on Bar from the Charts group.

Step 3: Select the Stacked Bar option from the 2-D Bar Charts. This should produce a figure such as Figure 13.9.

Step 4: Right-click on the chart you just created and select Move Chart from the pop-up menu. Select the New Sheet option so that the chart will be moved to a new Excel worksheet. Name the sheet Gantt Chart.

Step 5: In order to reverse the order in which the early start times and activity durations (time in weeks) appear in each bar, you must click on one of the Early Start bars and then move up to the formula bar in Excel and change the very last number from a 2 to a 1.

Step 6: In order to make the early start portion of each bar not visible, you must click on one of the Early Start bars, then right-click to get a menu of options. Select Format Data Series from the menu. Click on the Fill option in the left-hand frame of the dialogue box and then click the No Fill option in the right-hand frame of the dialogue box.

Step 7: You should now see a chart like the one in Figure 13.10. You may use other chart design features to customize the Gantt chart to your own specifications.

FIGURE 13.10   Gantt Chart in Excel

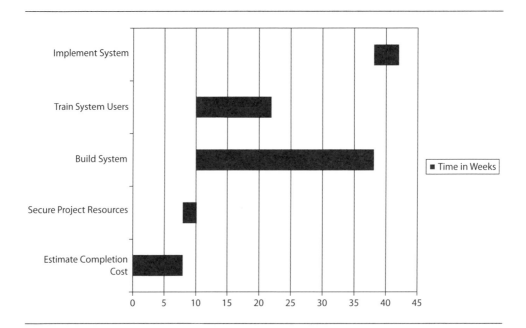

PROGRAM EVALUATION AND REVIEW TECHNIQUE

The *Program Evaluation and Review Technique (PERT)* offers an alternative to the critical path method (CPM) discussed earlier. With CPM, the activity durations are assumed to be known with certainty. For most projects, this is not the case. With PERT, a random variable is used to model the duration of each activity. PERT requires the project manager to estimate each activity's duration under the most favorable conditions (minimum estimated duration = *a*), the least favorable conditions (maximum estimated duration = *b*), and the most likely conditions (most likely estimated duration = *m*).

Often when PERT is employed, the network being evaluated is an activity-on-arc network. This means that the activities are on the arcs, not on the nodes as we have seen previously. In order to familiarize you with activity-on-arc networks, we have converted the network from our health care example (Figure 13.3) to an activity-on-arc network, and it is given in Figure 13.11. We will use this figure throughout this section on PERT.

Now that we have a network of activities on arcs, we can let $\mathbf{T}_{ij}$ be the random variable that represents the duration of activity (i,j). PERT requires the assumption that $\mathbf{T}_{ij}$ follows a beta distribution (Winston 2004). Although we did not discuss the beta distribution in detail in Chapter 5, what is important to note is that the beta distribution may be used to approximate a wide range of random variables.

If we want to know the expected duration of activity (i,j), we use the formula shown in Equation 13.1:

$$\text{expected duration} = \mathrm{E}\left(\mathbf{T}_{ij}\right) = \frac{\mathrm{a} + 4m + \mathrm{b}}{6} \tag{13.1}$$

FIGURE 13.11 Activity-on-Arc Network Diagram

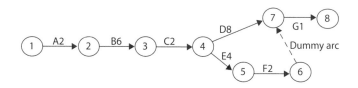

If we want to know the variance of the duration of activity (i,j), we use the formula shown in Equation 13.2:

$$\text{variance} = \text{var}\left(\mathbf{T}_{ij}\right) = \frac{(b - a)^2}{36} \tag{13.2}$$

PERT also requires the assumption that the durations of all activities are independent (Winston 2004). Using this assumption, for any path in the project network, the time required to complete the activities on the path is normally distributed.

Example from Health Care

Using the example presented in Figure 13.11, we can utilize Excel to perform relevant calculations for PERT. Figure 13.12 displays the Excel worksheet for the example, with most formulas for the top portion of the figure being determined in similar fashion as previously presented. Let us now examine how to determine the values for the "Expected Time" as well as those displayed in the lower half of the figure.

Recall that PERT requires the assumption that $\mathbf{T}_{ij}$ (the duration of activity i,j) follows a beta distribution. Thus, we calculate the values for the Expected Time column of Figure 13.11 using the formula in Equation 13.1, where a is the minimum estimated duration of the activity (optimistic), b is the maximum duration of the activity (pessimistic), and m is the most likely duration of the activity (most probable).

For the Critical Path column in the lower half of Figure 13.12, we recall that an activity is on the critical path if and only if it has a slack value of 0. Thus, we can use the formula for cell D14 of =IF(L3=0,1,0).

The IF statement in Excel tests to see if the condition tested is true. If the condition is true, it returns the value after the first comma. If the condition tested is not true, it returns the value after the second comma. We can copy this formula to cells D15 through D20.

The project completion column is used to indicate the cumulative time to get the current activity completed. The formula for cell E14 is given by =IF(D14=1, I3, 0). The IF conditional statement assigns either the activity's duration (from

FIGURE 13.12   PERT Example in Excel

	Activity	Activity Description	Precedence Activities	Optimistic	Most Probable	Pessimistic	Expected Time	ES	EF	LS	LF	Slack
1												
2	Activity	Activity Description	Precedence Activities	Optimistic	Most Probable	Pessimistic	Expected Time	ES	EF	LS	LF	Slack
3	A	collect relevant data	--	1	2	3	2.00	0.00	2.00	0.00	2.00	0.00
4	B	build forecsting model	A	4	6	8	6.00	2.00	8.00	2.00	8.00	0.00
5	C	model testing/validation	B	1	2	3	2.00	8.00	10.00	8.00	10.00	0.00
6	D	code development	C	5	8	11	8.00	10.00	18.00	10.00	18.00	0.00
7	E	interface development	C	3	4	5	4.00	10.00	14.00	12.00	16.00	2.00
8	F	user training	E	1	2	3	2.00	14.00	16.00	16.00	18.00	2.00
9	G	implementation	D, F	0.5	1	1.5	1.00	18.00	19.00	18.00	19.00	0.00
10									19.00			

	Activity	Activity Description	Precedence Activities	Critical Path	Project Completion	Variance	Project Variance
11							
12			Precedence	Critical	Project		Project
13	Activity	Activity Description	Activities	Path	Completion	Variance	Variance
14	A	collect relevant data	--	1	2.00	0.11	0.11
15	B	build forecsting model	A	1	8.00	0.44	0.44
16	C	model testing/validation	B	1	10.00	0.11	0.11
17	D	code development	C	1	18.00	1.00	1.00
18	E	interface development	C	0	0.00	0.11	0.00
19	F	user training	E	0	0.00	0.11	0.00
20	G	implementation	D, F	1	19.00	0.03	0.03
21					19.00		1.69
22							
23		Expected Project Completion Time	19.00				
24		Project Standard Deviation	1.30				
25							

column I) or a value of 0 (for noncritical activities) to each cell in column E. This formula should be dragged down and copied to cells E15 through E20.

The variance column displays the variance in the activity's length. Recall that the formula for variance is given by Equation 13.2. Thus, the formula we need to use for cell F14 is given by $= ((F3-B3)/6)^2$. Again, this formula can be copied to cells F15 through F20.

Only critical activities contribute to the overall project variance. For this reason, the project variance formula for cell G14 is $=IF(D14=1, F14, 0)$. Use of the IF conditional statement ensures that only the variances of critical activities are included.

IMPLEMENTATION

The concepts and tools presented in this chapter can enable effective and efficient project implementation. There are other factors to consider as well. These include but are not limited to budgeting and cost estimation, resource allocation, and monitoring and information systems.

Budgeting and Cost Estimation

Measures taken to improve project cost estimation are necessary, as a large majority of projects accomplished in industry are completed over budget. Many project managers fail to account for waste and spoilage. It may be necessary to budget for a small percentage of overstock in order to ensure that project progress is not delayed by a materials shortage.

It is generally the case that the resources needed for the project will have a change in their pricing during the life of the project, or perhaps before it even starts. For long-term projects, it is recommended to slightly increase the costs of resources by a percentage over time. A careful examination of historical figures and trends will enable one to be knowledgeable enough to use different inflators for different classes of labor and commodities.

It is also critical to be aware of when prices are falling. Costing projects too high can be problematic as well. Additionally, if any of the project workers leave during the course of a project, it may cost more to replace them than it did to put them on the project initially. This is due to both the learning curve and the rate at which salaries rise.

Resource Allocation

This chapter has discussed the issues of project crashing, resource leveling, and resource smoothing. Other resource allocation issues include assembling a project team, resource availability, and resource utilization.

The composition of a project team may change over time. It is important to make sure the right mix of both technical and professional skills is available on the team. Ensuring that the team members are in positions that give them the authority to make things happen that are necessary to keep the project on track can also save time and reduce frustration.

Resource availability is often overlooked when scheduling a project. Personnel and equipment may be obligated to other tasks or unavailable for some other reason. Before a project schedule is finalized, resource availability should be investigated and confirmation of availability should be received in writing.

Another issue to consider is resource utilization. When optimizing the performance of machines, it may be possible to seek very high utilization rates, such as 95 to 98 percent. People, however, may not function well at that rate of utilization. There are standards in place to make sure that health care providers, such as doctors and nurses, do not work too many consecutive hours without a break. When scheduling project work, one must consider the type of work being done and be realistic when estimating personnel utilization. There are some tasks a person may be able to perform at a high level for a number of hours, whereas other tasks may require a break every hour or two.

Monitoring and Information Systems

Some of the earliest business applications for computers were project management information systems (PMIS) (Meredith and Mantel 2000). The current versions of such software are capable of handling projects of large size and can even link multiple projects together for a business. Due to today's global market, the software now is designed to allow for easy sharing (via local networks or the Internet) of project data and progress reports. Basic features of PMIS software and selection criteria for determining a fit of software type for your company's needs are discussed in detail in Meredith and Mantel (2000).

SUMMARY

This chapter began with an examination of methods by which a decision maker may be guided to clarify his or her priorities for multiple, competing objectives a project may have. This prioritization enables proper trade-offs to be made to ensure high-priority objectives are met. Project planning and control were then introduced in an effort to inform the reader about tools that can aid in planning and control tasks. This was followed by a section on project scheduling, with additional detailed sections on the critical path method that provided explanations and examples of project crashing, resource leveling, and resource smoothing.

The chapter discussed Gantt charts and provided details on how to develop a Gantt chart in Excel. It also included information on Project Evaluation and Review Technique. Throughout, the chapter included examples from health care and provided details of problem solving in Excel. It closed with a section on implementation that presented an overview of factors contributing to project implementation.

KEY TERMS

critical path method (CPM)

Gantt chart

Program (or Project) Evaluation and Review Technique (PERT)

project control

project crashing

project management

project planning

resource leveling

resource smoothing

DISCUSSION QUESTIONS

1. Compare and contrast direct ranking methods and weighting methods. Provide a situation in which one approach would be preferred and explain why.

2. Conduct a SWOT analysis of your performance in a course. Are there any opportunities that you listed that you will take advantage of?

3. Think of a large project you have been involved with at work or at school. Create a work breakdown structure for the project.

4. Given the following data, perform a critical path analysis in Excel to determine the project's critical path. Your spreadsheet should indicate the early start schedule, late start schedule, and slack.

Activity	Duration	Predecessors
A	3 weeks	—
B	15 weeks	A
C	5 weeks	B
D	3 weeks	C
E	6 weeks	B
F	4 weeks	E
G	2 weeks	D, F

5. Draw a network diagram for the project described in question 4.

6. Use the results of question 4 to crash the project on activity B. Assume the cost of one additional resource applied to activity B will cost $100 per week

and will cut a week of the completion time of activity B. Also assume that exceeding a project total duration of over 26 weeks is penalized at a rate of $125 per week.

7. Use the results of question 4 and assume that the same resource is required to perform activity C and activity F. Use Excel to determine the best approach for resource leveling.

8. Use Excel to create a Gantt chart of the project given in question 4.

9. Using the provided data values for minimum expected activity durations and maximum expected activity durations, use Excel to provide a PERT analysis of the project given in question 4. Include all calculations demonstrated in Figure 13.12.

Activity	Minimum Duration	Maximum Duration
A	2	4
B	12	18
C	3	7
D	2	4
E	4	8
F	3	5
G	1	3

10. Convert the diagram you created for question 5 into an activity-on-arc diagram.

MINICASE: IMPLEMENTING ELECTRONIC MEDICAL RECORDS AT ST. HAMPTON'S HOSPITAL

Assume that you are the project manager at St. Hampton's Hospital, located in a large city in the Midwest area of the United States. Your project team has been tasked with implementing electronic medical records (EMR) at St. Hampton's. The information technology infrastructure is in place and the EMR software has been purchased. Your project focuses on implementation and adoption of EMR across the entire hospital (15 departments).

Explain how you would determine appropriate objectives and trade-offs for this project and how you might employ a weighting method to assist with this task.

How might use of a SWOT analysis play a role?

What role might benchmarking play?

Assume that the network for this project is provided in Figure 13.13. Also assume that it is not possible to accomplish tasks A, D, and E any faster than the durations provided in Figure 13.13.

What other data would be needed in order to determine if project crashing can occur?

If we now add in the assumption that activity D and activity F require the same person (resource), then we are faced with an example of resource leveling. Either D or F must be delayed.

How would we determine which resource leveling option is preferred?

FIGURE 13.13 Network for Electronic Medical Records Implementation

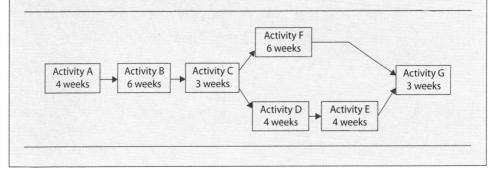

REFERENCES

Blanchard, B., and W. Fabrycky. 2006. *Systems Engineering and Analysis.* 4th ed. Upper Saddle River, NJ: Pearson Prentice Hall.

Chang, C. M. 2004. *Engineering Management—Challenges in the New Millennium.* Upper Saddle River, NJ: Pearson Prentice Hall.

Cleland, D. I., and R. Gareis. 2006. *Global Project Management Handbook.* Boston: McGraw-Hill Professional.

Goldratt, E. M. 1997. *Critical Chain.* Great Barrington, MA: North River Press.

Kros, J. 2011. *Spreadsheet Modeling for Business Decisions.* 3rd ed. Dubuque, IA: Kendall Hunt.

Meredith, J., and S. Mantel. 2000. *Project Management: A Managerial Approach.* 4th ed. New York: John Wiley & Sons.

www.microsoft.com/project/en/us/project-standard-2010-benefits.aspx.

Olson, D. L. 2004. *Information Systems Project Management.* 2nd ed. Boston: McGraw-Hill Irwin.

www.pmi.org/About-Us.aspx.

www.premierinc.com/safety/topics/guidelines/cms-guidelines-4-infection.jsp#HAC-PO.

Winston, W. 2004. *Operations Research Applications and Algorithms.* 4th ed. Belmont, CA: Thomson Learning.

CHAPTER 14

AGGREGATE PLANNING, SCHEDULING, AND CAPACITY MANAGEMENT IN HEALTH CARE

LEARNING OBJECTIVES

⫸ Understand the basics of aggregate/central planning and capacity planning.

(Continued)

⟶ Understand the role enterprise resource planning (ERP) systems play in health care.

⟶ Understand the importance of scheduling and capacity management within health care.

⟶ Understand what dispatching rules and scheduling methods are.

⟶ Understand the basics of facility location analysis including the center of gravity method.

AGGREGATE/CENTRAL PLANNING

Although service-based, large health care organizations do not differ from product-based organizations in that each organization must have aggregate planning and control. *Aggregate/central planning* is needed to determine what needs to be accomplished, while control ensures that the planned results are attained and resources used are properly accounted for.

Production control systems generally have three focal points for designing control functions (Bertrand et al. 1990):

1. Coordination between supply and demand (i.e., boundary control).

2. Aggregate control of flows (i.e., vertical stratification).

3. Production unit control of flows (i.e., horizontal stratification).

However, a health care organization is unique and in many ways contrasts with a manufacturing organization (e.g., manufacturers have homogeneous products or a focused factory).

Nevertheless, health care organizations are also characterized by planning and control systems at a high level. The following characteristics are typical:

- Coordination of demand that is typically larger than supply.

- Supply restrictions placed on the organization by contracting organizations (e.g., insurance companies, Medicare).

- High patient expectations on service quality constrained by organization resources (e.g., managing service quality while at the same time maximizing utilization of resources).

In managing the level of service quality, a health care organization should focus its planning and control efforts on eliminating patient waiting that exceeds predetermined levels.

In maximizing the utilization of resources, health care organizations must focus planning and control efforts on the most expensive resources (e.g., shared scarce resources such as specialist time).

Most health care facilities do not have the luxury of forecasting demand with any certainty. As the first characteristic mentioned, demand usually outstrips supply, and that demand tends to be variable, especially for facilities such as trauma I hospitals. Therefore, in most cases, planning and control are coordinated at the patient group level, with the health care organization broken up into focused business units such as pediatrics, emergency room (ER), rehab, and so on. For example, different control systems may be applied by different patient groups to achieve efficient overall planning (e.g., the ER may use different waiting list management procedures than the walk-in clinic).

In sum, a planning and control hierarchy does exist in a health care facility that is somewhat similar to that in a manufacturing setting. However, actual patient groups tend to drive the planning and control system in a health care facility more than a broad aggregate production plan drives a manufacturing facility. A close analogy could be made to a job shop that produces many unique products, some that are as unique as one-time-only production. Figure 14.1 displays the typical planning and control hierarchy in a health care setting.

Organization-Wide Planning/Control and Strategic Planning

Organization-wide patient planning/control and strategic planning would be at the top of the aggregate planning hierarchy. This level of planning and control is

FIGURE 14.1 **Aggregate Planning Hierarchy in a Health Care Organization**

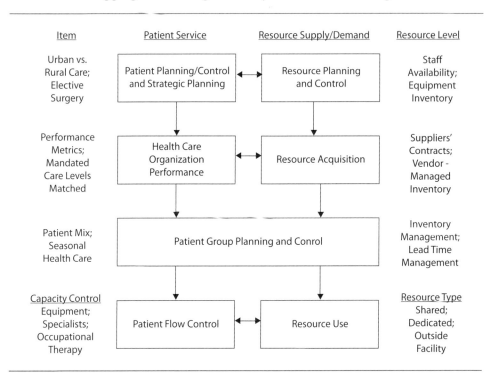

typically coupled with resource planning and control (discussed next). Items contained in this top level include the range of services provided (e.g., bariatric surgery or plastic surgery), markets (e.g., urban versus rural care), long-term resource requirements, and target service levels.

At this level, the organization's management is responsible for making arrangements with outside agencies on the total amount of output required at annual levels, and for securing the amount of resources available at the organization level that is sufficient to allow for treating the number of patients agreed on. In turn, this level is where the trade-off is made between service level and resource utilization level for the hospital as a whole.

RESOURCE PLANNING AND CONTROL

As organization-wide planning/control activities are set, the amount of resources of each type of service, market, and service level for a defined period of time must be determined. At this level the resources required by the different services are matched with the total amount of each type of resource that is available for the organization as a whole.

Another function at this planning level is that many resources are shared and that it will be necessary to manage resources that need to be made available to another service area at the time required. Also, staff availability, such as specialists, will be roughed out at this level. Organization-wide planning/control and resource planning and control usually are simultaneous activities (e.g., refer to the double-headed arrows in Figure 14.1 between the two high-level boxes).

Organization Performance and Resource Acquisition

Organization performance ties directly into service-level planning and resource planning and control. Resource acquisition and utilization represent another important perspective for developing control requirements and stem from the resources planning and control area. High-level performance metrics must be set at this stage so future planning and resource allocation can be made. These two areas should also have simultaneous activities, and both provide guidance for lower-level patient group planning and control as well as feedback to the higher-level activities.

Patient Group Planning and Control

The patient group planning and control level is where the determination of the items such as patient mix, urgency criteria, and acceptable waiting times occur. With regard to resource planning, the acquisition of the resources required for the patient group, the control of the patient flow, and the utilization of resources by the patient group occur here.

This level details patient flow control, and the progress of individual patients through associated health care procedures is tracked. The detailed control is at the level of the patient group and would involve checking the day-to-day scheduling of patients and matching/managing service requirements specified for the patient group as a whole. Any regulations on resource use imposed on the patient group are also a responsibility at this level.

Patient Flow Control and Use of Resources

Patient flow control and resource use are at the lowest aggregate planning level. At this level, actual health care services are provided and staff scheduling on an hour-by-hour or even minute-by-minute time frame is accomplished. This level is literally the day-to-day operations of a working health care organization (i.e., how many nurses are needed and where, how many surgeries are planned for the morning, what staff is needed and what equipment, etc.).

At this level, decisions may be made on an ad hoc basis to meet demand or shift resource capacity where needed (i.e., literal management of service levels at different units or patient groups). Staff schedules are developed, performance metrics are measured, and capacity management is carried out at this level.

To assist in coordinating all these activities, at both high level and low level, many manufacturing organizations use what is referred to as *enterprise resource planning (ERP)* software. ERP systems integrate functions such as *capacity planning*, staffing, and billing across the entire organization. ERP systems and their relationship to health care organizations are detailed next.

Enterprise Resource Planning Systems

Recently, large health care organizations have shown interest in ERP systems. However, as one would suspect, while the health care industry is intrigued with the concept of integrating major functions across their organizations, there is a question whether an application originally designed for the manufacturing sector can be transferred with any success to a health care setting. It is not an unreasonable question in that health care organizations primarily manage nurses, MDs, and other staff while providing clinical processes. However, this does not exclude the use of ERP systems within a health care organization. This section provides some insight into how health care organizations can apply ERP.

Patient Care versus Assembly Lines

Assembly-type processes focus on turning raw materials into finished goods. In a manufacturing organization, raw materials are turned into work in process and finally into finished goods, all while being coordinated with optimal production schedules and minimization of working capital. Sales forecasts usually drive the need for raw materials, which in turn drives the need for capital and labor.

Health care organizations, comparatively speaking, have a much more difficult time forecasting patient demand (compared to sales in a manufacturing organization). Costs are also difficult to predict, in that it may be unknown exactly what processes a patient will need when coming to the facility. In fact, the treatment of every patient varies to some degree in terms of processes, staffing needs, and delivery of services (e.g., the variation that might be seen in delivering a baby from natural birth to cesarean section to drugs administered to length of stay).

Labor as a Driver

Since most health care processes are labor intensive, the primary cost driver in a health care organization is labor. This is much different from a manufacturing setting where materials tend to be the primary cost driver. Since labor tends to be the main cost driver for health care organizations, scheduling staff and delivering care at a high service level are key functions that must be managed. In turn, any use of an ERP system must have these two functions in mind.

An ERP system applied to health care can assist as follows:

- Forecast staff workloads.

- Manage human resources and coordination across entities outside the health care facility itself (Medicare payments, specialists, etc.).

- Identify specific work flows for associated health care processes.

Variability in Health Care Processes

As mentioned before, many processes within a health care organization have substantially higher variability than processes within a manufacturing organization. However, this does not exclude the use of ERP within a health care organization. An ERP system can be used to create and maintain a common database of diagnostic and treatment procedures as well as the underlying bill of resources (BOR). A BOR can be created when patient services are rendered. A BOR is akin to a bill of materials (BOM) in a manufacturing setting. While a BOM contains the necessary materials and labor to build or assemble a unit or product, the BOR contains all processes and procedures that a patient will receive or has received, and incorporates both capacity and materials resources requirements. BORs may contain diagnosis-related groups (DRGs) and treat them like products or end items. Many procedures can be broken down this way (e.g., appendectomy).

Overall, there are many more stable processes (e.g., billing or materials management) within a health care organization that can also be brought under the ERP umbrella. The more variable processes can be planned and controlled on a more ad hoc basis. The next section discusses methods for planning and controlling more variable processes such as scheduling and capacity management.

SCHEDULING AND CAPACITY MANAGEMENT

The importance of *scheduling* within a health care organization is obvious. In being a service provider almost every process undertaken in a health care organization requires some form of labor (e.g., nurses to triage patients, MDs or physicians' assistants [PAs] to diagnose patients, lab technicians to run tests, etc.). For a health care organization to run efficiently, this labor must be available in the right place, at the right time, and in the right capacity (i.e., quantity).

Therefore, decisions regarding workforce scheduling beget decisions regarding capacity management. Health care organizations are continually faced with growing demand for care and higher expectations for improved service delivery in addition to standard or minimum resource levels (e.g., 2004 California legislation for a 6:1 nursing ratio on general wards).

However, budgets and overall labor constraints do not allow unlimited resources to be expended at all times. The conflict between service level and resource use forces health care organizations to investigate the balance between the level of service offered and the level of utilization of resources (e.g., beds, nursing staff). In short, it is those resources that determine the costs of service. This notion of resource allocation, especially in workforce scheduling, leads us to the next section on what scheduling problems exist within a health care organization.

WORKFORCE SCHEDULING

In general, workforce scheduling is a difficult, time-consuming managerial problem for any organization. Think about a manufacturing facility or a restaurant. However, health care has some very unique scheduling problems. Workforce scheduling is inextricably linked with determining total amount of labor resources needed within the organization (e.g., maximum nursing staff needed, maximum MD and PA requirements, etc.). Figure 14.2 displays a typical

FIGURE 14.2   Scheduling Framework for a Health Care Organization

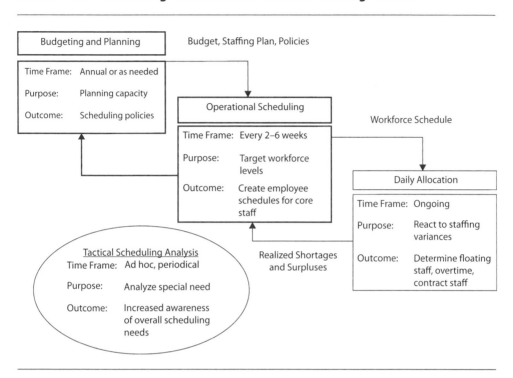

scheduling framework in a health care organization. There are two categories of scheduling that are discussed here: tactical and operational.

Tactical versus Operational Scheduling

Tactical scheduling tends to be non-employee-specific and to revolve around a minimum workforce needed to meet targets subject to rules or policies (e.g., being required to have three PAs on call each Friday evening). Tactical scheduling is done periodically almost in an ad hoc manner. Many times tactical scheduling is done for a special study or need. In can be said that within the health care industry there has been a lack of tactical scheduling and analysis performed.

Operational scheduling focuses on specific employees and is completed every two to six weeks. Workforce targets are the main purpose of operational scheduling, with employee schedules as the outcome. Operational scheduling leads directly to the daily allocation of health care staff and is a reaction to variation in demand and available resources. Outcomes can include the determination of floating staff or overtime hours, or the use of contract employees.

Difficulties within the Health Care Scheduling Framework

Health care scheduling presents difficult combinations of problems with conflicting objectives (e.g., high levels of service versus cost containment) and constrained resources (e.g., an organization can hire only so many nurses or PAs or afford only so many surgeons). Scheduling consumes costly managerial time and effort and is the main cause of employee dissatisfaction (e.g., "They make me work every Friday and Saturday night no matter how busy we are") and turnover. Overall, health care professionals want to do what they do best: assist patients with quality care.

In most cases health care professionals do not want to perform so-called office work, nor have they been trained to complete it. In reality, this statement applies to many industries (e.g., think of a top-rated chef at a top-rated restaurant preparing food versus scheduling staff). Many times those in charge of scheduling use ad hoc rules that are biased in favor of employee seniority or preferences over broad institutional needs. In turn, a commonly used rule is to err on the side of overstaffing in order maintain high levels of patient care. However, on one hand, overstaffing brings higher costs. On the other hand, understaffing impacts quality of care and patient satisfaction and in some cases may be illegal due to state or federal laws.

Approaches to Solving Scheduling Problems

Over time, a number of approaches to solving scheduling problems have sprung up. In fact, before the advent of computers and computer-based scheduling systems, much scheduling in every industry was completed by trial and error and on a day-to-day basis.

Smaller health care organizations may rely more on the trial-and-error method combined with some basic scheduling principles such as abiding by a simple set of management parameters (e.g., everyone will work four 10-hour days and we will have a minimum staff coverage of three nurses, one PA, and one MD). In most cases a master cyclical schedule is constructed and then modified as needed (e.g., Sue is out on vacation in the second week and she will trade with Stan).

For larger or more complex health care organizations, various specialized scheduling programs are available based on heuristics (i.e., rules of thumb) and presented within a computer algorithm. For many organizations these computer algorithms are created in-house or by a consultant and are spreadsheet based. A brief example of a spreadsheet-based scheduling algorithm is illustrated later in this chapter.

Higher-order solutions based on mathematical optimization models or artificial intelligence techniques also exist. Many of these are commercial packages and incorporate at least some of the aforementioned techniques or in many cases all of them. Table 14.1 displays a number of popular scheduling packages.

Health Care Operations and Supply Chain Management in Action: Scheduling an Emergency Department Using Excel

Many scheduling activities take place at a health care facility. However, much of the time scheduling is completed via an ad hoc method, and many times final schedules are made by handwritten methods. A large emergency department in North Carolina decided to develop and implement a better scheduling system via Excel.

TABLE 14.1   Workforce Scheduling Packages

ANSOS	www.per-se.com/forhospitals/h_onestaff.asp
ActiveStaffer	www.api-wi.com/products/activestaffer.asp
AtStaff	www.atstaff.com/Products/Products.htm
AcuStaf	www.acustaf.com/
Pathways Staff Scheduling	www.hboc.com/
Shiftwork Solutions	www.shift-schedules.com/
ShiftMaker	www.vastech.com/24–7/solutions/vastech24–7/247modules.htm
ESP eXpert	www.total-care.com/
InTime	www.intimesoft.com/
VSS Pro	www.abs-usa.com/index.epl
Kronos	www.kronos.com/
ScheduleSource	www.schedulesource.com/content/scheduling/default.asp
ORBIS	www.sieda.com/features_e.htm
Various packages	www.hr-software.net/pages/217.htm
StaffSchedule.com	www.staffscheduling.com/schedule.htm

In all, the emergency department (ED) staff, head nurse, and unit secretary spent excessive time on a complex six-week manual self-scheduling system. The large amounts of worker time, plus the inevitable errors and staff dissatisfaction, resulted in an initiative to automate elements of the scheduling process using Microsoft Excel. The implementation of this initiative included:

- Common coding of all 8- hour and 12-hour shifts, with each 4-hour period represented by a cell.

- Creation of a six-week master schedule using the COUNTIF function of Excel based on current staffing guidelines.

- Staff time-off requests processed by the department secretary.

- Fine-tuning accomplished by the head nurse, with staff input, to provide even unit coverage.

Numerous advantages appeared from the computerized schedule. Here are a few:

- Decrease in the amount of time the head nurse spent on scheduling; approximate time savings, 51 percent.

- Better visibility to all the staff from the introduction of the master track feature (e.g., if staff desired a particular day off when staffing was low, they now negotiated with other staff members in advance).

- Master schedule feature benefited nursing leadership since it allowed for future planning.

- Computerized schedules were clearer and easier to read, providing benefits to staff and in the preparation of payroll.

Ultimately, the automated self-scheduling method was expanded to the entire 700-bed hospital.

Basic Classes of Health Care Scheduling Problems

There are many classes of scheduling problems. In fact, the class of scheduling problem really depends more on what your time frame is (e.g., shift, day, week, monthly schedules) and your personnel goals (e.g., overtime use, length of work-day—four 10-hour days versus five 8-hour days, etc.). Three basic classes of health care scheduling problems are days-off scheduling, shift scheduling, and tour scheduling.

Days-Off Scheduling

Days-off scheduling is usually specified in a daily time frame. Within that daily time frame, standard shifts and day of week are recognized. In turn, the goal is to find the minimum staff size to meet coverage and other constraints such as weekends worked. Many times this is referred to as traditional scheduling.

Shift Scheduling

Shift scheduling refers to a specific short-term time frame, such as a workday and the number of hours in that day. Staffing requirements are then specified for the shift during that day. This method tends to be time consuming, as it has to be completed each time period (e.g., each hour of each day).

Tour Scheduling

Tour scheduling is a combination of days-off and shift scheduling over some planning cycle. The planning cycle tends to be longer (e.g., one or more weeks at a time) than in days off or shift scheduling. However, countless specific variations exist depending on organization size, health care service provided, legal impacts, or hours of operation.

DISPATCHING RULES

Dispatching rules are also referred to as job sequencing rules. They refer to the order in which certain jobs will be completed. Although each patient who enters a health care facility may have unique needs, many of the services performed in the facility are common (e.g., patients must check in first before going to triage, but after triage one patient may be moved ahead of another due to acuity). In a sense, triage itself is a dispatching rule.

In fact, the day-to-day activities being conducted within a health care facility are very similar to job shop scheduling problems. A job shop can be defined as an organization of work in a manufacturing organization by job functions such as welding, machining, and finishing. Although providing a service, health care facilities are akin to job shops. For example, nursing activities tend to be organized by function such as triage, preliminary health check (blood pressure, temperature), and discharge. Dispatching rules are the policy according to which the processing priorities of activities are determined. For the case of nursing activities, the nursing activities with higher priority would be handled first.

JOB SEQUENCING

An important aspect of scheduling is job sequencing. Whereas scheduling allocates jobs to relevant health care activities or centers, job sequencing specifies the order in which jobs are to be carried out. The simplest sequencing problem involves deciding in what order jobs are to be processed in a single facility (e.g., which x-ray request should be processed first—most likely first come, first served).

But should all jobs be assigned on a first-come, first-served basis? Perhaps jobs should be assigned based on a priority basis, with the most urgent jobs being given preference. The total time for processing all jobs will not change regardless of their places in the queue. However, different job sequencing can affect delivery speed and reliability as well as patient satisfaction.

A job's completion (or flow) time is the time it takes for the job to flow through the system; processing time or *duration* is the length of time it takes to process a job. The job's *due date* is the required date of delivery to the patient, while *lateness* is defined as the job's actual completion date minus its due date. Since lateness cannot be negative, jobs that finish ahead of schedule are assigned a lateness value of zero. The ratio of total job processing time to total flow time is called *utilization*. The reciprocal of utilization is called the *average* number of jobs in the system. The process of prioritizing jobs is usually made on the basis of a set of dispatching or priority rules. The most common of these rules require only details of a job's duration and due date:

- *First come, first served (FCFS)*. The first job to arrive is the first job to be processed. Think about the x-ray example given earlier. The vast majority of the time, FCFS is used to process x-ray jobs.

- *Shortest processing time (SPT).* The shortest jobs are completed first, with the longest jobs being placed last in the queue. An example of SPT being used could be when final paperwork is being submitted and longer jobs are pushed to the back so shorter and simpler jobs can be processed, taken out of the system, and closed out (i.e., think about a stack of paperwork that must be done; it might be better to knock out all the simple ones first and then tackle the tougher ones).

- *Earliest due date (EDD).* The job with the earliest due date is processed first. This rule usually improves delivery reliability, but some jobs may have to wait a long time. An example of EDD being used would be scheduling labor and delivery for pregnant mothers.

- *Longest processing time (LPT).* This rule is the opposite of SPT. The longer jobs are often bigger and more important and should therefore be completed first. An example of using LPT might be processing a more complicated claim form that pays a bigger claim, and in turn the organization receives compensation sooner.

JOHNSON'S RULE

The material presented next illustrates *Johnson's rule*. Johnson's rule is used when jobs must be sequenced through multiple work centers. For example, suppose that patients are assigned to a medical clinic for treatment and all arrive at the same time. Assuming there are no life-threatening illnesses or injuries and all patients need to go through the same treatment centers, then in what order should they be treated?

This type of scheduling problem occurs at many clinics and has been studied in the past. S. M. Johnson in 1954 developed a very efficient algorithm, called Johnson's rule, to solve sequencing problems that cover two-activity situations. In general the jobs or patients must pass through each facility or activity center in the same order. The rule finds the correct sequencing that will minimize the total processing time for all jobs/patients. Johnson's rule involves the following five steps:

1. List the time required for each job/patient to complete each process. Set up a one-dimensional horizontal matrix to represent the desired sequence, with the number of slots equal to the number of jobs/patients.

2. Select the smallest overall completion time. If that time is for the first process, put the job/patient as near to the beginning of the sequence as possible.

3. If the smallest time occurs on the second process, put the job/patient as near to the end of the sequence as possible.

4. Remove that job/patient from the list.

5. Repeat steps 2 to 4 until all slots in the matrix are filled and all jobs/patients are sequenced.

In using Johnson's rule, two objectives are achieved. First, the processes will all be completed in the minimum amount of time; second, the amount of idle time will also be minimized. Let's take a look at an example. Table 14.2 contains a set of patients who must be processed through a clinic at the end of their stay.

Johnson's Rule Steps

Table 14.2 lists five patients who must accomplish the two back-to-back processes of completing paperwork and then checking out and paying. Johnson's rule will be used to sequence the patients.

1. Draw a one-dimensional horizontal matrix with five slots, one for each job/ patient (see Figure 14.3).

2. Choose Colbert due to the overall smallest completion time of three minutes for checking out and paying. Since the time is for the second process, the patient Colbert is positioned at the end of the sequence. Figure 14.4 displays this step.

TABLE 14.2 Johnson's Rule Example

Patient	Complete Paperwork (Minutes)	Check Out and Pay (Minutes)
Allstot	6	8
Barnes	11	6
Colbert	7	3
Dunn	9	7
Eggbert	5	10

FIGURE 14.3 One-Dimensional Horizontal Matrix with Five Job/Patient Slots

FIGURE 14.4 Johnson's Rule First Iteration

				Colbert

FIGURE 14.5 Johnson's Rule Second Iteration

Eggbert				Colbert

FIGURE 14.6 Johnson's Rule Third Iteration

Eggbert	Allstot			Colbert

3. Patient Colbert is crossed off the list and the next smallest completion time is chosen, which corresponds to patient Eggbert (refer to Table 14.2, which shows five minutes for Eggbert completing paperwork). Since the time is for the first process, the patient Eggbert is positioned at the beginning of the sequence. Figure 14.5 displays this step.

4. Patient Eggbert is crossed off the list and the next smallest completion time is chosen, which corresponds to either patient Allstot or patient Barnes (refer to Table 14.2, which shows six minutes for Allstot completing paperwork and six minutes for Barnes checking out and paying). Since both jobs have the same duration, chose one and move forward. Patient Allstot is chosen and since the time is for the first process, the patient Allstot is positioned as near the beginning of the sequence as possible (i.e., after Eggbert). Figure 14.6 displays this step.

FIGURE 14.7 Johnson's Rule Fourth Iteration

Eggbert	Allstot		Barnes	Colbert

FIGURE 14.8 Johnson's Rule Fifth and Final Iteration

Eggbert	Allstot	Dunn	Barnes	Colbert

5. Patient Allstot is crossed off the list and the next smallest completion time is chosen, which corresponds to patient Barnes (refer to Table 14.2 and six minutes for Barnes checking out and paying). Since the time is for the second process, the patient Barnes is positioned as near the end of the sequence as possible (i.e., before Colbert). Figure 14.7 displays this step.

6. At this juncture, the only patient left is Dunn, and only one slot remains in our matrix. Therefore, Dunn is sequenced in the third slot. Figure 14.8 displays the final patient sequence.

Therefore, we can see that the most efficient manner to queue up the patients (i.e., the quickest time to process all patients through the system) is to complete Eggbert first, followed by Allstot, Dunn, Barnes, and finally Colbert. The solution using Johnson's rule ensures that the total processing time required for the five patients will be the minimum. No other sequence will result in a smaller processing time. The Johnson's rule solution also guarantees the smallest amount of idle time for the system (e.g., the clerk at the check out and pay window sitting and waiting for the next patient to process).

Johnson's Rule in Excel

Although Johnson's rule assisted us in finding the sequence in which patients should be processed, it does not assist in finding total time for all patients to be processed through the system, nor does it give idle time. To illustrate how to find total processing time and idle time, Figure 14.9 displays a sample spreadsheet for our patient sequencing problem. The spreadsheet calculates total time in the system and idle time for all patients. Take a look at cells C9 to I9 in Figure 14.9 for the Johnson's Rule solution to the scheduling problem presented earlier.

FIGURE 14.9   Spreadsheet to Accompany Johnson's Rule Patient Processing Problem

	A	B	C	D	E	F	G	H	I	J	K	L
1		1-Complete Paperwork (CP)	2-Check Out and Pay (CO&P)		Original Sequence	1-CP Time	1-Earliest Start Time	1-Earliest Finish Time	2-CO&P Time	2-Earliest Start Time	2-Earliest Finish Time	Idle
2	Allstot	6	8		1 Allstot	6	0	6	8	6	14	6
3	Barnes	11	6		2 Barnes	11	6	17	6	17	23	3
4	Colbert	7	3		3 Colbert	7	17	24	3	24	27	1
5	Dunn	9	7		4 Dunn	9	24	33	7	33	40	6
6	Eggbert	5	10		5 Eggbert	5	33	38	10	40	50	0
7										Total Time	50	
8											Total Idle	16
9			Johnson'S Rule	Eggbert	Allstot	Dunn		Barnes		Colbert		
10			Sequence									
11												
12				Johnson's Rule Sequence	1-CP Time	1-Earliest Start Time	1-Earliest Finish Time	2-CO&P Time	2-Earliest Start Time	2-Earliest Finish Time	Idle	
13				1 Eggbert	5	0	5	10	5	15	5	
14				2 Allstot	6	5	11	8	15	23	0	
15				3 Dunn	9	11	20	7	23	30	0	
16				4 Barnes	11	20	31	6	31	37	1	
17				5 Colbert	7	31	38	3	38	41	1	
18									Total Time	41		
19										Total Idle	7	
20												
21				Gantt Chart								
22				Sequence	1-CP Time	Sequence	2-CO&P Time					
23				Eggbert	5	Idle 1	5					
24				Allstot	6	Eggbert	10					
25				Dunn	9	Allstot	8					
26				Barnes	11	Dunn	7					
27				Colbert	7	Idle 4	1					
28						Barnes	6					
29						Idle 5	1					
30						Colbert	3					
31												

Table 14.3 contains the formulas for the spreadsheet. It must be noted that this is a sample problem and although Johnson's Rule can be applied to any sequencing problem, the spreadsheet presented here is specific to this example. With that said, the underlying spreadsheet can be modified for problems that contain more patients or different processing times.

A good way to depict total system processing time and idle time is to plot these via a Gantt chart. The next section discusses Gantt charts.

Gantt Charts

The total processing time and idle time can be illustrated with what is referred to as a Gantt chart. Gantt charts were introduced in the project management

TABLE 14.3 Formulas and Brief Explanatory Notes for Figure 14.9

Cells	Formula	Action/Note
A1 to C6	—	Original data from Table 14.2 is entered into cells A1 to C6.
E1 to L1	—	Self-explanatory headers.
E2	=A2	Copy down to E6.
F2	=B2	Copy down to F6.
G2	0	Earliest start time for entire sequence is time zero.
G3	=H2	Copy down to G6.
H2	=G2+F2	Copy down to H6.
I2	=C2	Copy down to I6.
J2	=H2	Earliest start time for check out and pay area (i.e., first patient must be done with paperwork area to be able to move on).
K2	=J2+H2	Copy down to K6.
J3	=IF(H3>K2, H3, K2)	Copy down to J6 (this is a check to make sure patient is finished with paperwork area).
L2	=H2	Idle time at check out and pay area for the first patient is equal to the patient's time in the first process.
L3	=IF(J3=K2, 0, J3-K2)	Copy down to L6 (this command compares earliest start times for the current patient to earliest finish times for the former patient—if they match, there is no idle time; if they do not match, then there is idle time).
K7	=K6	This is total time in the system.
L7	=SUM(L2:L6)	This is total system idle time.
E12 to L19	—	Copy cells E1 to L8 to cells E12 to L19 and then make the following adjustments.
E13 to E17	—	Using the sequence created using Johnson's rule, link cells E13 to E17 to their proper cells A2 to A6 (e.g., cell E13 is =A6).
F13 to F17	—	Using the sequence created using Johnson's rule, link cells F13 to F17 to their proper cells B2 to B6 (e.g., cell F13 is =B6).
I13 to I17	—	Using the sequence created using Johnson's rule, link cells I13 to I17 to their proper cells C2 to C6 (e.g., cell I13 is =C6).
E23	=E13	Copy down to E27.
F23	=F13	Copy down to F27.
G23	Idle 1 (type this in)	There will be idle time on the second process in the sequence.
G24	=E13	
G25	=E14	No idle time for second patient (refer to cell L14).

TABLE 14.3 (*Continued*)

Cells	Formula	Action/Note
G26	=E15	No idle time for third patient (refer to cell L15).
G27	Idle 4 (type this in)	There is idle time between the third and fourth patients (refer to cell L16).
G28	=E16	
G29	Idle 5 (type this in)	There is idle time between the fourth and fifth patients (refer to cell L17).
G30	=E17	
H23	=L13	Idle time for check out and pay area to start the sequence.
H24	=I13	Copy down to H26.
H27	=L16	
H28	=I16	
H29	=L17	
H30	=I17	

chapter, Chapter 13. We provide a brief overview here, but encourage the reader to reread the section on Gantt charts in Chapter 13.

Gantt Charts and Excel

The Johnson's rule methodology presented here works very well for smaller projects. However, the process becomes unwieldy for larger projects with numerous entities that must be scheduled. For large projects, commercial software packages, such as MS Project or a proprietary scheduler like those listed in Table 14.1, are a must. One of the benefits of using commercial project management software is the graphical output the software produces. One type of graphical output common to these software packages is a Gantt chart.

Gantt charts are a popular means for displaying a set of scheduled activities. Gantt charts are very useful for visualizing activity start times, activity end times, and the length of the scheduled activities. Figure 14.10 displays the final formatted Gantt chart for the sequential scheduling problem presented in Table 14.3.

From Figure 14.10, it is very obvious that, if all start times are met, the patients will all be through the paperwork and payment processes in 41 minutes (refer to the bar graph in Figure 14.10 labeled 2-CO & P Time). It is also very easy to see when the check out and pay area will have idle time. Using Johnson's

FIGURE 14.10   Gantt Chart for Patient Scheduling Problem

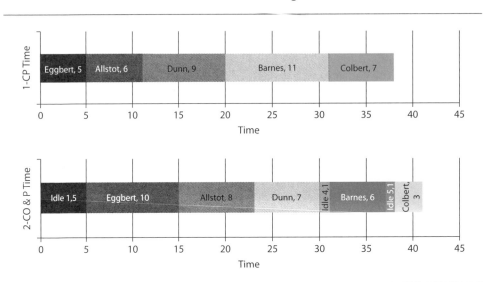

rule minimizes total idle time (seven minutes total for the check out and pay area), but it must be noted idle time is not eliminated. Figure 14.10 displays idle time of five minutes at the start of the process (refer to Idle 1,5 in Figure 14.10), one minute of idle time between patients Dunn and Barnes (refer to Idle 4,1 in Figure 14.10), and one minute of idle time between Barnes and Colbert for the check out and pay area (refer to Idle 5,1 in Figure 14.10).

Drawbacks to Gantt Charts

Although very useful as a visual aid, Gantt charts do have some drawbacks. Gantt charts do not show interdependencies between activities. Gantt charts, as a result of their inability to show interdependencies, do not answer questions easily regarding delay of activities.

Creating Gantt Charts in Excel

The Gantt chart in Figure 14.10 is fairly simple to create in a spreadsheet program such as Excel. The chart is a stacked horizontal bar chart. These are the steps for creating a Gantt chart in Excel:

1. From Figure 14.9 select cells E22 to F27.

2. Select the Insert tab in the Excel ribbon and click on Bar in the Charts group. Choose the Stacked Bar option (see Figure 14.11).

3. A screen such as Figure 14.11 will appear including the bar graph (see area from rows 13 to 28 and columns C to J in Figure 14.12—the bar graph was created by the actions in Step 2). Right click on the bar graph and choose the Select Data option in the menu in Figure 14.12.

4. A screen resembling Figure 14.13 will appear. This is the Select Data Source menu. From this menu click on the Switch Row/Column button and click OK. A figure that resembles Figure 14.14 will appear. This is the preliminary Gantt chart for the complete paperwork area (i.e., 1-CP Time).

5. Go back to Figure 12.9 and now select cells G22 to H30. We do this since we must create a bar chart for the second step of the process (i.e., check out and pay).

FIGURE 14.11 Stacked Bar Option

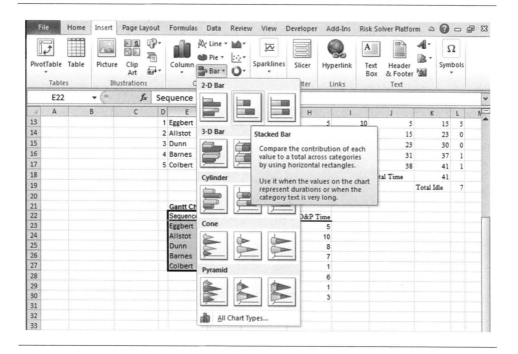

FIGURE 14.12 Initial Bar Chart for Gantt Chart Creation

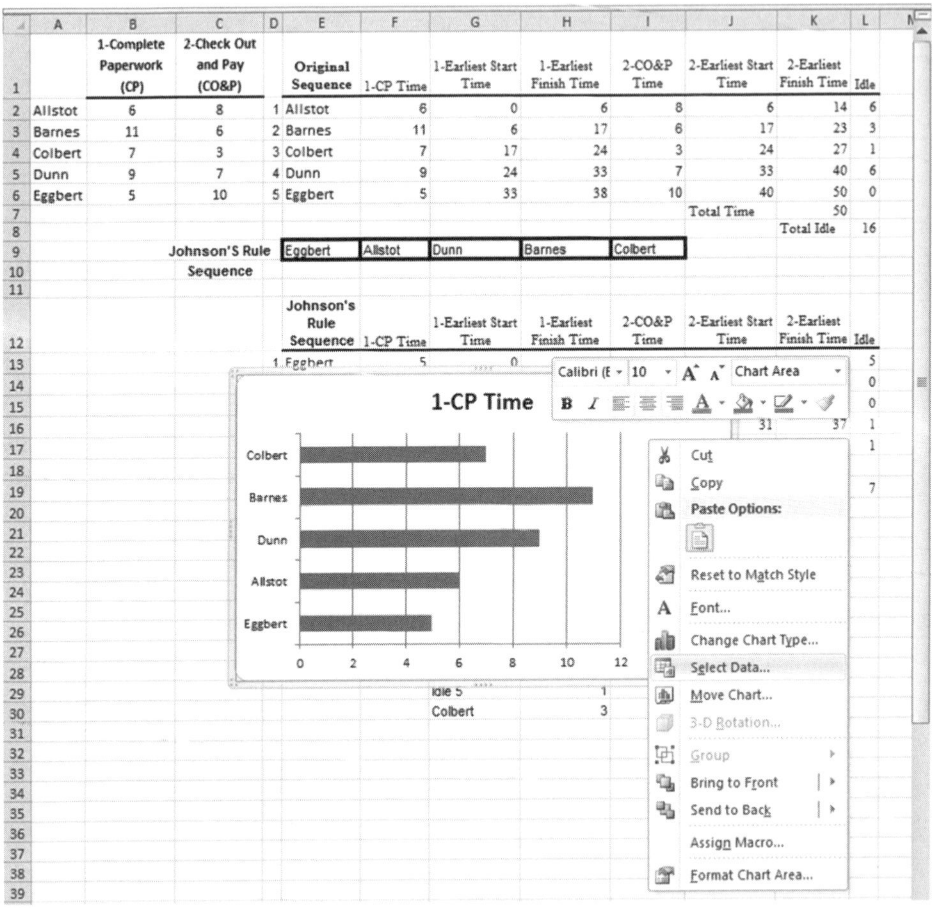

6. Select the Insert tab in the Excel ribbon and click on Bar in the Charts group. Choose the Stacked Bar option (refer to Figure 14.11). This is the step to insert the second bar chart for the second process, check out and pay.

7. Another bar graph that resembles the bar graph in Figure 14.12 will appear but this bar graph is the bar graph for the second process check out and pay. Right click on the bar graph and choose the Select Data option in the menu in Figure 14.12 just as was done in Step 3 earlier.

8. A screen resembling Figure 14.13 will appear. This is the Select Data Source menu. From this menu click on the Switch Row/Column button and click

FIGURE 14.13 **Data Option Menu**

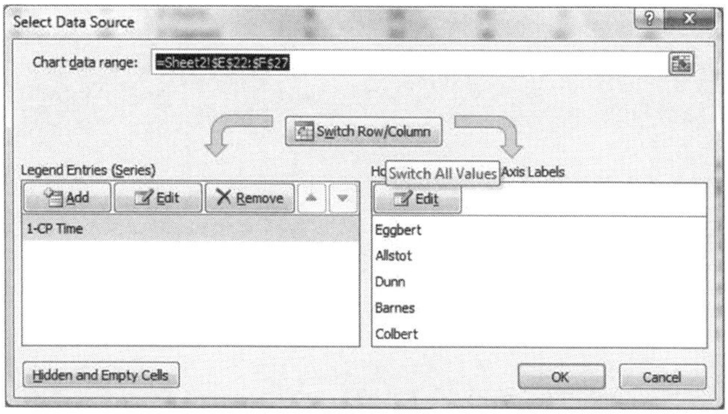

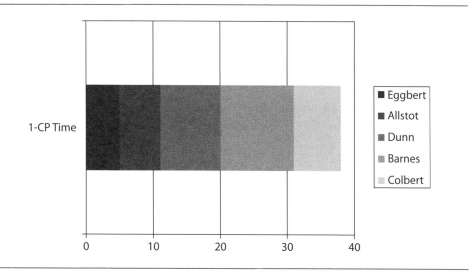

FIGURE 14.14 **Preliminary Gantt Chart for First Process Complete Paperwork**

OK. A figure that resembles the bottom bar chart in Figure 14.15 will appear. This is the preliminary Gantt chart for the check out and pay area.

The Gantt chart can now be customized, as the creator deems appropriate, using standard Excel charting commands. For brevity, the series of steps to format Figure 14.14 to appear as Figure 14.15 is not given here. Those steps are left up to the individual reader.

FIGURE 14.15 Formatted Gantt Chart

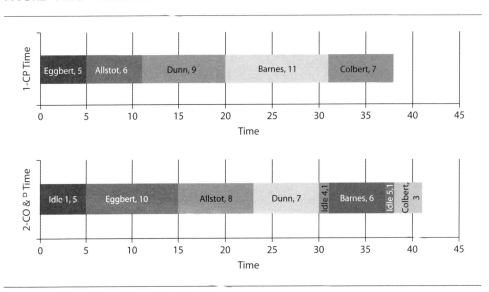

Scheduling is an important task for any organization. So is the job of locating new facilities or other stand-alone entities. For health care organizations, the choice of location for off-site emergency departments or outpatient clinics plays a key role in servicing patients and entire communities. The next section discusses facility location in the service industry and provides one method of solving location problems.

SERVICE FACILITY LOCATION ANALYSIS

Many times the objective for industrial facility *location analysis* is a minimization of costs, either shipping or processing. The main objective for service facility location analysis is either the maximization of revenue or the maximization of service levels. These different objectives tend to stem from the difference in business focus of manufacturing organizations and service organizations. Costs (e.g., labor, raw materials, shipping) associated with different locations tend to vary greatly for manufacturing firms, and those firms wish to choose locations that minimize those costs. By contrast, service-based firms find that location has more to do with revenue streams and customer service levels than cost.

Volume of customers can be said to drive service-based firms' choices of facility locations. Five major components for customer volume in a health care organization are:

1. Need of the customer base (e.g., rural versus urban hospitals).

2. Competition in the area or lack of competition in the area.

3. Quality of competition.

4. Uniqueness of locale (e.g., again think rural facilities assisting underserved communities).

5. Operating policies or requirements of the firm—at times requirements are set down by local or state entities for coverage requirements.

In the case of a large health care organization, part of its mission may be to provide care to underserved communities. In turn, it must locate facilities in areas where none exist or must locate in an area central to many smaller communities to pool resources and attempt to provide the largest reach for its services.

Methods of Evaluating Location Alternatives

A number of methods exist for solving location problems. Factor rating, locational break-even analysis, and the center of gravity method are a few. This chapter introduces the center of gravity method and provides an example of its use in a spreadsheet.

CENTER OF GRAVITY METHOD

Although an objective of the *center of gravity method* is to minimize cost, the method is often used to locate heath care facilities. However, in the case of a rural medical facility the objective could be to minimize the combination of volume and distance between numerous small communities that seek health care–related services. The method takes into account the volume of services demanded, location of that demand, and the distance from that demand to the facility location.

Center of Gravity Solution Steps

The following is a list of the steps involved with using the center of gravity method:

1. Place the demand locations (most likely small towns or geographic locales) on an *x-y* coordinate system (i.e., use a map and latitude/longitude, or center one town on the 0,0 point and align the other towns accordingly). The scale of the coordinate system can be arbitrary as long as the relative distances are correct.

2. Identify the demand at each of the demand locales (e.g., this could be simply based on population).

3. The center of gravity is determined by Equations 14.1 and 14.2:

$$x\text{-coordinate of the center of gravity} = \frac{\sum_{i=1}^{n} d_{ix} Q_i}{\sum_{i=1}^{n} Q_i} \qquad (14.1)$$

$$y\text{-coordinate of the center of gravity} = \frac{\sum_{i=1}^{n} d_{iy} Q_i}{\sum_{i=1}^{n} Q_i} \qquad (14.2)$$

where
d_{ix} = *x*-coordinate of location i
d_{iy} = *y*-coordinate of location i
Q_i = demand for services at location i
n = number of demand locales

The method assumes that the combination of volume and distance must be minimized. The best location is one that minimizes weighted distance between demand locales where the distance is weighted by demand itself.

The two equations contain the term Q_i, the demand for services at location i. Since the demand for services impacts the volume/distance relationship, it must be included (i.e., in our example, if all towns had equal demand, then all would equal out, but in most cases larger towns will have larger demand). From the two equations, the x-y coordinate pair is transferred back to the original x-y coordinate system and a location then deduced. A spreadsheet example is given next.

Center of Gravity Example

Let's consider two counties that have received a grant to set up an outpatient clinic (e.g., a clinic that provides checkups, gives minor medical treatment, writes prescriptions, etc.). The counties, Bartie and Hartford, have decided that the outpatient clinic needs to be centrally located so that all incorporated cities have access. However, they also know that the bigger cities may try to claim the clinic as theirs since they are just bigger. Therefore, the two counties have decided to use the center of gravity method, which balances distance as well as volume of demand (based predominantly on population) to determine where the clinic might be placed.

Table 14.4 displays the demand for the clinic by incorporated city. Demand is derived from the population base of each city.

TABLE 14.4   Demand Locale Data for Outpatient Clinic

Demand Locale	Health Care Demand (Based on Population)	d_{ix} x-Coordinate	d_{iy} y-Coordinate
Ahoskie	4,785	5.62	6.29
Askewville	163	6.29	2.41
Aulander	888	3.70	5.04
Cofield	347	6.74	7.82
Colerain	200	8.84	4.40
Como	74	5.27	11.00
Harrellsville	93	8.50	6.64
Kelford	222	2.06	3.94
Lewiston/Woodville	413	2.76	2.70
Murfreesboro	2,415	3.93	9.69
Powellsville	359	6.40	4.95
Roxobel	240	1.75	4.45
Windsor	2,783	6.21	0.00
Winton	956	6.41	8.68
Total	13,939		

FIGURE 14.16 Coordinate Locations for the County Demand Locales

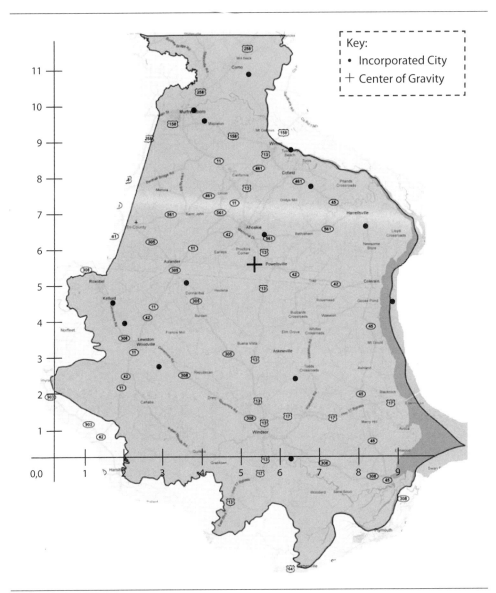

Figure 14.16 displays the coordinate locations for the demand locales in the two counties. Per step 1 in the center of gravity walk-through section, Figure 14.16 acts as the coordinate system for the clinic example.

The demand for each locale is displayed in Table 14.4. Therefore, the center of gravity is determined as follows:

$$= \frac{\begin{array}{c} 5.62(4785) + 6.29(163) + 3.7(888) + 6.74(347) + 8.84(200) \\ + 5.27(74) + 8.5(93) + 2.06(222) + 2.76(413) + 3.93(2415) \\ + 6.4(359) + 1.75(240) + 6.21(2783) + 6.41(956) \end{array}}{13,938}$$

$$= 5.29$$

$$= \frac{\begin{array}{c} 56.29(4785) + 2.41(163) + 5.04(888) + 7.82(347) + 4.40(200) \\ + 11(74) + 6.64(93) + 3.94(222) + 2.70(413) + 9.69(2415) \\ + 4.95(359) + 4.45(240) + 0.00(2783) + 8.68(956) \end{array}}{13,938}$$

$$= 5.49$$

The method minimizes the combination of volume and distance. The coordinates (5.29, 5.49) are then the center of gravity for the two-county outpatient clinic problem. The large "+" in Figure 14.16 denotes the center of gravity. These coordinates are near the cities of Ahoskie, Aulander, and Powellsville. Using the center of gravity method, the outpatient clinic could be located in or around any of these cities. Most likely, since Ahoskie has the largest population and associated infrastructure, the clinic would be built close to it (e.g., somewhere like Proctors Corner just on the outskirts of Ahoskie).

Center of Gravity Spreadsheet Example

Figure 14.17 displays the center of gravity method within a spreadsheet. Table 14.5 contains the formulas that accompany Figure 14.17.

Health Care Operations and Supply Chain Management behind the Scenes: Determining Emergency Medical Services Vehicle Locations

Many cities across the United States must determine what services should be delivered, by what entity, via what number and types of equipment, and sited at which locations. These decisions are particularly important for emergency medical services (EMS).

Generally, cities wish to provide the maximum amount of service to their citizens but must stay within budget. For the EMS situation, cities must

FIGURE 14.17   Excel Spreadsheet for Center of Gravity Method

	A	B	C
1	**Demand Locales**	**Healthcare Demand (based on population)**	
2	Ahoskie	4785	
3	Askewville	163	
4	Aulander	888	
5	Cofield	347	
6	Colerain	200	
7	Como	74	
8	Harrellsville	93	
9	Kelford	222	
10	Lewiston/Woodville	413	
11	Murfreesboro	2415	
12	Powellsville	359	
13	Roxobel	240	
14	Windsor	2783	
15	Winton	956	
16			
17			
18	**Demand Locales**	d_{x} = **x-Coordinate**	d_{y} = **y-Coordinate**
19	Ahoskie	5.62	6.29
20	Askewville	6.29	2.41
21	Aulander	3.70	5.04
22	Cofield	6.74	7.82
23	Colerain	8.84	4.40
24	Como	5.27	11.00
25	Harrellsville	8.50	6.64
26	Kelford	2.06	3.94
27	Lewiston/Woodville	2.76	2.70
28	Murfreesboro	3.93	9.69
29	Powellsville	6.40	4.95
30	Roxobel	1.75	4.45
31	Windsor	6.21	0.00
32	Winton	6.41	8.68
33			
34			
35	*x*-coordinate of center of gravity =	**5.29**	
36			
37	*y*-coordinate of center of gravity =	**5.49**	
38			

TABLE 14.5   Formulas to Accompany Spreadsheet in Figure 14.17

Cells	Formulas
A2 through B15	Data from Table 14.4
A19 through C32	Data from Table 14.4
B35	=SUMPRODUCT(B19:B32, B2:B15)/SUM(B$2:B$15)
B37	=SUMPRODUCT(C19:C32, B2:B15)/SUM(B$2:B$15)

determine the number and location of vehicles to deploy so as to provide quality of services to the city population at a reasonable cost.

Facility Location Techniques

The city of Austin, Texas, tackled this problem using facility location techniques (Eaton et al., 1985). A variety of deterministic location optimization models was considered.

A maximum covering model (one of the underpinnings to basic center of gravity methods) was chosen by the EMS staff since they preferred a coverage objective. The model allowed analysis of a variety of policy options, including changes in the number of vehicles, the response time used to define coverage, and the allowable candidate vehicle locations. Each option could be assessed in terms of its ability to serve a variety of call-based and population surrogates for demand.

Results of the Model

The EMS deployment plan developed provides equitable service, in that the system covers over 80 percent of critical and noncritical calls within five minutes. Preferential service is provided to those segments of the population most likely to require emergency medical care. For example, within a five-minute response time the current EMS system can reach a larger fraction of the elderly than of the general population.

In all, determining sites for EMS facilities is always a process of choice. In this project, facility location techniques enhanced traditional methods for making decisions. Optimization techniques were used to calculate benefits and costs and to assess opportunity costs of a number of policies, but not to select a mathematically optimal answer. The model provided a platform for sensitivity analysis and further discussion.

SUMMARY

Although service-based, large health care organizations do not differ from product-based organizations in that each organization must have aggregate planning and control. This chapter has discussed the basics of aggregate/central planning coupled with capacity planning. For further information on resource planning applied to health care, see Bretthauer and Murray 1998, Hershey et al. 1974, Hershey et al. 1981, Smith-Daniels et al. 2008, and Vissers et al. 2001.

That discussion led to the role that enterprise resource planning (ERP) systems play in health care organizations. Healthcare ERP 2001, Jenkins and Christenson 2001, and van Merodea et al. 2004 provide excellent articles on health care ERP systems. Working down the planning hierarchy, the chapter presented the importance of scheduling through a single queue. Refer to Abernathy et al. 1973, Cheng et al. 2007, Irvin and Brown 1999, Isken and Hancock 1998, and Warner et al. 1991 for further reading on health care scheduling. Finally, it discussed the basics of facility location and illustrated the center of gravity method.

KEY TERMS

aggregate/central planning

capacity planning

center of gravity method

dispatching rules

enterprise resource planning (ERP)

Johnson's rule

location analysis

scheduling

DISCUSSION QUESTIONS

1. What does an ERP system do, and how does it benefit a health care organization?

2. Table 14.6 contains eight laboratory jobs (listed by job number) that must complete the two back-to-back processes of heating and then extraction. The times in minutes are listed for the heating and extraction processes for each job. Use Johnson's rule to sequence the jobs. State the final job sequence, idle time, and total time to complete all jobs.

3. Create a Gantt chart for question 2.

4. What is the difference between tactical and operational scheduling?

5. Table 14.7 contains 12 billing inquiries that had errors and must go through two validation processes (balance check and DRG match). For some billing inquiries, the balance check is as easy as matching two numbers on the forms, whereas other times the inquiry must be checked via a

TABLE 14.6 Laboratory Jobs Processing Times

Job	Heating	Extraction
R451	60	89
R462	101	67
R773	57	31
R673	37	43
R351	19	87
R262	91	27
R873	49	71
R551	25	100

TABLE 14.7   Billing Inquiry Processing Times

Inquiry #	Balance Check	DRG Match
22	8	20
62	10	5
73	15	3
67	15	3
51	5	20
27	25	25
17	50	5
33	15	10
91	1	20
21	25	1
87	5	5
55	15	10

computer system that takes extra time to access and is not very user friendly. The DRG match follows in about the same vein. Some DRG matches are resolved quickly (e.g., the DRG was written improperly or digits transposed); other times the inquiry must be verified via telephone with accounting, and that adds time. The inquiries are screened in batches of 12 (hence the 12 listed in the table), and the approximate time requirements in minutes are listed for each process for each inquiry. At present the staff completes the claims using a first-come, first-served (FCFS) sequencing rule. However, there is an idea that this method creates too much idle time and does not process the inquiries in the fastest time. Compute the total time to complete the jobs using FCFS and using Johnson's rule, and compare how each method performs with regard to idle time and total time to complete all jobs.

6. Create Gantt charts for both the FCFS and Johnson's rule methods in question 5.

7. Discuss three job sequencing rules and give health care examples when you would want to use one versus another.

8. Blairville's city council is deciding on where to position a new emergency management services (EMS) station. The city has 10 landmark senior/community centers that play a large role in the city's health plan (i.e., many go to the senior/community centers for advice, counseling, transportation, etc.).

TABLE 14.8   Senior/Community Center Location Data

Senior/Community Center	Usage (Visits per Month)	d_{ix} x-Coordinate	d_{iy} y-Coordinate
Elm Street Center	385	3.2	1.9
Bernard James Center I	163	2.9	1.1
Bernard James Center II	1,888	11	7.5
Catherine Stas Senior Center	1,122	12.6	3.9
Mark Clem Center	313	3.7	2.7
River Road Senior Center	1,115	6.3	9.9
George Wilson Community Center	359	4.4	4.5
Chuck Jorgensen Community Center	140	7.5	4.5
Sports and Courts Center	883	8.1	0
Harley Huff Senior Center	1,956	2.1	8.6
Total	8,324		

The new EMS station needs to be centrally located but must serve a dispersed and unevenly distributed population. Table 14.8 contains the senior/community center locales, overall usage numbers, and map coordinates. Use the center of gravity method to find a location for the new EMS station.

9. For question 8, graph the center of gravity solution along with the coordinates for the senior/community center locations. Comment on what you see with regard to the center of gravity solution and the senior/community center locations. If this is an urban setting, what implications does the center of gravity method solution bring with it?

10. Dawgton has received a grant to build a blood bank center. The city has 25 health care–related facilities that need to be included in the location plan. Some of the health care facilities demand more blood than others. Table 14.9 contains the health care facility locations, overall blood bank transaction demand, and map coordinates. Use the center of gravity method to find a location for the new blood bank facility.

11. Dawgton has just learned it actually received a grant to build three smaller blood bank centers instead of one large one. Create a graph of the center of gravity solution along with the coordinates for the health care facility locations included (use the data in Table 14.9).

TABLE 14.9 Health Care Facility Location Data

Health Care Facility Location	Blood Bank Transaction Demand	$d_{ix,}$ x-Coordinate	$d_{iy,}$ y-Coordinate
5th and State	403	0.8	4
Fort Street Clinic	242	3.2	4
Blair Memorial	2,634	6	4.5
Children's	1,454	6.8	2.5
State Road Clinic	783	9	4
Fort Calhoun Surgi Center	1,597	2.5	7
Med Direct I	711	3.9	5.2
Med Direct II	885	5	10
Washington County Clinic	1,399	8	7
EastSide Center	461	0.8	16
James Bernard Community Hospital	2,849	1	15
Eastern Surgi Center	1,581	3	13
PCMH	1,150	4	10
Bertie Clinic	1,443	6.5	14.5
Burt County Surgical	986	8	12
Denny Sellon Blood Center	853	11	15
Hillcrest Clinic I	983	5	16
Hillcrest Clinic II	2,378	4.8	18
J&J Health Center	2,010	3.8	20
Jensen Healthcare Systems	725	4	24
Trimark Care	1,465	6	21
JMK Health Center	1,154	5.5	27
Triple J Senior Care Center	293	7	18
ReadyReady Surgi Center	892	9	20
Desoto Health Care Center	2,611	9.5	24
Total	31,942		

It has been proposed that the city divide up the facilities into three areas by north-south direction (y-coordinates on the center of gravity graph). The suggestion is to group any facility that has y-coordinates from 0 up to 8 together, group facilities with y-coordinates above 8 up to 17 together, and then group facilities with y-coordinates above 17 together.

Regroup the health care facilities and rerun the center of gravity method on the three subgroups. Report on your results and compare to your answer to question 10.

12. In another proposal, City Councilman Chris Jensen has suggested that grouping by north-south is maybe not the best solution. He is suggesting that the grouping be made based on the east-west direction. His groupings would be along these x-coordinates: 0 up to and including 4, above 4 up to and including 6, and above 6. Regroup the health care facilities and rerun the center of gravity method on the three subgroups. Report on your results and compare your answer to questions 10 and 11.

REFERENCES

Abernathy, W. J., N. Baloff, J. C. Hershey, and S. Wandel. 1973. "3 Stage Manpower Planning and Scheduling Model: Service Sector Example." *Operations Research* 21 (3): 693–711.

Bertrand, J. W. M., J. C. Wortmann, and J. Wijngaard. 1990. *Production Control: A Structural and Design Oriented Approach.* New York: Elsevier Science.

Bretthauer, Kurt M., and J. Murray. 1998. "A Model for Planning Resource Requirements in Health Care Organizations." *Decision Sciences* 29 (1).

Cheng, Mingang, Hiromi Itoh Ozaku, Noriaki Kuwahara, Kiyoshi Kogure, and Jun Ota. 2007. "Nursing Care Scheduling Problem: Analysis of Staffing Levels." *Proceedings of the 2007 IEEE International Conference on Robotics and Biomimetics*, December 15–18, Sanya, China.

Eaton, David J., Mark S. Daskin, Dennis Simmons, Bill Bulloch, and Glen Jansma. 1985. "Determining Emergency Medical Service Vehicle Deployment in Austin, Texas." *Interfaces* 15 (1): 96–108.

"Healthcare ERP and SCM Information Systems: Strategies and Solutions." Healthcare Information and Management Systems Society (HIMSS) White Paper, HIMSS website, July 2011.

Hershey, J. C., W. J. Abernathy, and N. Baloff. 1974. "Comparison of Nurse Allocation Policies—A Monte Carlo Model." *Decision Sciences* 5:58–72.

Hershey, J. C., W. Pierskalla, and S. Wander. 1981. "Nurse Staffing Management." In *Operational Research Applied to Health Services*, edited by D. Boldy, 189–220. New York: St. Martin's Press.

Irvin, Stephen A., and Hazel N. Brown. 1999. "Self-Scheduling with Microsoft Excel." *Nursing Economics* 17, no. 4 (July/August): 201–206.

Isken, M. W., and W. M. Hancock. 1998. "Tactical Staff Scheduling Analysis for Hospital Ancillary Units." *Journal of the Society for Health Systems* 5 (4): 11–23.

Jenkins, Elizabeth, and E. Christenson. 2001. "ERP Systems Can Streamline Healthcare Business Functions." *Healthcare Financial Management*: 48–52.

Smith-Daniels, Vicki L., Sharon B. Schweikhart, and Dwight E. Smith-Daniels. 2008. "Capacity Management in Health Care Services: Review and Future Research Directions." *Decision Sciences* 19:889–919.

van Merodea, Godefridus G., Siebren Groothuisb, and Arie Hasman. 2004. "Enterprise Resource Planning for Hospitals." *International Journal of Medical Informatics* 73:493–501.

Vissers, J. M. H., J. W. M. Bertrand, and G. De Vries. 2001. "A Framework for Production Control in Health Care Organizations." *Production Planning & Control* 12 (6): 591–604.

Warner, D. M., B. J. Keller, and S. H. Martel. 1991. "Automated Nurse Scheduling." *Journal of the Society of Health Systems* 2 (2): 66–68.

CHAPTER 15

INVENTORY

MANAGEMENT

LEARNING OBJECTIVES

➠ Understand the purpose of inventories.

➠ Know what factors influence the cost of inventories.

➠ Be able to differentiate independent demand from dependent demand.

➠ Understand and be able to apply the formula for economic order quantity.

➠ Comprehend the basic concepts of periodic review systems and continuous review systems.

➠ Know what is meant by ABC inventory management and how it can assist in overall inventory management.

(Continued)

⟶ Become aware of different types of inventory management technology and the advantages and disadvantages of each.

INTRODUCTION

We are all familiar with the concept of inventory. No doubt at some point in your life you have become frustrated to learn that the item you came to the store to purchase or the item you tried to order from an online catalog is out of stock. You may also run into inventory issues at your job, perhaps needing a new notepad and box of staples, only to find out that none are available.

There are numerous factors that influence the amount of inventory a business keeps on hand and several key concepts that play a role in managing that inventory. This chapter introduces key inventory management concepts and provides detailed examples in Excel to help further enhance understanding of those concepts. After explaining the purpose of inventories, the chapter examines costs of inventories. It introduces and explains a fundamental concept, the economic order quantity (EOQ), and provides an Excel example of determining the proper EOQ. Different types of demand (independent and dependent) are described as well. The chapter explains how to monitor inventory via a periodic or continuous review system. It provides details on the concept of ABC inventory management, along with an example that utilizes Excel. The chapter closes with an introduction to three types of inventory management technology.

PURPOSE OF INVENTORIES

Inventory can be defined as the stock of physical goods that contain value held at a specific location at a specific time. Each item in the inventory is referred to as a stock-keeping unit (SKU), and each SKU has a quantity associated with it, which is the number of units in stock. A stock point is a location where inventory is held. Inventories exist because demand for physical goods and their corresponding supply cannot be matched identically.

In a health care setting, there are many types of items held in inventory. There must always be ample supply of medications held at the pharmacy. Items used by the cleaning staff (mops, rags, cleaners, etc.) must be kept in inventory since infection control is such an important consideration for health care facilities. Items used by doctors and nurses (syringes, gauze, bedpans, etc.) must also be kept in inventory.

Maintaining sufficient inventories in a health care setting is much more critical than in retail settings. If Office Depot runs out of the toner you want to buy for your printer, the result is that you will probably go somewhere else to buy it. If a hospital runs out of an item, the consequences could be serious. Safety stock refers to a level of extra inventory maintained to diminish the risk of stock-outs (inability to fulfill a demand with current inventory) due to uncertainties in supply and demand. Adequate safety stock enables a business to proceed with its planned daily operations.

Inventory in Health Care for Disaster Preparedness

Hospitals and other health care facilities are often a first line of defense or recovery when disaster strikes. For this reason, such facilities are obligated to maintain certain levels of inventories for disaster preparedness. The website of the Centers for Disease Control and Prevention (CDC) provides separate documentation on disaster preparedness for hospitals, long-term care facilities, outpatient clinics and urgent care centers, physicians' offices, and pediatricians' offices (www.bt.cdc.gov/healthcare).

Disaster used to mean natural disasters such as hurricanes and earthquakes. Today, the word has the additional meaning of other chemical, biological, radiological, nuclear, and explosive (CBRNE) events (Cook 2007). Planning for needed inventories to cover disaster response is not a simple task.

It is critical for a hospital to create a network within its community of possible sources of medical supplies in the event of a disaster. By locating alternative sources of equipment and supplies, it may be possible to reduce the on-hand quantity of supplies needed for disaster preparedness. It is also possible to conduct predisaster contracting for some items. An example of this would be for a hospital to have a contract with the local school system so that school buses could be used as transport vehicles in response to a disaster.

Another step that must be taken is to investigate the internal supply chain of the hospital to identify areas that might be closed in the event of a disaster (Cook 2007). It is important to have a plan for how to divert supplies from closed areas to areas with high need in a disaster-recovery situation. Hospitals must also work with distributors in their supply chains to determine how much the distributors can supply in a short turnaround time. In addition, it is critical for hospitals and other emergency facilities to maintain a list of alternate suppliers in case the main supplier is inaccessible in an emergency.

COSTS OF INVENTORIES

There is a cost associated with inventories. Obviously, space is needed for storing items in inventory. Additionally, a system must be put into place to ensure that perishable items or items with a shelf life are used in order of age and are not put into circulation if they are out of date. This becomes especially important in health care settings in relation to medications, blood, and other items that are put into patients.

The cost of inventories is heavily impacted by the safety stock a business keeps on hand. Too much safety stock can lead to excessive inventory holding costs, and for health care facilities, too little safety stock can result in suboptimal treatment being given to one or more patients. This leads to consideration of another factor that plays a role in the cost of inventories: order quantity. Not only do companies need to determine when to order more of a product, but they must also determine how much to order. When to order and how much to order are related to the economic order quantity (EOQ), which is the level of inventory a facility should maintain in order to minimize total inventory holding costs and ordering costs. Details of the EOQ are provided in a later section of this chapter.

Order cost is based on the frequency with which orders are placed. Usually, order cost has two components. There is a fixed cost, K, that is incurred independent of order size and a variable cost, c, incurred on a per unit basis. K is also referred to as setup cost, while c is also known as the proportional order cost. The components of K include clerical costs associated with placing orders, the vendor-required fixed cost for an order, the cost of generating an order, and receiving and handling costs (Nahmias 2009).

Holding cost, also known as carrying cost, is also pertinent to decisions of when and how much to order. Obviously, the amount of inventory a business decides to hold will impact its cash flows. For example, if the out-of-pocket cost of an item is $25 per unit and if the company borrows money at a 20 percent interest rate, then the cost to hold/carry each additional unit of the item is $5.00.

Stock-out costs are very difficult to measure (Narasimhan, McLeavey, and Billington 1995). A stock-out occurs when there is no inventory to meet demand for a particular item. If the item is critical, then additional clerical and expediting costs will most likely be incurred in order to obtain the item in a timely manner.

In a health care setting, ordering costs, holding costs, and stock-out costs are treated differently than in a manufacturing setting. As previously mentioned, running out of an item has the potential to have a much greater impact in a health care setting. However, it is still possible and recommended to utilize historical data and appropriate formulas when making ordering decisions.

In order to make decisions about costs, we must be able to model them. The following example uses a small set of variables to model an inventory problem. The problem is solved in the subsequent section on economic order quantity (EOQ).

Hospital Gowns Order Quantity Problem

A children's hospital wants to know the number of hospital gowns it should purchase in order to minimize annual costs. Currently, the hospital is ordering 500 gowns per order. As a first step, we define all of the variables of the problem:

P = purchase cost

D = annual demand

H = holding cost

K = setup cost

Q = order quantity

D/Q = orders per year

$Q/2$ = average annual inventory

Now, based on information from the hospital, we assign values to some variables:

$P = \$2.00$

$D = 10,000$ units per year

$H = 10$ percent of the purchase price per year

$K = \$50$

$Q = 500$

Some basic calculations will give us values for annual purchase cost, annual holding cost, and annual setup cost:

$$\text{Annual purchase cost (APC)} = P \times D = \$2 \times 10,000 = \$20,000$$
$$\text{Annual holding cost (AHC)} = P \times H \times Q/2 = \$2 \times 0.10 \times (500/2) = \$50$$
$$\text{Annual setup cost (ASC)} = K \times D/Q = \$50 \times (10,000/500) = \$1,000$$

Now, combining these costs will give us total annual cost (TAC). So we have:

$$\text{Total annual cost} = \text{APC} + \text{AHC} + \text{ASC}$$
$$= (P \times D) + (P \times H \times Q/2) + (K \times D/Q)$$
$$= \$21,050$$

In order to determine what value of Q will minimize total annual cost, we must now move to a discussion of the economic order quantity.

ECONOMIC ORDER QUANTITY

The *economic order quantity* (EOQ) is the level of inventory that minimizes total inventory holding costs and setup costs. The EOQ model provides the foundation for all the inventory control models. Developed in 1915, the model considers the trade-off between setup costs, which are fixed, and holding costs, which are variable (Nahmias 2009).

As we did in the hospital gown example in the previous section, we will let H represent the holding cost per unit and K represent the setup cost. The order quantity that minimizes cost per unit time is $Q = 2KD/H$, where D is the annual demand. This quantity is known as the economic order quantity (EOQ).

The formula for EOQ provides an accurate approximation for the optimal order quantity when demand is uncertain, which is often the case in health care settings. We note that this formula for the EOQ could be derived by setting the formula for total annual cost equal to 0 and solving for Q.

Hospital Gowns Example in Excel

Our first task is to enter all of the variable values into Excel and then enter the formulas to calculate APC, AHC, ASC, and TAC. Figure 15.1 shows one way to do this. Values for P, D, H, K, and Q are simply typed into the spreadsheet. Formulas for the cost calculations are given in Figure 15.2.

So, using an order quantity of 500, the total annual cost is $21,050. Let us now modify the spreadsheet and use the calculated value of EOQ for Q. Figure

FIGURE 15.1 Spreadsheet Model Using Given Value of Q

	A	B	C
1			
2	P	Purchase Price	$2.00
3			
4	D	Annual Demand	10,000
5			
6	H	Holding Cost Per Unit	10%
7			
8	S	Setup Cost	$50.00
9			
10	Q	Order Quantity	500
11			
12	APC	Annual Purchase Cost	$20,000.00
13			
14	ACC	Annual Holding Cost	$50.00
15			
16	ASC	Annual Setup Cost	$1,000.00
17			
18	TAC	Total Annual Cost	$21,050.00
19			

FIGURE 15.2   Cost Formulas for Figure 15.1

Cost	Formula
Annual Purchase Cost	= C2*C4
Annual Holding Cost	= C2*C6*C10/2
Annual Setup Cost	= C8*C4/C10
Total Annual Cost	= C12 + C14 + C16

FIGURE 15.3   Spreadsheet Model Using Formula to Calculate Economic Order Quantity

	A	B	C
1			
2	P	Purchase Price	$2.00
3			
4	D	Annual Demand	10,000
5			
6	H	Holding Cost Per Unit	10%
7			
8	S	Setup Cost	$50.00
9			
10	Q	Order Quantity	2,236
11			
12	APC	Annual Purchase Cost	$20,000.00
13			
14	ACC	Annual Holding Cost	$223.60
15			
16	ASC	Annual Setup Cost	$223.61
17			
18	TAC	Total Annual Cost	$20,447.21
19			

15.3 shows one way to do this. Values for P, D, H, and K are left as they were in the original spreadsheet of Figure 15.1. Formulas for the cost calculations also remain the same. The only cell to modify is cell C10.

We know from before that the formula we need to work with is $Q = \sqrt{2KD/H}$.

The square root function in Excel is given by SQRT( ). We will need to make sure we enter the correct formula in the ( ) next to the SQRT function. The tricky part is our denominator. In our spreadsheet, we have used a percentage to indicate holding cost. In our formula for Q, we will need to convert H to a cost. This means our denominator becomes $(H{*}P)$.

If we entered the formula =SQRT(2*C8*C4/(C6*C2)) into cell C10, we would get a value of 2,236.068. However, the hospital cannot purchase a partial gown, so we need to find the integer portion of the value we calculated. The function INT( ) in Excel returns the integer portion of a calculated value. Thus, the formula we need to enter in cell C10 in order to get the correct value for Q is =INT(SQRT(2*C8*C4/(C6*C2))). The resulting value, 2,236, tells us that the optimal order quantity for hospital gowns is 2,236.

By changing its ordering quantity from 500 to 2,236, the hospital will reduce its total annual cost by $602.79 per year. Simple subtraction leads to this conclusion.

$$\text{TAC with } Q \text{ of } 500 - \text{TAC with } Q \text{ of } 2,236$$
$$= \$21,050.00 - \$20,447.21$$
$$= \$602.79$$

INDEPENDENT VERSUS DEPENDENT DEMAND

If demand for an item is not dependent upon the demand for another item, it is referred to as *independent demand*. If, in contrast, the demand for an item is related to the demand for another item, then we refer to it as *dependent demand*. The idea of classifying demand in this way was developed in the mid-1960s (Snyder 1982) and reported in Orlicky (1970). Let us consider an example from health care using a hospital setting.

Suppose we are able to forecast the patient count for each floor (ward) for a given week. These patients represent independent demand items. Using that forecast, hospital administrators can develop an aggregate plan based on the demand forecast and existing hospital policies. These policies may relate to employee work hours, patient safety, nurse-to-patient ratios, and other types of standards. Such policies must be considered, as they directly influence the hospital's ability to meet demand.

Using forecasted demand and length of stay estimates, an operations plan is developed indicating the number of patients to be served by each floor for the given time period. If we have a forecast for the number and types of patients on each floor, then we can determine the number of tests, surgeries, and treatments that will be needed. These tests, surgeries, and treatments are considered dependent demand items.

Using the dependent demand relationship will allow for the correct sequencing and lead times to be associated with the test, surgery, and treatment procedures. This will enable better planning and controlling of both the patients and the care providers (doctors and nurses) (Snyder 1982). If the demand exceeds the available capacity, revision of the master schedule must occur. In some instances, it may be possible to make more capacity available, such as in the case of scheduling additional doctors or nurses. In other cases, this may not be possible. For example, hospitals have a fixed number of operating rooms, and if demand for surgeries exceeds this capacity, some surgeries will be forced to be rescheduled.

There is another level of dependent demand, in that the tests, surgeries, and treatments require items kept in inventory such as needles, gauze, gloves, and so on. Maintaining inventories of these types of items will be discussed in several of the following sections.

Other characteristics of demand that play a role in how the item's inventory is managed include whether the demand is constant or variable and whether the demand is known or random. For example, at a hospital emergency department, the demand for bedsheets may be constant but the demand for pints of B+ blood may be highly variable.

PERIODIC REVIEW SYSTEMS

Under a *periodic review system*, the level of inventory is known only at discrete points in time.

Suppose a facility's policy is to place an order every T days and to order a quantity Q that brings the inventory up to a desired stock level S. If we assume the order has a lead time of L days, the cycles of our periodic inventory system will behave as shown in Figure 15.4.

The periodic review system was used more often prior to the advent of computers. This type of review system required inventory personnel to check levels of inventory periodically and place orders based on their findings. Now computers have made it possible to maintain continuous inventory records, which enable businesses to maintain lower values of safety stock. Continuous review systems are discussed in the next section.

FIGURE 15.4 Cycles in a Periodic Review System

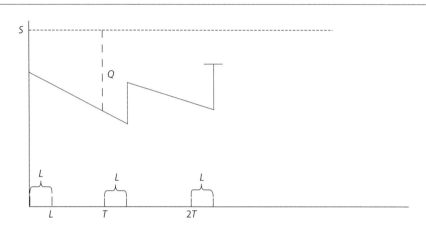

CONTINUOUS REVIEW SYSTEMS

With a *continuous review system*, the level of inventory on hand is known at all times. Computer systems are used to maintain inventory information. When the level of on-hand inventory falls to some level, *R*, an order for *Q* units is generated automatically. Continuous review systems are often referred to as (*Q,R*) systems since those two variables' values drive the actions of the system.

A continuous inventory review system allows a company to maintain its inventory records via a systematized documenting process that is in agreement with the physical inventory. Each time an item is removed from inventory, the continuous inventory review system adjusts to reflect the reduction in physical inventory. This type of system makes it easy to know when to reorder products. In many manufacturing settings, there is a supply manager who oversees the continuous review system. That manager is responsible for ensuring that the physical and computerized inventories remain in sync.

Periodic versus Continuous (i.e., Perpetual) Inventory Systems: An Example

As previously presented, health care organizations can use two basic systems to maintain inventory records: periodic and continuous (also referred to as perpetual).

Periodic systems are generally used by smaller organizations that have minimal inventories (e.g., an old-school local pharmacy with low levels of in-store inventory). Continuous systems are used by most large health care organizations using computerized record-keeping systems that tie together inventory held and services provided as the service is administered.

To illustrate how a periodic system differs from a continuous system, an example is developed next. The best manner to illustrate this difference in systems is to highlight the accounts used and the accounting entries made in each system and how they differ. In essence, the manner in which the inventory is accounted for contains the differences between the two systems. Overall, Table 15.1 summarizes these differences.

Next we present the accounting entries that accompany each inventory system to illustrate the differences documented in Table 15.1.

Periodic System

In using the periodic inventory system, physical counts of inventory are conducted from time to time or periodically, and then accounts are brought up to date. The example presented uses the same transactions as will be used in the continuous system example:

TABLE 15.1 Differences between Periodic and Continuous Inventory Systems

Activity or Transaction	Periodic System	Continuous System
Inventory purchases are debited . . .	To purchases	To inventory
Freight, discounts, and returns/allowances are debited . . .	To individual accounts (e.g., transportation, discount, or returns/allowances)	To inventory
Cost of good is recorded . . .	At the end of the period	At the time of each sale with a debit to cost of goods sold
Physical inventory count is completed . . .	At least once a year and maybe more often if current information is available	At least once a year to account for discrepancies occurring from breakage, errors, or thefts

- Purchase of 2,000 units on account at $10 each = $20,000.

- Sale of 1,000 units on account at $23 each = $23,000.

Figure 15.5 displays the journal entries for Health Care Corp., and Figure 15.6 displays the formulas behind Figure 15.5. Now the same set of transactions is illustrated using the continuous inventory system.

Continuous System

When employing the continuous inventory system, inventory and cost of goods sold are recorded following an up-to-date (really an up-to-transaction) running balance. The example below shows the journal entries in a continuous system for the same transactions as presented earlier:

- Purchase of 2,000 units on account at $10 each = $20,000.

- Sale of 1,000 units on account at $23 each = $23,000.

In turn, it can be seen from Figure 15.7 that there is no need to make an entry at the end of the period in order to bring the inventory and cost of goods sold accounts up to date. The continuous method already shows the correct balance. Figure 15.8 displays the formulas in Excel for Figure 15.7.

FIGURE 15.5 Periodic Review Journal Entries for Health Care Corp.

◇	A	B	C	D	E	F
1	Journal Entries Health Care Corp.					
2	Date	Account Title—Notes		Ref.	Debit	Credit
3	April 21, 20XX	Purchases			$20,000	
4		Accounts Payable				$20,000
5		Purchase of 2,000 units @ $10 per				
6	April 22, 20XX	Accounts Receivable			$23,000	
7		Sales				$23,000
8		Sale of 1,000 units @ $23 per				
9	April 30, 20XX	Inventory (ending − 1,000 × $10)			$10,000	
10		Cost of Goods Sold (1,000 × $10)			$10,000	
11		Purchases				$20,000
12		End-of-Period Entry				

FIGURE 15.6 Formulas for Figure 15.5

◇	A	B	C	D	E	F
1	Journal Entries Health Care Corp.					
2	Date	Account Title—Notes		Ref.	Debit	Credit
3	April 21, 20XX	Purchases			=2000*10	
4		Accounts Payable				=2000*10
5		Purchase of 2,000 units @ $10 per				
6	April 22, 20XX	Accounts Receivable			=1000*23	
7		Sales				=1000*23
8		Sale of 1,000 units @ $23 per				
9	April 30, 20XX	Inventory (ending — 1,000 × $10)			=1000*10	
10		Cost of Goods Sold (1,000 × $10)			=1000*10	
11		Purchases				=2000*10
12		End-of-Period Entry				
13						

FIGURE 15.7 Continuous Review Journal Entries for Health Care Corp.

◇	A	B	C	D	E	F
1	Journal Entries Health Care Corp.					
2	Date	Account Title—Notes		Ref.	Debit	Credit
3	April 21, 20XX	Inventory			$20,000	
4		Accounts Payable				$20,000
5		Purchase of 2,000 units @ $10				
6	April 21, 20XX	Accounts Receivable			$23,000	
7		Sales (1,000 × $23 per)				$23,000
8		Cost of Goods Sold (1,000 × $10)			$10,000	
9		Inventory				$10,000
10		Sale of 1,000 units @ $23 per				

In the case in which a difference does exist between the continuous balance and the physical count balance, then an adjustment should be made. For a physical count that is lower than the continuous inventory balance, a journal entry is made debiting an "inventory over and short" account and crediting inventory. In contrast, for a physical count showing more inventory on hand than what the continuous balance shows, then the inventory account is debited and the "inventory over and short" account is credited. In sum, when using the periodic system, an end-of-period entry must be made to bring the inventory and cost of goods sold accounts up to date. As previously mentioned, no end-of-period entry is needed with the continuous system. It must be noted that the example provided assumed that there was no beginning inventory.

FIGURE 15.8   Formulas for Figure 15.7

◇	A	B	C	D	E	F
1	Journal Entries Health Care Corp.					
2	Date	Account Title — Notes		Ref.	Debit	Credit
3	April 21, 20XX	Inventory			=2000*10	
4		Accounts Payable				=2000*10
5		Purchase of 2,000 units @ $10 per				
6	April 21, 20XX	Accounts Receivable			=1000*23	
7		Sales (1,000 × $23 per)				=1000*23
8		Cost of Goods Sold (1,000 × $10)			=1000*10	
9		Inventory				=1000*10
10		Sale of 1,000 units @ $23 per				

ABC INVENTORY MANAGEMENT

ABC inventory management is a method for classifying items according to their relative importance. Many times the phrase "separating the vital few from the trivial many" is used. This phrase refers to the idea that in any group of items that contribute to a common effect a relatively few contributors account for the majority of the effect.

In a manufacturing setting, all customers and all stock-keeping units (SKUs) are not equally important. A company's most valuable customers and the SKUs whose inventories tie up a significant amount of money are considered high priority. Under the ABC system of inventory planning, 20 percent or less of the SKUs account for approximately 70 to 75 percent of the dollar value in inventory and are classified as A's. In turn, 20 to 30 percent of the SKUs account for approximately 20 percent of the cumulative dollar value and are classified as B's. Finally, the remaining 50 to 70 percent of the SKUs account for 5 to 10 percent of the cumulative dollar value and are classified as C's. The classification categories and associated percentages are approximate, but the general idea is that A's make up a low amount of items but contain the lion's share of cumulative dollar value, C's make up many items but contain a small amount of cumulative dollar value, and, finally, the B's make up the middle.

Example: Suppose we take a typical pharmacy at a health care facility: the annual consumption of drugs and cost for those drugs whose SKUs are 1–10. The dollar volume is determined by multiplying annual demand by cost for each

SKU (see Table 15.2). The SKUs are then ranked based on this dollar volume (see Table 15.3).

Under the ABC system, 20 percent or less of the items, representing between 70 percent and 80 percent of the dollar value, are selected to be A items. For our example, SKU 3 and SKU 1 are A items. In a similar manner, 20 to 30 percent of the items are categorized as B items. In the example, SKUs 4, 5, and 8 are identified as B items. The remainder of the items are C items. For the example, SKUs 2, 7, 9, 6, and 10 are C items. Thus, we have approximately the following scenario for the ABC inventory system:

Item Type	% SKUs	% Value
A	20%	70.5%
B	30%	19.2%
C	50%	10.3%

ABC Inventory Management in Excel

Now we will explore an example similar to the previous one and will utilize Excel to perform all necessary calculations.

Suppose we know the annual demand and cost for items whose SKUs are 1 to 10. We can determine the dollar volume (by multiplying annual demand times cost) for each SKU (see Figure 15.9), determine the percentage of total dollar volume for each SKU (see Figure 15.10), and then rank the SKUs based on this

TABLE 15.2 Inventory Data

SKU	Annual Consumption	Cost	Dollar Volume
1	21,000	$11	$231,000
2	4,000	$15	$60,000
3	100,000	$12	$1,200,000
4	20,000	$7	$140,000
5	10,000	$13	$130,000
6	175	$100	$17,500
7	800	$75	$60,000
8	1,000	$120	$120,000
9	160	$350	$56,000
10	1,200	$14	$16,800
Total			$2,031,300

TABLE 15.3   Percent Total Dollar Volume Data

ABC Classification	SKU	Annual Consumption	Cost	Dollar Volume	Cumulative % Dollar Volume	Cumulative % SKU
A	3	100,000	$12	$1,200,000	59.1%	10%
A	1	21,000	$11	$231,000	70.5%	20%
B	4	20,000	$7	$140,000	77.3%	30%
B	5	10,000	$13	$130,000	83.7%	40%
B	8	1,000	$120	$120,000	89.7%	50%
C	2	4,000	$15	$60,000	92.6%	60%
C	7	800	$75	$60,000	95.6%	70%
C	9	160	$350	$56,000	98.3%	80%
C	6	175	$100	$17,500	99.2%	90%
C	10	1,200	$14	$16,800	100%	100%
	Total			$2,031,300		

FIGURE 15.9   Inventory Data

◇	A	B	C	D
1	SKU	Annual Consumption	Cost	Dollar Volume
2	1	21,000	$ 11.00	$ 231,000
3	2	4,000	$ 15.00	$ 60,000
4	3	100,000	$ 12.00	$ 1,200,000
5	4	20,000	$ 7.00	$ 140,000
6	5	10,000	$ 13.00	$ 130,000
7	6	175	$ 100.00	$ 17,500
8	7	800	$ 75.00	$ 60,000
9	8	1,000	$ 120.00	$ 120,000
10	9	160	$ 350.00	$ 56,000
11	10	1,200	$ 14.00	$ 16,800
12	Totals			$ 2,031,300

percentage of total dollar volume and assign labels of A, B, and C as appropriate (see Figure 15.11).

To create the table presented in Figure 15.9, SKUs, annual consumption, and cost figures are loaded in based on data given. Since dollar volume is calculated by multiplying annual consumption and cost, the formula for cell D2 is =B2*C2. This formula can be dragged down to calculate values for cells D3 through D11. Cell D12 provides the total dollar volume for all 10 SKUs. The formula for cell D12 is =SUM(D2:D11).

FIGURE 15.10   Percent Total Dollar Volume Data

◇	A	B	C	D	E
1	SKU	Annual Consumption	Cost	Dollar Volume	% Dollar Volume
2	1	21,000	$ 11.00	$ 231,000	11.4%
3	2	4,000	$ 15.00	$ 60,000	3.0%
4	3	100,000	$ 12.00	$ 1,200,000	59.1%
5	4	20,000	$ 7.00	$ 140,000	6.9%
6	5	10,000	$ 13.00	$ 130,000	6.4%
7	6	175	$ 100.00	$ 17,500	0.9%
8	7	800	$ 75.00	$ 60,000	3.0%
9	8	1,000	$ 120.00	$ 120,000	5.9%
10	9	160	$ 350.00	$ 56,000	2.8%
11	10	1,200	$ 14.00	$ 16,800	0.8%
12	Totals			$ 2,031,300	

FIGURE 15.11   Sorted Data

◇	A	B	C	D	E	F	G
1	SKU	Annual Consumption	Cost	Dollar Volume	Cumulative % Dollar Value	Cumulative % SKU	ABC Classification
2	3	100,000	$ 12.00	$ 1,200,000	59.08%	10%	A
3	1	21,000	$ 11.00	$ 231,000	70.45%	20%	A
4	4	20,000	$ 7.00	$ 140,000	77.34%	30%	B
5	5	10,000	$ 13.00	$ 130,000	83.74%	40%	B
6	8	1,000	$ 120.00	$ 120,000	89.65%	50%	B
7	2	4,000	$ 15.00	$ 60,000	92.60%	60%	C
8	7	800	$ 75.00	$ 60,000	95.55%	70%	C
9	9	160	$ 350.00	$ 56,000	98.31%	80%	C
10	6	175	$ 100.00	$ 17,500	99.17%	90%	C
11	10	1,200	$ 14.00	$ 16,800	100.00%	100%	C
12	Totals			$ 2,031,300			

To create the table presented in Figure 15.10, we can use the results from Figure 15.9 for SKU and dollar volume values.

As a last step, we can sort the data of Figure 15.10 to determine which of our SKUs are item type A, which are item type B, and which are item type C. To sort, we need to highlight all but the last row of what is displayed in Figure 15.10 and then use Excel's sort feature to sort based on % Dollar Volume, with largest to smallest being our sort order.

Once the data are sorted, the ABC classifications can be made. Figure 15.11 displays the ABC classifications. In order to calculate the values in column E, we divide the dollar volume for each SKU by the total dollar volume that we calculated (which is in cell D12 of Figures 15.9, 15.10, and 15.11) and for a cumulative sum. For % Dollar Volume, our formula for cell E2 would be =D2/$D$12. The Cumulative % Dollar Value begins in cell E3, and the formula would be =(D3/$D$12)+D2. This formula can be copied to cells E4 through E11.

In order to calculate the values in column F, we use the formula =1/count(A$2:A$11) for cell F2. In turn, to calculate the Cumulative % SKU starting in cell F3, the same formula is used plus the cell above in the spreadsheet (e.g., =(1/COUNT(A$2:A$11))+F2). This formula can be copied to cells F4 through F11. As a check, we should get "100%" in cell F11 (see Figure 15.11).

As was previously discussed, it can be seen from Figure 15.11 that SKUs 3 and 1 are classified as A's, SKUs 4, 5, and 8 are classified as B's, and the other SKUs are then classified as C's.

INVENTORY MANAGEMENT TECHNOLOGY

In today's world of globalized supply chains, there are a number of technology tools that can be used to assist with inventory management. Some of the most common forms of inventory management technology are highlighted here.

Radio-Frequency Identification

Radio-frequency identification (RFID) technology uses radio waves to identify and track objects. The object must have an RFID label (or tag) attached to it. Data are transferred from the object through a reader.

RFID technology has numerous applications, including tracking and managing inventory and assets, both machine and human. The health care industry utilizes RFID to reduce time spent counting items and auditing items. The technology has also been used to track doctors and nurses, in order to reduce time wasted searching a large hospital ward when a specific care provider is needed.

There are two major types of RFID tags, active and passive. An active tag has a battery that can serve to power the tag's circuitry and antenna (www.technovelgy.com/ct/Technology-Article.asp?ArtNum=21). Some but not all active tags utilize replaceable batteries. A major advantage of an active RFID tag is that it can be read at distances of 100 feet or more.

Active RFID tags have several disadvantages (www.technovelgy.com/ct/Technology-Article.asp?ArtNum=21):

- They have a limited lifetime since they cannot function without battery power.

- They are usually more expensive than passive tags.

- Their larger physical size may limit applications where they can be used.

- Their battery outages can result in costly misreads.

A passive RFID tag contains no battery; power is supplied by the reader. Passive tags offer several advantages over their active counterparts. They have a useful life of 20 years or more and are usually much less expensive to manufacture. Also, because passive tags are much smaller, they have the potential to be used in countless applications.

A major disadvantage of a passive RFID tag is that it cannot be read from a distance. However, in terms of distance from which it can be read, RFID is superior to bar coding. With bar coding, like we typically see on items at a grocery store, the reader device must be shown the label. Also, unlike bar codes, RFID tags can be read hundreds at a time.

Third-Party Logistics (3PL)

Sometimes, it is advantageous for a business to outsource some or all of its supply chain management functions. Third-party logistics (3PL) providers are companies that offer the services to do this. They specialize in all aspects of supply chain management, from warehousing to transportation and logistics.

Hertz and Alfredsson (2003) describe four categories of 3PL providers:

1. *Standard providers* perform activities such as pick and pack, warehousing, and distribution.

2. *Service developers* offer advanced value-added services such as tracking, tracing, cross-docking, packaging, and security.

3. *Customer adapters* come in at the request of the customer and basically take over control of the company's logistics activities.

4. *Customer developers* integrate themselves with customers and take over their entire logistics functions.

Vendor-Managed Inventory

Vendor-managed inventory (VMI) is a way to improve supply chain performance by making the manufacturer responsible for maintaining the distributor's inventory. Downstream, perhaps at a health care facility, the distributor maintaining the facility's inventory is also considered VMI. The distributor will be given access to the facility's inventory data and will be responsible for generating purchase orders (www.vendormanagedinventory.com/definition.php).

Using a vendor-managed inventory model, the distributor receives electronic data (typically via the Internet) regarding the facility's use of goods and stock levels. The distributor can view every item stocked at the facility. The distributor is responsible for creating and maintaining an effective inventory plan (www .vendormanagedinventory.com/definition.php).

SUMMARY

In this chapter, we have examined numerous aspects of inventory management. The chapter began by explaining the purpose of inventories, with some coverage of inventories for disaster preparedness. We discussed costs of inventories, and presented an example from health care to demonstrate how Excel can be used to solve economic order quantity problems. Two types of demand, independent and dependent, were considered, along with two types of inventory review systems, periodic and continuous.

We explained ABC inventory management using a health care example with Excel. The chapter closed with an introduction to types of inventory management technology, including radio-frequency identification (RFID), third-party logistics (3PL), and vendor-managed inventory (VMI).

KEY TERMS

ABC inventory management	*independent demand*
continuous review system	*inventory*
dependent demand	*periodic review system*
economic order quantity	*vendor-managed inventory*

DISCUSSION QUESTIONS

1. Explain how inventories in a health care setting differ from inventories in a manufacturing or production setting.

2. What factors contribute to the cost of inventories? What strategies can be employed to lower these costs?

3. Explain the difference between independent demand and dependent demand.

4. Given the following data, calculate the EOQ by hand.

   Setup cost = $200

   Holding cost = 5 percent per item

   Item purchase price = $20

   Annual demand = 5,000

5. A medical supply store wants to know the number of stethoscopes it should purchase in order to minimize annual costs. Currently, the store is ordering 1,000 stethoscopes per order. Formulate a model in Excel to determine the EOQ for the store. Include all of the variables and calculated examples from Figure 15.1 in order to determine the cost of the store's current plan. Use a separate worksheet to determine the EOQ, and report on the savings the store would have if it changed its order quantity for stethoscopes to the EOQ.

   Problem data:

   P = purchase cost = $65

   D = annual demand = 15,000

   H = holding cost = 10 percent per item

   K = setup cost = $250

6. Explain the difference between periodic review systems and continuous review systems.

7. For the given inventory data that follows, determine which items are type A, type B, and type C.

Part Line Number	Average Weekly Sales	Cost ($ Value)	Dollar Volume
1	21,000	$1.00	$21,000
2	4,000	$40.00	$160,000
3	1,600	$3.00	$4,800
4	12,000	$1.00	$12,000
5	1,000	$100.00	$100,000
6	50	$50.00	$2,500
7	800	$2.00	$1,600
8	10,000	$3.00	$30,000
9	4,000	$1.00	$4,000
10	5,000	$1.00	$5,000
11	250	$2.00	$500
12	1,900	$55.00	$104,500

8. Choose one of the types of inventory management technology discussed in the last section of the chapter (RFID, 3PL, VMI) and discuss its advantages and disadvantages. Also conduct Internet research to find out the leading companies that provide the technology. Discuss those companies.

REFERENCES

www.bt.cdc.gov/healthcare.

Cook, A. 2007. "The Dangers of Stockpiling: Planning Rules Change as Hospitals Brace for Potential Disasters." *Materials Management in Health Care* 9:52–54.

Hertz, S., and M. Alfredsson. 2003. "Strategic Development of Third Party Logistics Providers." *Industrial Marketing Management* 32 (2): 139–149.

Nahmias, S. 2009. *Production and Operations Analysis.* 6th ed. Boston: McGraw-Hill Irwin.

Narasimhan, S., D. McLeavey, and P. Billington. 1995. *Production Planning and Inventory Control.* 2nd ed. Upper Saddle River, NJ: Prentice Hall.

Orlicky, J. A. 1970. "Requirements Planning Systems: Cinderella's Bright Prospects for the Future." *Proceedings of the 13th International Conference of APICS.*

Snyder, C. 1982. "A Dependent Demand Approach to Service Organization Planning and Control." *Academy of Management Review* 7 (3): 455–466.

www.technovelgy.com/ct/Technology-Article.asp?ArtNum=21.

www.vendormanagedinventory.com/definition.php.

INDEX